A Profile of Health and Disease in America

Respiratory and Infectious Disease

A Profile of Health and Disease in America

Respiratory and Infectious Disease

Wrynn Smith, Ph.D.

Facts On File Publications
New York, New York • Oxford, England

A Profile of Health and Disease in America: Respiratory Disease

First Published in the United States of America by Facts On File, Inc., 460 Park Avenue South, New York, New York 10016.

Library of Congress Cataloging-in-Publication Data
Smith, Wrynn.
Respiratory disease.

(A Profile of health and disease in America)
Bibliography: p.
Includes index.
1. Respiratory organs—Diseases—Statistics.
I. Title. II. Series: Smith, Wrynn. Profile of health and disease in America. [DNLM: 1. Communicable Diseases —occurrence—United States. 2. Respiratory Tract Diseases—occurrence—United States. WF 140 S664r]
RC732.S57 1987 614.5'92'0021 87-5396
ISBN 0-8160-1458-2

ISBN 0-8160-1558-0 (7 volume set)

Series design: Jo Stein

Printed in the United States of America

10 9 8 7 6 5 4 3 2 1

CONTENTS

Preface

Just a few decades ago, treating the sick was a simple affair. The local family doctor, equipped with a small array of poultices and a sympathetic manner, did his best to fight disease. Knowledge, medicines, instrumentation, and surgical procedures developed slowly. Today, however, in the era of proliferating biotechnology, specialization, third-party financing, hospices, and surgicenters, medical school professors seem to relish telling their students that 50% of what they are learning will be obsolete five years after graduation.

The flow of information crossing the desk of busy health-care professionals trying to keep abreast of ever-accelerating developments in disease diagnosis, treatment, and prevention, as well as in the financing, organization, and delivery of health care, is often overwhelming. Clearly, the need to keep up is critical. To be informed, health-care professionals—be they practitioners, hospital administrators, health-care planners, policy makers, insurers, or hospital or pharmaceutical supply executives—must attend to material from many disconnected sources. These sources might include current editions of classic texts, weekly and monthly professional journals, current research papers presented at colloquia, and a steady stream of government bulletins and study publications from the Centers for Disease Control, NIH, the Center for Health Statistics, and foundation reports. As with the proverbial forest that can't be seen for the trees, the voluminous and fragmented form of this information often obscures the major changes and trends rapidly occurring in the health-care field.

The task of a grant applicant to locate and collate statistical information when framing the need for his work is a research project in itself. The same is true of a researcher defining a hypothesis, a physician determining the current utilization of a particular therapy regimen or a hospital administrator projecting bed needs.

To help such workers and investigators, I decided to gather data from many sources into one comprehensive coordinated source, this series entitled *A Profile of Health and Disease in America*, that will serve as a handy and definitive resource tool for health professionals.

Each volume contains both historical and current statistics on the incidence, prevalence, and mortality of major diseases within one of the major medical specialties. I've presented data for different geographic areas within the United States as well as international data. I've also included information on the use of various medicines and surgical procedures. Treatment costs and the length of a hospital stay and how it varies geographically or for patients based on sex are included as are discussions of major controversies. Thus, the reader will easily find data on flu viruses, changes in virus strains, current fertility rates of American teenagers, changes in the obesity level of Americans, and the latest incidence of pertussis, with a discussion of the pros and cons of the pertussis vaccine and of how many men suffer from toxic shock syndrome. Those readers interested in digestive disease can find recent information from government surveys on problems as diverse as ulcers and hemorrhoids. The volume on mental disease provides a wealth of data on depressive symptomatology, drug usage, alcoholism, and homicide and puts the recent increase of teenage suicide in historical perspective.

Data sources include the 1983 Symposium on Cancer Treatment; Public Health Reports; the National Natality Survey; the NHANES Surveys; publications of the Atlanta Centers for Disease Control; and NIH publications, as well as those of the American Heart, Lung, and Blood Institute, The American Cancer Institute, and the Institute For Allergy and Infectious Disease. Published research articles are discussed and referenced, and each volume includes a bibliography that can be used by those seeking to go beyond initial review of pertinent health data. These comprehensive volumes on so many health topics need not be the last source consulted, but I think for those owning them they will always be the first.

Introduction

While advances in medicine and surgical techniques already discussed in this series describe statistically the progress made against disease within the last one hundred years, no volume contains more success stories than this one on Respiratory and Infectious Disease.

At the turn of the present century, pneumonia and influenza (P & I), which often occur together, were among the most common causes of death. During the 1918 influenza pandemic, the death rate for P & I in the United States was 588 per 100,000. Although the incidence of influenza is still closely monitored each year, the death rate from P & I in the 1980s is only about 23 per 100,000.

The threat of these diseases has not only been mitigated by antimicrobial agents that can prevent secondary infections but also by vaccines for various strains of influenza and pneumonia. The types of isolates identified in the 1980s, their incidence nationally, and the morbidity and mortality due to influenza in recent years are reviewed in this volume.

Another killer, often of young people in their prime, was tuberculosis. But past efforts to isolate victims, the introduction of new antituberculosis drugs and mass screening of the population has reduced the number of new cases reported nationally in the 1980s to about 25,000. However, both a large influx of Asian refugees in the early 1980s and the failure of many patients to complete their treatment regimen has slowed the rate of decline in incidence, which the United States has enjoyed for more than a decade. Intensified efforts to monitor outpatients, to trace the contacts of reactivated and drug-resistant patients, and to introduce new 6-month regimens using a combination of drugs have seemingly reversed this trend. But analysts remain cautious in their pronouncements about the future of tuberculosis in the United States, especially in light of the growing prevalence of acquired immunodeficiency syndrome (AIDS). These victims with impaired immunity will be more susceptible to tuberculosis, and many old cases may become reactivated.

Pertussis, also known as whooping cough, is another disease that used to claim the lives of many children. But it has claimed dramatically fewer lives during the last several decades as a result of the development of a vaccine. Administered in combination with vaccines for diphtheria and tetanus, the vaccine is commonly called the DPT vaccination. However, in 1974, English authorities began to report side effects of the vaccine including coma and brain damage leading to death in a small percentage of the children vaccinated. This concern arose more recently in the United States and has led to an ongoing controversy about the safety of the pertussis vaccine.

Some members of the medical community do not believe that the supposed side effects are caused by the vaccine. But other evidence from the Netherlands seems to indicate that the whole-virus vaccine may be related to serious vaccination sequelae. Based on these data, critics of the vaccine estimate the risk of permanent brain damage as 1 in every 350,000. At the same time that the controversy has flared, questions have been raised about the vaccine's efficacy. Because many parents may be avoiding the vaccine, the number of pertussis patients and pertussis mortality has risen in both the United States and England.

The incidence of diphtheria has dropped from 1.2 per 100,000 in 1955 to less than 0.1 per 100,000 in 1983. Cases occurred in Washington state in the 1970s but all were cutaneous nonrespiratory cases.

A new but feared disease, Legionnaires' disease, has been identified only as of the late 1970s. Medical experts believe that it accounts for 52,000 cases of *Legionella pneumophilia* annually in the United States; the mortality rate is about 12%. The key to survival is early diagnosis, prompt treatment with erythromicin, and attention to risk factors—especially hospitalization. The infection is frequently found in hospitalized patients and identified as hospital-caused or as a nosocomial infection.

The gains in conquering and identifying these acute respiratory infections have been offset to some extent by the increasing prevalence and mortality of several chronic respiratory illnesses. They include bronchitis, emphysema, and chronic obstructive pulmonary disease (COPD). Changes in disease classification have obscured the increases in emphysema. But when these changes are kept in mind, the trend is unmistakable. The age-adjusted death rate for emphysema in 1982 was 12.6 per 100,000. The combined rate of emphysema and COPD rose to 31.3 per 100,000 by 1977. These diseases are associated with cigarette smoking and occur more often among members of lower-income groups. The role of pollution is as yet not clearly defined, but it is suspected cause in the growing prevalence of these diseases as well.

By 1979, asthma was the seventh leading chronic condition causing limitation of activity. Approximately 9 million Americans suffer from asthma, and the prevalence rate is climbing. It has increased from 8.1 per 1000 in 1969 to 15 per 1000 in 1984. Another 15 million who are not asthmatic suffer from allergic rhinitis. One-third of them are children. In 1975, those suffering from allergic rhinitis lost 3.5 million work days, which cost them $154 million in wages.

In addition to genetically related chronic diseases, such as asthma and allergic rhinitis, government observers estimate that about 100,000 people die in the United States from occupationally related lung disease, in particular pneumoconiosis, "black lung" disease. In a study of coal miners with varying lengths of service in the mines, 38% of those with long-term exposure to coal dust reported persistent cough compared to only 2.3% among those working in the mines just a short time. Current estimates of black lung disease among coal miners place the prevalence between 5 to 15%.

Just as anti-dust measures can and do lower the incidence of black lung disease, many other disorders have been controlled in the United States by vigilant preventive measures. They include complete cooking of meats, storage of food under refrigeration, and proper sanitary food handling conditions. Such measures have led to a sizable decline in the incidence of trichinosis, but other enteric infections are increasing perhaps due to a lapse in precaution or better reporting. The latter include nontyphoid salmonellosis, botulism, and shigellosis infections: In 1982, 19,380 cases of food-borne disease, including cholera, were reported in the United States; the number is increasing.

The incidence of sexually transmitted diseases has also risen during the late 1970s and early 1980s as sexual activity becomes less monogamous and less selective. Authorities believe that 10 million people annually exhibit symptoms of venereal disease in the United States. A particularly disturbing trend is the increased incidence of syphilis in women during their childbearing years, the widespread incidence of herpes in the same group, and the runaway incidence of chlamydia. Between 1950 and 1978, the number of gonorrhea cases increased from 192 to 468 cases per 100,000. A common result of both chlamydial and gonorrheal infections, salpingitis (inflammation of the fallopian tubes), has been a cause of infertility which poses concern to observers as well.

The newest venereal disease, AIDS, has been spreading rapidly in Africa and to a lesser extent in the United States and Europe. But in the United States, projections of the number of people who will have been exposed to the HTLV III/LAV (HIV) virus have been of epidemic proportion. Authorities are not optimistic that a vaccine can be perfected within the next one or two years. Thus, thoughts are turning to prevention and education of the public as well as those who care for AIDS patients. So far, the five-year survival rate of AIDS victims is about zero. As of March 1986, 18,406 cases of AIDS were reported in the United States and the incidence is still rising.

Other infections causing concern are nosocomial, or hospital-related infections, which have been increasing in recent years as well. The rate of infection in each type of hospital studied—from small nonteaching to large teaching—has been highest on the surgical service and lowest on the neonatal and pediatric services where infection control measures may be followed more methodically. In 1983, the most common infection was urinary and the most common pathogen was *Escherichia coli*.

With the development of vaccines, the incidence of several other dreaded infectious diseases has declined greatly in the 1980s. These diseases include polio, measles, rubella, and mumps. The incidence of rabies in man in the United States is very low today due to prevention efforts, and mortality has been reduced because of treatment. The same is true of tetanus, but cases of bubonic plague and leprosy have been increasing. The incidence of leprosy has been increasing because of emigration by peoples from areas where leprosy is indigenous; U.S. military personnel returning from the Far East who contracted malaria also account for increases in the United States of this disease.

The increases have fortunately been in diseases which are not endemic to the United States; the incidence declines have been in diseases that were widespread throughout the United States, such as polio and measles. Thus, the gains in understanding, preventing, and treating infectious diseases still outweigh the recent loss of ground to several chronic diseases. Current attempts to educate the public about smoking, venereal disease, occupational disease, and the proper handling of food should promote additional health gains reportable in future data.

Acute Respiratory and Infectious Disease 1

RESPIRATORY DISEASE

Acute and chronic lung diseases are among the leading causes of death and disability in the United States annually. Each year there are about 100 million cases of influenza, pneumonia, and acute bronchitis. This does not include the common cold and other viral or bacterial infections of the upper respiratory tract or chronic respiratory problems afflicting an estimated one in five persons in the United States. At least 16 million Americans suffer from chronic bronchitis, asthma, and emphysema.

Lung diseases are the chief cause of death for 240,000 persons annually and a contributory cause for an equal number of deaths.

The National Ambulatory Care Survey conducted in 1975 and 1976 gathered extensive data on utilization of health-care resources by those afflicted with both acute and chronic respiratory diseases. The information was obtained from a national sample of office-based physicians in the continental United States. One item of interest was the number of office visits to private physicians made because of respiratory problems.

The survey revealed that respiratory diseases accounted for 14% of all physician office visits annually, leading all other disease categories. Respiratory disease was the reason for 28% of all office visits made by children under age 15 years. The estimated number of office visits attributed to care for respiratory disease determined in the study totaled 163.4 million.

TABLE 1–1. Number and Percentage of Office Visits for All Diagnostic Classes and for Diseases of the Respiratory System, by Patient, Sex, Race, and Age: United States, 1975–76

SEX, RACE, AND AGE	ALL ICDA Diagnostic classes* Number of Visits (in thousands)	ALL ICDA Diagnostic classes* Visits (%)	Diseases of the Respiratory System* Visits (in thousands)	Diseases of the Respiratory System* Visits (%)
All visits	1,155,900	100.0	163,401	14.1
Sex and race:				
Female	697,727	100.0	87,464	12.5
White	625,201	100.0	76,850	12.3
Black and all other races	72,525	100.0	10,614	14.6
Male	458,174	100.0	75,937	16.6
White	413,320	100.0	67,947	16.4
Black and all other races	44,853	100.0	7,990	17.8
Age (years)				
Under 15	209,005	100.0	58,036	27.8
15–24	174,974	100.0	21,833	12.5
25–34	171,827	100.0	20,532	12.0
35–44	122,805	100.0	15,001	12.2
45–54	147,082	100.0	16,552	11.3
55–64	143,060	100.0	16,362	11.4
65 and over	187,148	100.0	15,086	8.1

*Based on the *Eighth Revision International Classification of Diseases, Adapted for Use in the United States* (ICDA). Source: *Vital and Health Statistics*, Series 13 Number 42

OFFICE VISITS

Table 1–1 summarizes the number of respiratory-related office visits for people with various age, race, and sex characteristics compared to the office visits undertaken for all diseases. As the data show, visits for respiratory conditions were more common among children younger than age 15 than among any other age group. Respiratory disease was also determined to be the most common diagnosis for persons in this age range. This finding squares with known generalizations that children are more susceptible to viral illnesses including the common cold because of the limited exposure history that young people have compared to those who have lived longer.

Interestingly, women made 12 million more visits for a respiratory problem than did men. But the percentage of total visits made by women due to respiratory problems was lower than for men. This accords with the fact that women visit office-based physicians for female conditions throughout life, and therefore the proportion of all their visits accounted for by respiratory problems is lower than it is for males.

The discrepancy between the number of visits made by whites compared to blacks is large, as one would expect when it is remembered that blacks constitute only 12% of the general population. On the other hand, the office visits made by blacks for respiratory problems constitutes a slightly greater proportion of all visits undertaken by them than by whites. The difference, however, is so small that it may reflect chance variation in the data more than any real difference between racial groups.

MEDICATIONS

In 1980, the National Center for Health Statistics surveyed office-based physicians about the medications given or recommended to their patients. Responses by those treating respiratory patients are presented in the following tables and figures. Some show once again the number of respiratory-related office visits, but the numbers differ drastically in most cases from those gathered in the 1975-76 survey. Part of the reason is that some classifications, such as acute respiratory infections, encompassed fewer ICDA code illnesses than did the earlier survey.

Another possible reason for the divergence is the variability of viral respiratory illnesses from year to year. However, some illnesses that are not viral, such as asthma, were reported as accounting for approximately one-half as many office visits in 1980 as in 1975-76. Aside from possible changes in survey design, this variation may be partly due to the declining size of the population younger than age 15 who constitute the majority of asthmatics and partly to better forms of treatment in 1980 that may have prevented flare-ups of chronic disease.

The drug mention rate (the number of times physicians listed a drug as one prescribed or given) during office visits for respiratory patients compared to patients with other illnesses is shown in Figure 1–1. After ischemic or coronary heart disease, the diagnoses with the highest drug mention rates were acute bronchitis and asthma followed closely by acute upper respiratory infections and all diseases of the respiratory system.

Table 1–2 lists the most frequently mentioned medications during respiratory disease-related office visits by their generic composition and therapeutic category reported in the 1980 National Health Survey. The five most commonly mentioned drugs by type were antihistamines, anti-infectives, central nervous system drugs, expectorants, and cough preparations.

Actifed and Dimetapp were the most widely mentioned antihistamines, whereas Phenergan expectorant with codeine was prominent in the cough preparation category. Over-the-counter drugs often mentioned included aspirin, Dimetane, Tylenol, Novahistine, Robitussin, Sudafed, and Triaminic. Actifed became available over the counter after 1980.

HOSPITAL STAYS AND MEDICAL PROCEDURES

The number and rate of hospital discharges for patients suffering from various select acute and chronic respiratory diseases classified according to geographic region, sex, and age in 1981 are shown in Table 1–3. Despite its milder climate, the South showed the most hospitalization for respiratory diseases.

TABLE 1–2. Number and Percent as a Distribution of Drug Mentions in Office Visits for Selected Respiratory Conditions by Most Frequently Mentioned Specific Drugs Described by Principal Generic Ingredient(s) and Principal Therapeutic Category: United States, 1980

PRINCIPAL DIAGNOSIS AND NAME OF DRUG	Drug Mentions		Principal Generic Ingredient(s)	Principal Therapeutic Category
	Number in thousands	Percent distribution		
Acute upper respiratory infections of multiple or unspecified sites (acute URI)	32,311	100.0	. . .	. . .
Pencillin	1,353	4.2	Penicillin	Antibiotics
Tetracycline	1,191	3.7	Tetracycline	Antibiotics
E.E.S.	1,124	3.5	Erythromycin	Antibiotics
Actifed	1,121	3.5	Triprolidine, pseudoephedrine	Antihistamine drugs
Dimetapp	1,107	3.4	Brompheniramine, phenylephrine, phenylpropanolamine	Antihistamine drugs
Phenergan expectorant with codeine	1,022	3.2	Promethazine, codeine, phenylephrine, guaiacolsulfonate	Expectorants and cough preparations
Ampicillin	978	3.0	Ampicillin	Antibiotics
Phenergan	878	2.7	Promethazine	Antihistamine drugs
Amoxicillin	767	2.4	Amoxicillin	Antibiotics
Dimetane	746	2.3	Brompheniramine	Antihistamine drugs
Amoxil	674	2.1	Amoxicillin	Antibiotics
Erythromycin	650	2.0	Erythromycin	Antibiotics
Rondec	615	1.9	Carbinoxamine, pseudoephedrine	Antihistamine drugs
Terramycin	529	1.6	Oxytetracycline	Antibiotics
Aspirin	523	1.6	Aspirin	Analgesics and antipyretics
Naldecon	465	1.4	Phenylpropanolamine, phenylephrine, phenyltoloxamine, chlorpheniramine	Antihistamine drugs
Novahistine	446	1.4	Phenylpropanolamine, chlorpheniramine	Antihistamine drugs

TABLE 1–2. (Continued)

PRINCIPAL DIAGNOSIS AND NAME OF DRUG	Drug Mentions		Principal Generic Ingredient(s)	Principal Therapeutic Category
Benylin Syrup	428	1.3	Diphenhydramine	Antihistamine drugs
E-mycin	407	1.3	Erythromycin	Antibiotics
Keflex	*374	*1.2	Cephalexin	Antibiotics
Tylenol	*359	*1.1	Acetaminophen	Analgesics and antipyretics
Drixoral	*341	*1.1	Pseudoephedrine	Antihistamine drugs
Robitussin	*329	*1.0	Guaifenesin	Expectorants and cough preparations
Sudafed	*323	*1.0	Pseudoephedrine, chlorpheniramine	Sympathomimetic drugs
Vibramycin	*308	*1.0	Doxycycline	Antibiotics
Triaminic	*305	*0.9	Phenylopropanolamine, pheniramine, pyrilamine	Antihistamine drugs
Residual	14,947	46.3	. . .	. . .
Acute pharyngitis or acute laryngitis and tracheitis	16,139	100.0	. . .	. . .
Penicillin	1,779	11.0	Penicillin	Antibiotics
Ampicillin	1,160	7.2	Ampicillin	Antibiotics
Aspirin	750	4.6	Aspirin	Analgesics and antipyretics
Pen-Vee-K	555	3.4	Penicillin	Antibiotics
Erythromycin	553	3.4	Erythromycin	Antibiotics
Tetracycline	452	2.8	Tetracycline	Antibiotics
V-cillin	447	2.8	Penicillin	Antibiotics
E.E.S.	430	2.7	Erythromycin	Antibiotics
Keflex	*377	*2.3	Cephalexin	Antibiotics
Celestone	*342	*2.1	Betamethasone	Adrenals
Amoxicillin	*304	*1.9	Amoxicillin	Antibiotics
Residual	8,990	55.7	. . .	. . .
Acute bronchitis and bronchiolitis or bronchitis, not specified as acute or chronic	16,349	100.0	. . .	. . .
Amoxicillin	759	4.6	Amoxicillin	Antibiotics
Phenergan	747	4.6	Promethazine	Antihistamine drugs
Ampicillin	740	4.5	Ampicillin	Antibiotics
Penicillin	678	4.1	Penicillin	Antibiotics
Tetracycline	615	3.8	Tetracycline	Antibiotics
Phenergan expectorant with codeine	583	3.6	Promethazine, codeine, phenylephrine, potassium guaiacolsulfonate	Expectorants and cough preparations
Erythromycin	432	2.6	Erythromycin	Antibiotics
Dimetane	421	2.6	Brompheneramine	Antihistamine drugs
E.E.S.	*368	*2.3	Erythromycin	Antibiotics
Robitussin	*342	*2.1	Guaifenesin	Expectorants and cough preparations
Residual	10,664	65.2	. . .	. . .

Source: *Vital and Health Statistics,* Series 13, No. 17

Table 1–4 presents information on the number and rate of procedures performed in short-stay hospitals for patients by age, sex, and geographic region in 1981.

Fig. 1–1. Drug mention rates per visit for selected diagnoses: United States, 1980

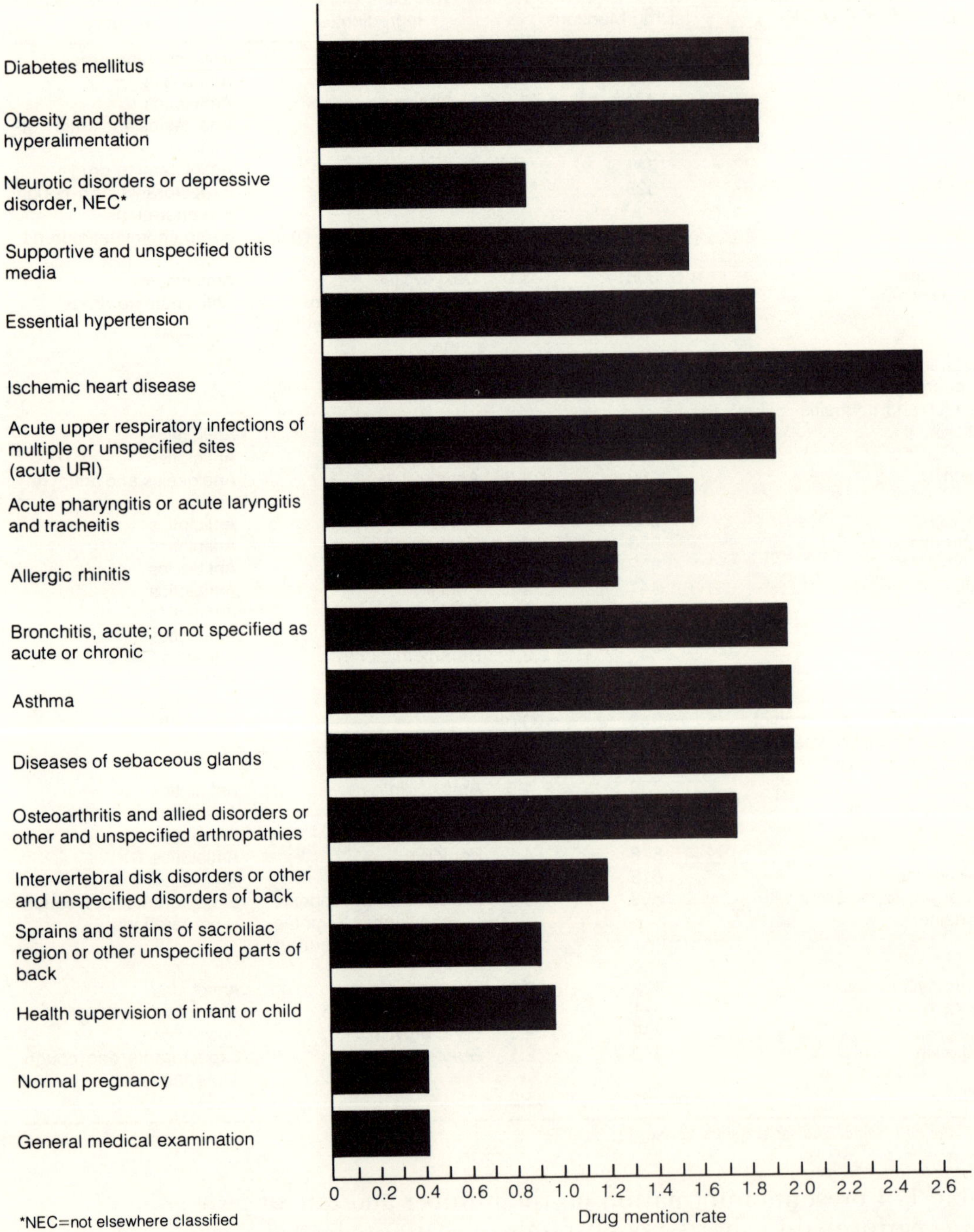

*NEC=not elsewhere classified

Source: *Vital and Health Statistics,* Series 13, No. 71

TABLE 1–3. Number* and Rate of Patient Discharges from Short-stay Hospitals by Geographic Region, Sex, and Age According to Respiratory Diagnosis, 1981

	RESPIRATORY DISEASE	ACUTE BRONCHITIS	ACUTE URI†	PNEUMONIA	ASTHMA
Total	3475	223	256	769	418
Northeast	620	36	43	119	95
North Central	1039	68	77	215	120
South	1307	93	109	330	133
West	509	27	27	105	69
Sex	No Rate	No Rate	No Rate	No Rate	No Rate
Male	1721 156.6	98 8.9	128 11.6	384 34.9	180 16.4
Female	1754 148.9	125 10.6	128 10.9	384 32.7	237 20.2
Age (years)					
15	1034	101	157	229	128
15–44	767	31	55	107	112
45–64	663	34	22	130	104
65 and older	1010	57	22	302	74

* In thousands
† Upper Respiratory Infection
Source: *Vital and Health Statistics*, Series 13, No. 72

The direct and indirect economic costs of respiratory illness are presented in Table 1–5. The direct costs of treatment were $5.9 billion, while the indirect costs were $15.8 billion.

Table 1–6 presents information on how respiratory disease per capita personal health-care expenditures rank compared to other kinds of disease according to patient age and sex for 1980.

MORTALITY AND MORBIDITY

At the turn of the 20th Century, the most common cause of death was pneumonia and influenza (P & I). But by 1950, these two

TABLE 1–4. Number and Rate of Procedures in Short-stay Hospitals by Age, Sex, and Geographic Regions, 1981

	TOTAL OPERATIONS		THORACENTESIS	
	Rate*	Number†	Rate	Number
Total	399.5	910	44.5	101
Male under 15 years	499.8	NA‡	39.5	NA
Female under 15 years	305.9	NA	49.1	NA
Both over 15 years	490.1	NA	56.4	NA
Northeast	462.1	227	58.7	29
North Central	437.8	257	43.0	25
South	329.3	251	38.8	30
West	400.0	175	40.2	18

* Rate per 100,000 population
† In thousands
‡ NA, not available
Source: *Vital and Health Statistics,* Series 13, No. 72

TABLE 1–5. Direct and Indirect Economic Costs of Illness, U.S., 1979

	Amount ($ Billions)				Percentage Distribution*			
			INDIRECT COSTS				INDIRECT COSTS	
DIAGNOSIS	Total	Direct Costs	Morbidity	Mortality	Total	Direct Costs	Morbidity	Mortality
Diseases of the respiratory system	21.8	5.9	10.6	5.2	5.8	3.3	17.6	3.8

* Percent of costs for all diseases
Source: *Health, U.S.* 1982

TABLE 1–6. Per Capita Personal Health-care Expenditures and Rank for Leading Medical Conditions, According to Age and Sex: United States, 1980

MEDICAL CONDITION	PERSONS YOUNGER THAN AGE 65 YEARS		PERSONS OLDER THAN AGE 65 YEARS	
	MALE	FEMALE	MALE	FEMALE
	Per capita amount ($)			
Circulatory diseases	67	61	674	848
Digestive diseases	110	143	213	223
Mental disorders	73	69	181	246
Injury and poisoning	86	61	105	203
Respiratory diseases	60	68	192	137
Neoplasms	30	50	244	178
Musculoskeletal system and connective tissue diseases	40	55	91	187
Genitourinary system diseases	21	82	128	70
Nervous system and sense organ diseases	57	69	168	176
Endocrine, nutritional, metabolic diseases	15	31	82	138
	Rank			
Circulatory diseases	4	7	1	1
Digestive diseases	1	1	3	3
Mental disorders	3	4	5	2
Injury and poisoning	2	6	8	4
Respiratory diseases	5	5	4	9
Neoplasms	8	9	2	6
Musculoskeletal system and connective tissue diseases	7	8	9	5
Genitourinary system diseases	9	2	7	10
Nervous system and sense organ diseases	6	3	6	7
Endocrine, nutritional, metabolic diseases	10	10	10	8

Note: Conditions are based on the *International Classification of Diseases, 9th Revision, Clinical Modification.*
Source: National Center for Health Statistics: Computed by the Division of Analysis from data compiled by the Health Care Financing Administration, the National Center for Health Statistics, and other organizations.

related acute respiratory diseases were the sixth leading cause of death, while chronic lung diseases—such as emphysema, bronchitis, and asthma grouped together as chronic obstructive pulmonary disease (COPD)—constituted the fifth leading cause of death (Table 1–7).

Another major respiratory illness in its pulmonary form, tuberculosis, was the second leading cause of death in 1900, but it became the eighth by 1950 and was no longer a major cause of death at all in 1980.

The two lung disease classifications of P & I and COPD encompass most major nonmalignant lung diseases. Together they accounted for 5.4% of all deaths in 1968 and 5.5% of all deaths in 1981 (Fig. 1–2). It should be noted, however, that although the rate for these two lung disease classifications combined has remained constant, there has been a decline in mortality due to P & I, which has been offset by an increase in the death rate due to chronic obstructive lung diseases referred to commonly as COPD.

The death rate for the major respiratory diseases including tuberculosis and unspecified malignancies of the respiratory system between 1960 and 1984 are shown in Table 1–8. As indicated, several respiratory diseases including tuberculosis, pneumonia, in-

TABLE 1–7. Ten Leading Causes of Death, U.S., 1900, 1950, 1960, 1970, 1980 (Unadjusted Rate per 100,000 Population and Rank)

CAUSES OF DEATH	1900		1950		1960		1970		1980	
	Rate	Rank	Rate	Rank	Rate	Rank	Rate	Rank	Rate	Rank
Diseases of the heart	137.4	4	355.5	1	369.0	1	362.0	1	343.0	1
Malignant neoplasms	64.0	8	139.8	2	149.2	2	162.8	2	186.3	2
Cerebrovascular diseases	106.9	5	104.0	3	108.0	3	101.9	3	76.6	3
Accidents	72.3	7	60.6	4	52.3	4	56.4	4	47.9	4
Chronic obstructive pulmonary disease	—*	—	—	—	—	—	17.4	8	25.1	5
Influenza and pneumonia	202.2	1	31.3	6	37.3	6	30.9	5	23.7	6
Diabetes mellitus	—	—	16.2	9	16.7	8	18.9	7	15.4	7
Cirrhosis of the liver	—	—	—	—	11.3	10	15.5	10	14.4	8
Arteriosclerosis	—	—	20.4	7	20.0	7	15.6	9	13.4	9
Suicide	—	—	—	—	—	—	—	—	12.7	10
Certain causes of mortality in early infancy	—	—	40.5	5	37.4	5	21.3	6	—	—
Congenital malformation	—	—	—	—	12.2	9	—	—	—	—
Tuberculosis	194.4	2	22.5	8	—	—	—	—	—	
Diarrhea, enteritis, and ulceration of the intestines	142.7	3	—	—	—	—	—	—	—	—
Nephritis	88.6	6	16.4	10	—	—	—	—	—	—
Senility	50.2	9	—	—	—	—	—	—	—	—
Diphtheria	40.3	10	—	—	—	—	—	—	—	—

* (—) Means below the ten leading causes of death
Source: National Center for Health Statistics

Fig. 1–2. Percentage distribution of causes of death, U.S., 1968 and 1981

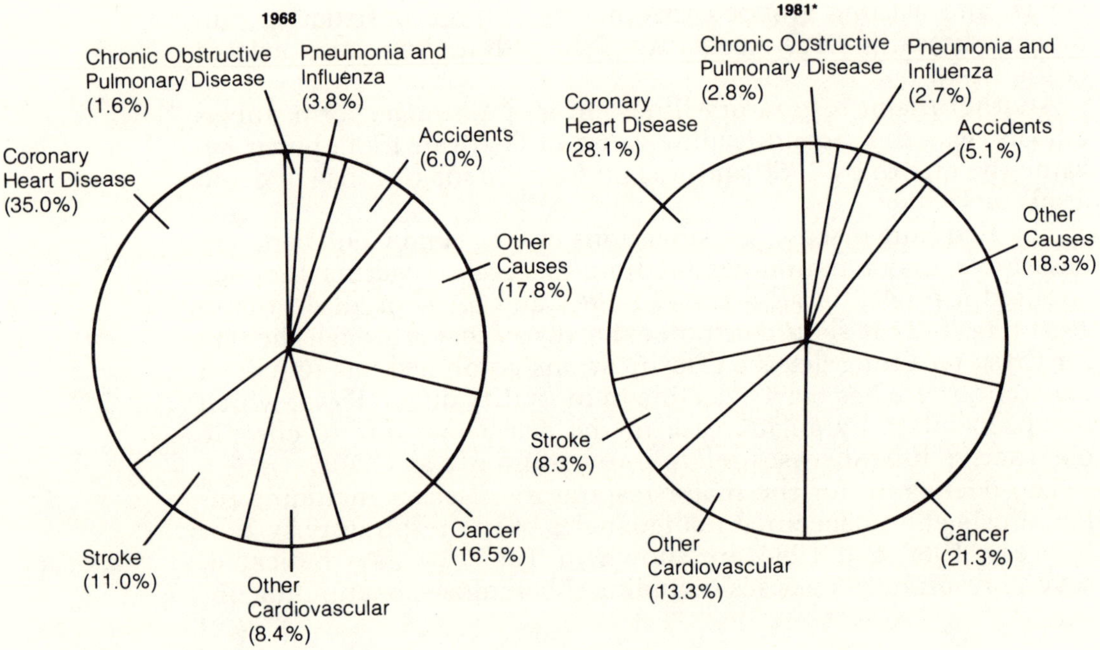

* Provisional and based on the *Ninth Revision of the International Classification of Diseases*, which assigns almost 100,000 fewer deaths to coronary heart disease and results in other less serious discontinuities of trends.
Note: Percentages may not add to 100% due to rounding. Source: National Center for Health Statistics.

fluenza, and even asthma are causing fewer deaths today than in 1960. On the other hand, malignancies of the lung, bronchitis[a], and emphysema and/or COPD continue to take their toll.

PNEUMONIA AND INFLUENZA

The story of the influenza epidemic of 1918 is among the most memorable in the annals of recorded disease. Spread around the world, this pandemic of influenza and pneumonia, which often occur together, killed over 10 million people and was responsible for a death rate of 588.2 per 100,000 in the United States in that year. Since then, with the exception of the epidemics of 1957–58 and 1968, the level of mortality due to P & I has been decreasing

[a] Recent bronchitis rate does not reflect a real decline; see discussion in Chapter 2, pp. 63–98.

steadily. As of August 1984, the death rate due to P & I was only 23.9 per 100,000.

Influenza cases in the United States vary in number and location from year to year. The cause of influenza is any of several related viruses referred to most commonly as types A, B, or C. The common subtypes or strains of type A are classified according to two antigens (substances that elicit immune response when introduced into the body). One is hemagglutinin—or (H) antigen—and the

TABLE 1—8. Death Rates for All Causes and for Diseases of the Respiratory System, Including Tuberculosis of Respiratory System, Malignant Neoplasm of Respiratory System, Asthma, and Other Specified Diseases of the Respiratory System: United States, 1960–84 (Numbers after causes of death are category numbers of the *Eighth Revision, International Classification of Diseases, Adapted for Use in the United States,* 1965 (ICDA). The asterisk before category number 519.3 indicates that the title to which this number corresponds was not included in ICDA but was introduced by the National Center for Health Statistics. Rates are based on deaths classified according to the *Seventh Revision* for 1960–67 and according to the *Eighth Revision* for 1968–77)

YEAR	All causes of death	Diseases of the Respiratory System, including Tuberculosis, Malignant Neoplasm of Respiratory System, and Asthma			
		Total	Tuberculosis of respiratory system (010–012)	Malignant neoplasm of respiratory system not specified as secondary (160–163)	Asthma (493)
	Rate per 100,000 population				
1984‡	862.8	—	0.8	52.0	1.5
1983	862.4	—	0.8	51.0	1.5
1982	857.6	—	0.8	49.2	1.4
1981	862.4	—	0.8	49.0	1.4
1980	874.1	—	0.8	47.5	1.1
1977*	878.1	96.1	1.1	44.0	0.8
1976*	889.6	100.0	1.1	42.5	0.9
1975*	888.5	94.5	1.2	40.7	0.9
1974*	915.1	92.5	1.3	39.5	0.9
1973*	940.2	95.3	1.4	37.8	0.9
1972†	943.2	94.4	1.7	37.0	1.1
1971*	934.7	89.5	1.7	35.4	1.0
1970*	945.3	91.7	2.0	34.2	1.1
1969	954.4	92.9	2.2	32.8	1.2
1968	967.9	96.3	2.5	31.8	1.3
1967	937.6	84.2	3.2	29.4	2.1
1966	952.6	86.9	3.6	28.1	2.2
1965	944.6	84.6	3.8	26.9	2.3
1964	940.7	81.2	4.0	25.7	2.3
1963	962.2	88.0	4.6	24.9	2.7
1962	945.6	79.9	4.7	24.0	2.6
1961	929.8	75.9	5.0	23.1	2.7
1960	954.7	83.3	5.6	22.2	3.0

TABLE 1–8 (Continued)

YEAR	Total	Chronic and unqualified bronchitis (490,491)	Emphysema and Chronic obstructive lung disease (492, *519.3)	Influenza (470–474)	Pneumonia (480–486)	Residual diseases of respiratory system
	OTHER SPECIFIED DISEASES OF RESPIRATORY SYSTEM					
	Rate per 100,000 population					
1984‡	—	1.5	25.9**	0.5	22.2	—
1983	—	1.5	25.3**	0.6	22.3	—
1982	—	1.5	22.9**	0.3	20.9	—
1981	—	1.7	22.8**	1.4	22.3	—
1980	—	1.7	21.8**	1.1	22.1	—
1977*	50.3	2.0	18.7	0.6	23.1	6.0
1976*	55.5	2.2	18.3	3.7	25.2	6.2
1975*	51.7	2.2	17.1	2.0	24.1	6.2
1974*	50.8	2.4	16.2	1.0	24.9	6.3
1973*	55.1	2.6	16.0	2.4	27.4	6.6
1972*,†	54.7	2.8	14.7	2.4	27.7	7.0
1971*	51.4	2.7	14.0	0.7	27.0	6.9
1970*	54.3	2.9	13.4	1.8	29.0	7.1
1969	56.7	2.9	12.7	3.0	31.0	7.1
1968	60.6	3.1	12.1	3.5	33.3	8.5
1967	49.5	2.7	10.6	0.7	28.1	7.4
1966	53.0	2.6	10.4	1.4	31.1	7.5
1965	51.6	2.5	9.6	1.2	30.8	7.4
1964	49.1	2.3	8.3	0.9	30.2	7.4
1963	55.9	2.3	8.0	3.8	33.8	8.0
1962	48.5	1.9	6.7	1.8	30.4	7.7
1961	45.1	1.7	5.6	1.2	29.0	7.7
1960	52.5	1.8	5.2	4.4	32.9	8.3

* Excludes deaths of nonresidents of the United States.
† Based on a 50-percent sample of deaths.
‡ As year ending in August 1984
** Rare for 519.3 classification NA rates used are for ICDA 492, 494–496
Source: *Vital and Health Statistics*, Series 20, No. 17

other is neuraminidase—or (N) antigen. Among these are five common strains of type A flu (H1, H2, H3, N1, and N2), which have caused widespread disease in the U.S. population. Asian flu is a variation of type A influenza.

Excess deaths due to P&I totalling 200,000 between 1968 and 1982 have been attributed mostly to influenza type A viruses. These deaths are typically among the elderly or chronically ill.

Type B influenza, which is more stable and shows less propensity to mutate into different strains, has been associated with excess deaths in the 1979–80 flu season and with Reye's syndrome in children and adolescents. Figure 1–3 shows the percentage of reported cases due to each of the main isolates between the 1977–78 flu season and the 1982–83 season.

Influenza is highly contagious and usually acute with sudden onset. Symptoms can be minimal, or the infection can lead to

Fig. 1–3. Isolates of influenza viruses reported to CDC by collaborating civilian and military laboratories — United States, 1977–1983

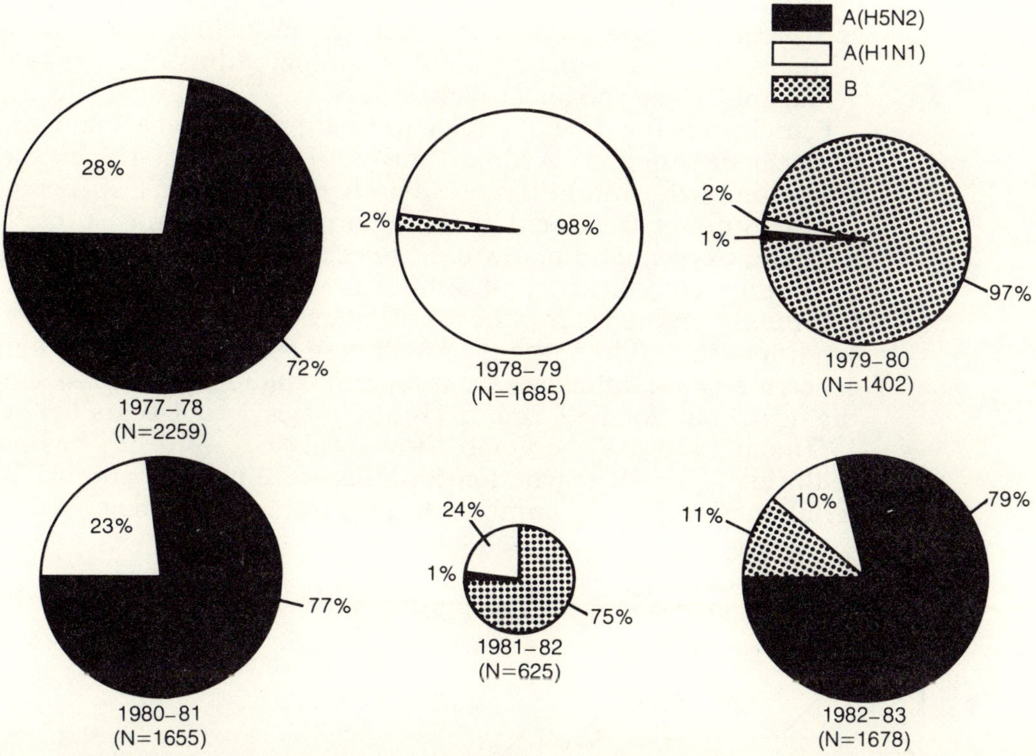

U.S. Department of Health and Human Services/Public Health Service

pneumonia and death. Most often symptoms include fever, headache, chills, malaise, cough, and sore throat. Treatment is usually symptomatic since viruses are not susceptible to antibiotic therapy. Antibiotics however, are useful if influenza becomes complicated by a bacterial infection in the sinuses or middle ear, or if a bacterial pneumonia develops in the lungs. Without complication, the disease is self-limiting and passes in two to seven days. Some patients, however, feel poorly for weeks following the acute stage.

In all, there are over 50 causes of pneumonia. They include viruses, bacteria, allergy, chemical irritants, and vegetable dusts. Viral pneumonia can be caused directly by the influenza virus, or bacterial pneumonia can occur secondarily to an influenza viral infection. Persons subject to a secondary pneumonia complication often have a history of upper respiratory infections, cigarette smoking, or alcohol abuse.

Viral pneumonia often begins with headache, fever, coryza (head cold), and myalgias (muscle pain). Sometimes rales may be heard in the chest. But diagnosis is made by observing alveolar and interstitial infiltrates on chest X-ray. The onset of bacterial pneumonia is accompanied by chills, fever, shaking, purulent sputum, and pleuritic chest pain. There may be bronchial chest sounds, dullness to percussion, and rales. Radiologic films often show alveolar infiltrates and air bronchograms.

Penicillin is the drug of choice to treat pneumococcal and streptococcal pneumonia. Without antibiotic treatment for bacterial pneumonia, the mortality rate has been as high as 30 percent. Other forms of treatment include comfort-giving measures, bed rest, and oxygen administration, if necessary.

Another complication of influenza is acute bronchitis. Less commonly, influenza may be followed by encephalitis or by Reye's syndrome in children (see p. 178). These sequelae are of pediatric concern because influenza is common in children. Figure 1–4 shows the death rate for P&I among children ages 1 to 4 years between 1950 and 1970. As the graph shows, this rate of death has been declining since 1950 when antibiotics were used to combat bacterial pneumonia, a common complication of influenza.

Fig. 1–4. Death rates for children 1 to 4 years of age due to influenza and pneumonia—United States, 1950–79

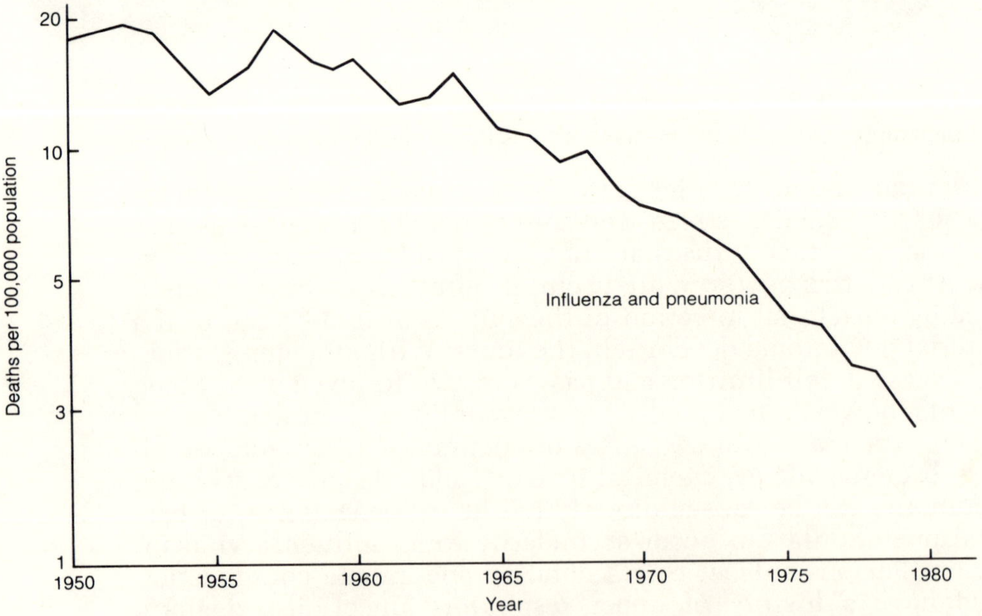

Note: Causes of death are assigned according to the International List of Causes of Death. Because of the decennial revisions and changes in rules for cause-of-death selection there may be some lack of comparability from one revision to the next. The beginning dates of the revision are 1949, 1958, 1968, and 1979.
Source: Health, U.S. 1982

MORTALITY IN RECENT SEASONS

Influenza occurs mostly during the winter and spring and varies annually, depending on what particular virus may be circulating and the immunity of the population from previous exposures.

In 1981 and 1982, the most common influenza viruses were types B and A(H1N1); however, 600 other strains were reported as well. As large as this number seems, 600 represents a decrease from the 1000 to 2000 strains identified in the 5 previous years. Of identified viruses, 74% were type B, which appeared first in the Southwest during January and February of 1981 and spread to the north and east. Influenza type A(H1N1) was isolated more in the Southwest and Pacific northwestern states throughout the season (Fig. 1–5).

Fig. 1–5. Influenza: reported isolate types, by state, United States, 1981–82 season up to June 1, 1982.

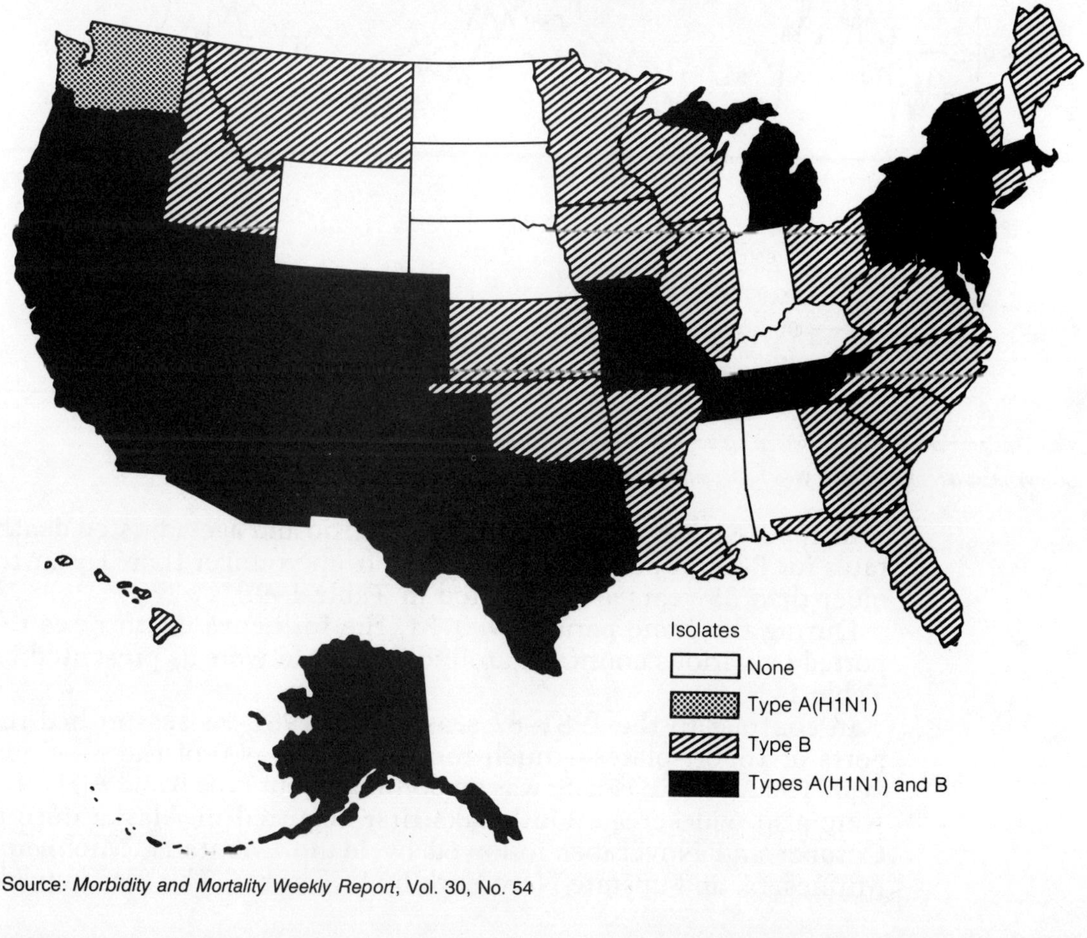

Source: *Morbidity and Mortality Weekly Report*, Vol. 30, No. 54

The mortality for P&I during the 1981–1982 season was not higher than expected although the death ratio was elevated for 13 weeks during the peak of the previous 1980–1981 flu season (Fig. 1–6). The observed cases depicted by the solid dark line was much higher than the expected number of cases depicted by the short dot dotted line between December 1980 and February 1981.

Fig. 1–6. Pneumonia/influenza: Observed and expected ratio of deaths attributed to pneumonia and influenza in 121 cities, as determined by the time series method, September 1979–August 1982

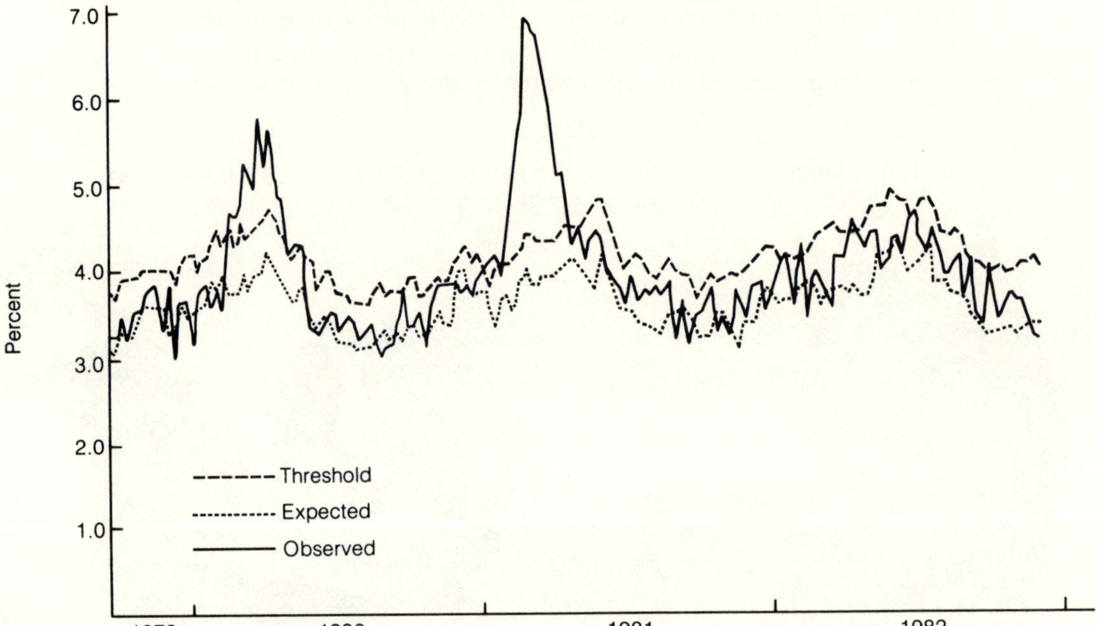

*Forecasts are made at 4-week intervals except during epidemic periods.

Source: *Morbidity and Mortality Weekly Report, Annual Summary* 1982

In 1980–81 and 1981–82, the age-specific and age-adjusted death rates for P&I for people in age groups from younger than 1 year to older than 85 years are presented in Table 1–9.

During the same period 1980–81, the influenza death rates reported by various countries around the world were as presented in Table 1–10.

In contrast to the 1981–82 season, the 1982–83 season had reports of 1650 isolates—much more than the 600 of the previous year. The A(H3N2) isolate was predominant, but type B and A(H1N1) were also widespread. Outbreaks first occurred in Alaska during October and November followed by Idaho, Montana, Michigan, Minnesota, and upstate New York by December. The season peak

Table 1–9. Age-specific and Age-adjusted Death Rates for 15 Leading Causes and Selected Components: United States, 1980 and 1981–1982 (Based on a 10% sample of deaths. Rate per 100,000 population in specified group)

	YEAR	AGE (YEARS) All ages	Under 1 year	1–14	15–24	25–34	35–44	45–54	55–64	65–74	75–84	85	AGE-AD-JUSTED RATE
Pneumonia influenza	1982	21.1	20.8	2.1	0.7	1.4	2.8	6.5	16.4	47.6	183.4	747.8	—
Pneumonia	1981	23.7	19.8	0.9	0.6	1.5	3.1	7.3	19.7	53.2	223.7	815.4	12.4
influenza...	1980	23.2	28.5	0.9	0.9	1.2	3.1	8.1	17.9	52.7	211.9	840.8	12.4

Source: Cause of death (Ninth Revision International Classification of Diseases, 1975), National Center for Health Statistics.

Table 1–10. Influenza and Pneumonia Death Rate Reported for 1980–81*

COUNTRY	INFLUENZA RATE	PNEUMONIA RATE	YEAR (19)
Australia	0.9	12.0	80
Austria	1.2	30.5	81
Bulgaria	3.5	52.8	81
Chile	4.5	38.5	80
France	1.9	9.0	80
Hungary	1.7	15.7	80
Japan	0.6	28.3	80
Poland	0.5	21.8	81
United Kingdom*†	1.3	109.0	81

*per 100,000
†United Kingdom includes only England and Wales

occurred in February with the outbreak subsiding in April.

The level of each of the three major isolates during 1982–83 is shown in Fig. 1–7.

MORBIDITY

During the 1982–83 season, a pilot program was initiated in which 150 primary-care physicians reported flu morbidity to the Atlanta Centers for Disease Control based on their office practices. Morbidity due to flu was defined as fever of 100° F or higher with at least a cough and sore throat. Reported results are shown graphically in Fig. 1–8.

Flu morbidity for the 1982–83 season reported geographically is shown in Fig. 1–9.

VACCINES

The major weapon against flu is the vaccine that has been avail-

Fig. 1–7. Laboratory surveillance of influenza virus — United States, 1982–83 season

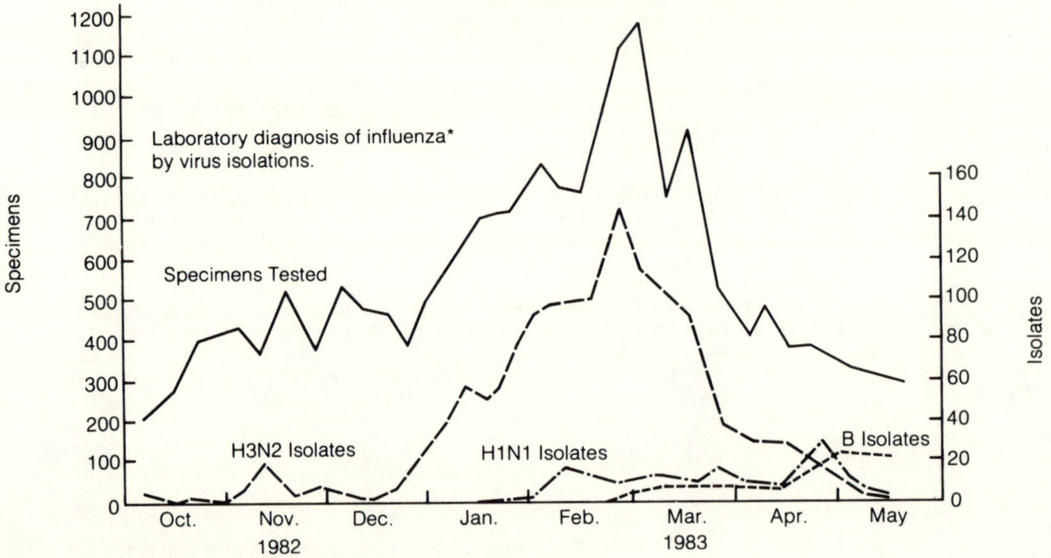

*Reported to CDC by WHO collaborating laboratories (including military sources).

Source: *Weekly Morbidity and Mortality Report*, Vol. 32, No. 29

able in the United States for several years. Immunity to the hemagglutinin antigens of type A flu effects the greatest reduction of infection because type A(H) influenza has been the most widespread. Mutation of the virus or "antigen drift" can lessen the effectiveness of vaccines from time to time. But these changes are generally followed by corresponding vaccine adjustment. For example, U.S. influenza vaccines have included an A(H3N2) strain identified in Bangkok in 1979 since 80% of U.S. influenza in recent years has been of the A(H3N2) type. But, as of 1982, an Asian variation called A/Philippines/2/82 has accounted for an increasing proportion of the H3N2 strains in Asia. This variation has not been combatted well by animal sera with A/Bangkok/79 immunity. Since immunity to the Philippine variation does seem to extend to Bangkok flu, authorities planned in 1983 to substitute the Philippine component in the vaccine for the Bangkok.

Vaccination has been strongly recommended for the elderly, especially those older than age 65 years; those with other illness of the respiratory track, such as asthma; those with heart disease, chronic renal disease with azotemia (increased blood levels of urea), or nephrotic syndrome, diabetes, other metabolic disorders, or

Fig. 1–8. Family practice-based morbidity surveillance for influenza virus (preliminary analysis) — United States, 1982–83 season

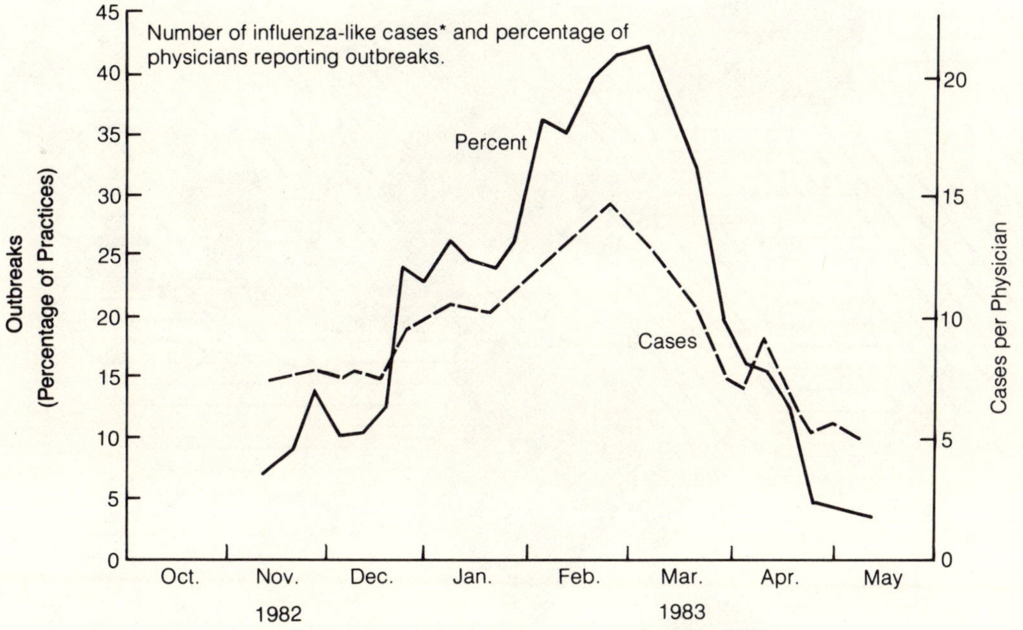

Source: *Weekly Morbidity and Mortality Report*, Vol. 32, No. 29

chronic anemia; and those with impaired immunity. Some communities have also urged vaccination of those who are health-care workers.

Vaccine side effects can include malaise and muscle aches; they occur most often in those with no previous exposure to the influenza virus, e.g., children. Some patients experience a sensitivity reaction on their arm if they are allergic to eggs since the vaccine contains egg protein residue left from its preparation process. Those anaphylactically (deathly) allergic to eggs should avoid taking the flu vaccine.

In 1976, cases of Guillain-Barré syndrome were reported within 10 weeks of the administration of the A/New Jersey/76 (swine) influenza vaccine at a rate of 10 cases per 1 million persons vaccinated. This was five to six times as high as the reported incidence of this syndrome in nonvaccinated persons. Surveillance since 1978 has not shown any increased incidence of this syndrome with the administration of other influenza vaccines. Thus, authorities consider the danger posed by flu infection in high-risk

Fig. 1–9. Highest level of influenza morbidity reported by state — United States, December 1982–June 1983

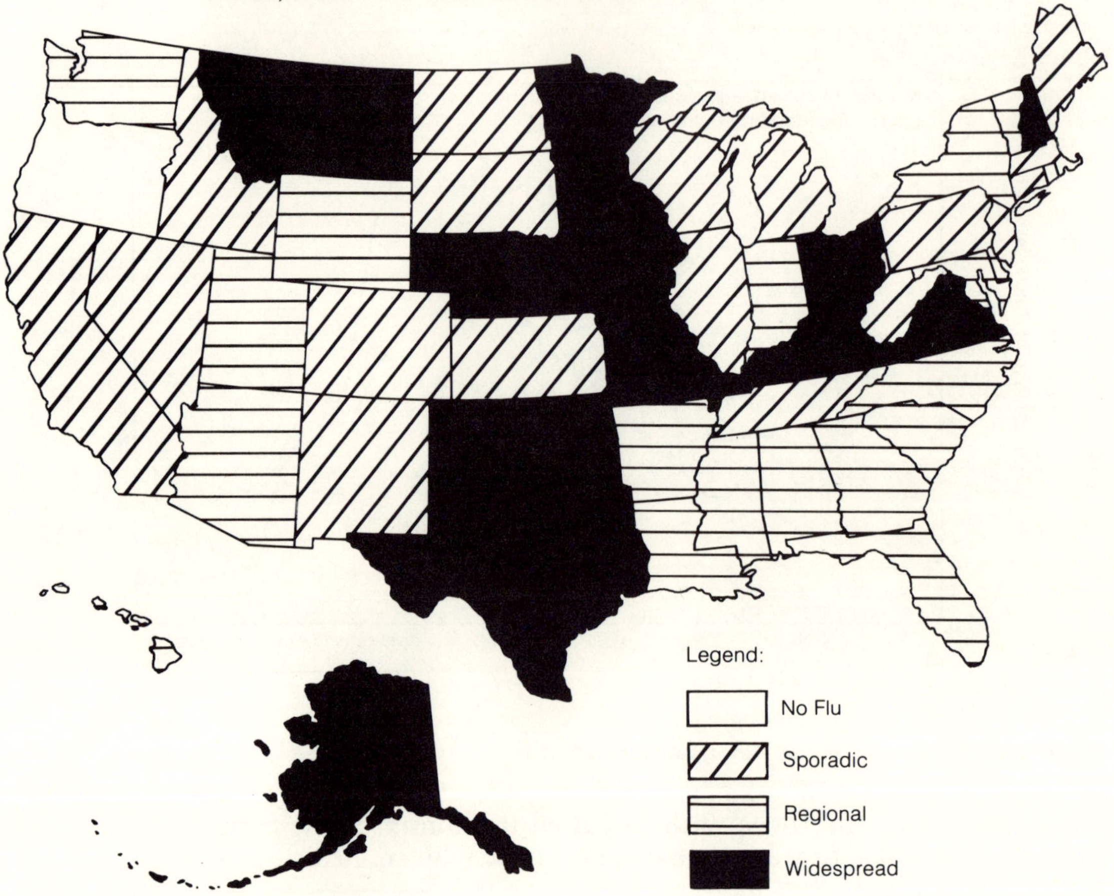

Source: *Weekly Morbidity and Mortality Report*, Vol. 32, No. 29

groups to exceed the risk of developing Guillain-Barré syndrome.

Another prophylactic measure is the administration of amantadine hydrochloride, an antiviral drug that seems to help prevent type A flu infection in persons who have not been vaccinated but who are living in an outbreak area. Its administration is not common, however, and not recommended as an alternative to vaccination.

In the absence of widespread vaccination against pneumonia, prevention of flu is also a mainline deterrent to the development of pneumonia. Federal and state authorities seek to reduce the number of pneumonia cases from 182 cases per 100,000 in 1978 to 115 per 100,000 in 1990. The goal was set with the introduction of a multivalent vaccine that appears to be 90% effective in preventing common young-adult pneumonia. Study of a pneumococcal vaccine has shown it to be 60% effective. It uses only 70% of the strains accounting for invasive pneumonias and has not been used widely by physicians although the Immunization Practices Committee of the Public Health Service has recommended it for high-risk groups. Meanwhile, efforts to improve available vaccines go on and patients primarily protect themselves through lifestyle precautions, including avoidance of excessive alcohol intake and other risk factors for respiratory disease, such as smoking.

TUBERCULOSIS

One of the most feared and widespread diseases that has ever threatened human survival is tuberculosis. It is this disease in its respiratory form that was written of by poets because it often struck the young as they approached their prime, rendering them thin and pale until they were consumed by it and died.

The organism that causes tuberculosis is a bacterium called *Mycobacterium tuberculosis.* Because it is aerobic and acid-fast, it thrives best in those parts of the body that are highly oxygenated, such as the lungs, kidney, and epiphyses of the long bones, but it

Table 1–11. Tuberculosis Cases by Form of Disease, States, 1982

STATE	TOTAL CASES	PULMONARY		EXTRAPULMONARY		CASES WITH BOTH PULMONARY AND EXTRAPULMONARY DISEASE	
		Number	Percent	Number	Percent	Number	Percent
United States	25,520	21,396	83.8	4,124	16.2	898	3.5
Alabama	631	556	88.1	75	11.9	7	1.1
Alaska	96	84	87.5	12	12.5	5	5.2
Arizona	300	246	82.0	54	18.0	22	7.3
Arkansas	412	362	87.9	50	12.1	46	11.2
California	3,606	3,079	85.4	527	14.6	100	2.8
Colorado	113	87	77.0	26	23.0	3	2.7
Connecticut	155	116	74.8	39	25.2	5	3.2
Delaware	55	44	80.0	11	20.0	4	7.3
District of Columbia	228	179	78.5	49	21.5	8	3.5
Florida	1,467	1,308	89.2	159	10.8	33	2.2
Georgia	830	671	80.8	159	19.2	18	2.2
Hawaii	252	225	89.3	27	10.7	3	1.2
Idaho	31	21	67.7	10	32.3	1	3.2
Illinois	1,653	1,397	84.5	256	15.5	85	5.1
Indiana	399	344	86.2	55	13.8	17	4.3

Table 1–11. (Continued)

STATE	TOTAL CASES	PULMONARY Number	PULMONARY Percent	EXTRAPULMONARY Number	EXTRAPULMONARY Percent	CASES WITH BOTH PULMONARY AND EXTRAPULMONARY DISEASE Number	CASES WITH BOTH PULMONARY AND EXTRAPULMONARY DISEASE Percent
Iowa	73	56	76.7	17	23.3	0	0.0
Kansas	92	78	84.8	14	15.2	5	5.4
Kentucky	605	544	89.9	61	10.1	15	2.5
Louisiana	471	398	84.5	73	15.5	4	0.8
Maine	57	46	80.7	11	19.3	0	0.0
Maryland	540	438	81.1	102	18.9	39	7.2
Massachusetts	503	376	74.8	127	25.2	5	1.0
Michigan	864	703	81.4	161	18.6	22	2.5
Minnesota	157	123	78.3	34	21.7	9	5.7
Mississippi	333	284	85.3	49	14.7	11	3.3
Missouri	390	330	84.6	60	15.4	6	1.5
Montana	37	24	64.9	13	35.1	4	10.8
Nebraska	32	30	93.8	2	6.3	4	12.5
Nevada	67	56	83.6	11	16.4	3	4.5
New Hampshire	33	25	75.8	8	24.2	3	9.1
New Jersey	804	612	76.1	192	23.9	19	2.4
New Mexico	122	82	67.2	40	32.8	10	8.2
New York	2,268	1,838	81.0	430	19.0	94	4.1
North Carolina	806	696	86.4	110	13.6	16	2.0
North Dakota	16	14	87.5	2	12.5	0	0.0
Ohio	621	526	84.7	95	15.3	13	2.1
Oklahoma	325	280	83.6	55	16.4	7	2.1
Oregon	194	146	75.3	48	24.7	10	5.2
Pennsylvania	1,080	884	81.9	196	18.1	41	3.8
Rhode Island	34	24	70.6	10	29.4	3	8.8
South Carolina	513	419	81.7	94	18.3	18	3.5
South Dakota	36	30	83.3	6	16.7	2	5.6
Tennessee	747	664	88.9	83	11.1	24	3.2
Texas	2,045	1,799	88.0	246	12.0	89	4.4
Utah	51	36	70.6	15	29.4	5	9.8
Vermont	13	9	69.2	4	30.8	0	0.0
Virginia	672	557	82.9	115	17.1	31	4.6
Washington	301	230	76.4	71	23.6	16	5.3
West Virginia	162	151	93.2	11	6.8	3	1.9
Wisconsin	208	163	78.4	45	21.6	10	4.8
Wyoming	10	6	60.0	4	40.0	0	0.0
American Samoa*	4	4	100.0	0	0.0	0	0.0
Guam*	49	41	83.7	8	16.3	0	0.0
Northern Mariana Is.*	75	69	92.0	6	8.0	0	0.0
Puerto Rico*	473	440	93.0	33	7.0	2	0.4
Trust Terr. Pacific Is.*	209	149	71.3	60	28.7	10	4.8
U.S. Virgin Is.*	0	0	0.0	0	0.0	0	0.0

*Not included in totals.

Notes:

(1) Cases with form of disease not specified were distributed proportionately for the U.S. and Puerto Rico.

(2) Cases with both pulmonary and extrapulmonary disease were included in the pulmonary or extrapulmonary count according to predominant site.

Source: U.S. Dept. of Health and Human Services pub. No. (CDC)84-8249

can affect any organ. As indicated in Table 1–11, which shows the number of cases affecting various parts of the body in the 50 states in 1982, most cases are confined to the lung. In 1982, there were 4,124 cases of nonpulmonary tuberculosis (TB) nationwide, representing 16.2% of the 25,520 reported cases in that year. Conversely, 83.8% of all cases were of the pulmonary form.

The mode of disease transmission in previously healthy persons is typically through inhalation of the tubercle bacillus into the bronchioles and alvioli. Having traveled this far, the bacilli multiply and invade tissue. When the organism reaches the bloodstream and lymph nodes, the infected person begins to mount specific immunity defenses for several weeks. With defenses mobilized, the body reaches a stage whereby infected tissue shows caseation necrosis (cheese-like mass of dead tissue). This greatly reduces the number of bacilli. The lesion then begins to heal through calcification and fibrosis. When this does not occur as in 10% of active cases, the disease can spread to other parts of the body. Symptoms include a cough, chest pain, and hemoptysis (coughing blood).

Those who recover have immunity to subsequent exposure to the bacillus, but they remain at risk of reactivation of their infection since the healing process of their original lesion involved a walling off of live bacilli that remain in the body. An outbreak can develop when immunity is diminished for any reason. Seven percent of TB cases in the United States are reactivated ones.

Detection of TB is often initiated by tuberculin screening skin tests administered widely to the general population. If a positive red flare reaction develops on the skin about the site of the skin puncture, follow-up diagnosis can be made through stain or—more effectively—through a culture of the patient's sputum to detect the bacilli. Chest films will show cavitary lesions and infiltrates in the lung when active tuberculosis is present. Cases diagnosed through bacteriologic identification in 1982 for pulmonary and nonpulmonary cases are shown in Tables 1–12 and 1–13. Nonpulmonary cases without bacteriologic identification are about twice as frequent as unidentified pulmonary cases.

There are other kinds of mycobacteria, the most well known of course is *Mycobacterium leprae* which causes Hansen's disease, or leprosy. But nontubercular mycobacteria can cause tuberculosis-like disease in man and may account for some of the unidentified bacteriologic cases reported.

CASE RATE

The incidence of TB in the 1980s is very slight compared to what

Table 1–12. Pulmonary Tuberculosis Cases by Bacteriologic Status: Cities of 250,000 or More Population, 1982

CITIES	TOTAL PULMONARY CASES	CASES WITH BACTERIOLOGIC RESULTS								CASES WITH BACTERIOLOGY NOT KNOWN	
		Total		Culture positive		Smear only positive		Negative			
		Number	Percent	Number	Percent	Number	Percent	Number	Percent	Number	Percent
Albuquerque, N.M.	18	17	94.4	10	58.8	1	5.9	6	35.3	1	5.6
Austin, Tex.	37	32	86.5	30	93.8	0	0.0	2	6.3	5	13.5
Baltimore, Md.	170	160	94.1	113	70.6	7	4.4	40	25.0	10	5.9
Birmingham, Ala.	62	62	100.0	56	90.3	3	4.8	3	4.8	0	0.0
Boston, Mass.	116	87	75.0	87	100.0	0	0.0	0	0.0	29	25.0
Buffalo, N.Y.	38	37	97.4	29	78.4	3	8.1	5	13.5	1	2.6
Charlotte, N.C.	49	49	100.0	37	75.5	0	0.0	12	24.5	0	0.0
Chicago, Ill.	930	870	93.5	383	44.0	321	36.9	166	19.1	60	6.5
Cincinnati, Ohio	61	60	98.4	54	90.0	1	1.7	5	8.3	1	1.6
Cleveland, Ohio	106	102	96.2	79	77.5	3	2.9	20	19.6	4	3.8
Columbus, Ohio	39	37	94.9	35	94.6	0	0.0	2	5.4	2	5.1
Dallas, Tex.	162	155	95.7	123	79.4	1	0.6	31	20.0	7	4.3
Denver, Colo.	41	39	95.1	34	87.2	0	0.0	5	12.8	2	4.9
Detroit, Mich.	252	247	98.0	145	58.7	76	30.8	26	10.5	5	2.0
El Paso, Tex.	68	62	91.2	53	85.5	5	8.1	4	6.5	6	8.8
Ft. Worth, Tex.	62	62	100.0	49	79.0	0	0.0	13	21.0	0	0.0
Honolulu, Hawaii	119	118	99.2	49	41.5	0	0.0	69	58.5	1	0.8
Houston, Tex.	567	529	93.3	418	79.0	10	1.9	101	19.1	38	6.7
Indianapolis, Ind.	77	71	92.2	50	70.4	8	11.3	13	18.3	6	7.8
Jacksonville, Fla.	83	79	95.2	73	92.4	2	2.5	4	5.1	4	4.8
Kansas City, Mo.	32	32	100.0	29	90.6	1	3.1	2	6.3	0	0.0
Long Beach, Cal.	84	77	91.7	59	76.6	7	9.1	11	14.3	7	8.3
Los Angeles, Cal.	579	554	95.7	493	89.0	10	1.8	51	9.2	25	4.3
Miami, Fla.	218	214	98.2	209	97.7	4	1.9	1	0.5	4	1.8
Milwaukee, Wisc.	52	50	96.2	39	78.0	1	2.0	10	20.0	2	3.8
Minneapolis, Minn.	24	22	91.7	15	68.2	0	0.0	7	31.8	2	8.3
Newark, N.J.	94	89	94.7	64	71.9	1	1.1	24	27.0	5	5.3
New Orleans, La.	95	95	100.0	94	98.9	0	0.0	1	1.1	0	0.0
New York, N.Y.	1,288	1,240	96.3	1,226	98.9	5	0.4	9	0.7	48	3.7
Norfolk, Va.	47	44	93.6	43	97.7	0	0.0	1	2.3	3	6.4
Oakland, Cal.	29	29	100.0	28	96.6	0	0.0	1	3.4	0	0.0
Oklahoma City, Okla.	41	41	100.0	34	82.9	4	9.8	3	7.3	0	0.0
Omaha, Nebr.	12	12	100.0	12	100.0	0	0.0	0	0.0	0	0.0
Philadelphia, Pa.	274	263	96.0	228	86.7	10	3.8	25	9.5	11	4.0

Table 1–12. (Continued)

CITIES	TOTAL PULMONARY CASES	CASES WITH BACTERIOLOGIC RESULTS: Total		Culture positive		Smear only positive		Negative		CASES WITH BACTERIOLOGY NOT KNOWN	
		Number	Percent	Number	Percent	Number	Percent	Number	Percent	Number	Percent
Phoenix, Ariz.	79	79	100.0	76	96.2	0	0.0	3	3.8	0	0.0
Pittsburgh, Pa.	58	57	98.3	43	75.4	5	8.8	9	15.8	1	1.7
Portland, Ore.	54	54	100.0	47	87.0	0	0.0	7	13.0	0	0.0
Sacramento, Cal.	80	72	90.0	63	87.5	0	0.0	9	12.5	8	10.0
St. Louis, Mo.	47	47	100.0	44	93.6	1	2.1	2	4.3	0	0.0
St. Paul, Minn.	21	21	100.0	11	52.4	0	0.0	10	47.6	0	0.0
San Antonio, Tex.	111	109	98.2	102	93.6	4	3.7	3	2.8	2	1.8
San Diego, Cal.	107	104	97.2	81	77.9	5	4.8	18	17.3	3	2.8
San Francisco, Cal.	253	226	89.3	136	60.2	4	1.8	86	38.1	27	10.7
San Jose, Cal.	94	91	96.8	75	82.4	1	1.1	15	16.5	3	3.2
Seattle, Wash.	73	70	95.9	61	87.1	0	0.0	9	12.9	3	4.1
Tampa, Fla.	76	74	97.4	60	81.1	2	2.7	12	16.2	2	2.6
Toledo, Ohio	23	22	95.7	17	77.3	2	9.1	3	13.6	1	4.3
Tucson, Ariz.	31	31	100.0	27	87.1	1	3.2	3	9.7	0	0.0
Tulsa, Okla.	25	24	96.0	21	87.5	0	0.0	3	12.5	1	4.0
Virginia Beach, Va.	13	11	84.6	10	90.9	0	0.0	1	9.1	2	15.4
Washington, D.C.	179	173	96.6	156	90.2	8	4.6	9	5.2	6	3.4
Wichita, Kans.	21	21	100.0	18	85.7	3	14.3	0	0.0	0	0.0
Total: 52 cities	7,271	6,923	95.2	5,528	79.8	520	7.5	875	12.6	348	4.8
San Juan, P.R.	72	66	91.7	40	60.6	13	19.7	13	19.7	6	8.3
Counties*											
Atlanta-Fulton Co., Ga.	171	162	94.7	141	87.0	6	3.7	15	9.3	9	5.3
Louisville-Jefferson Co., Ky.	91	84	92.3	69	82.1	10	11.9	5	6.0	7	7.7
Memphis-Shelby Co., Tenn.	77	77	100.0	32	41.6	35	45.5	10	13.0	0	0.0
Nashville-Davidson Co., Tenn.	73	73	100.0	72	98.6	1	1.4	0	0.0	0	0.0
Total: 4 counties	412	396	96.1	314	79.3	52	13.1	30	7.6	16	3.9

*Counties which include a principal city of 250,000 or more population; data for principal city were not available separately.
Source: U.S. Dept. of Health and Human Services, Pub. No. (CDC) 84–8249

Table 1–13. Extrapulmonary Tuberculosis Cases by Bacteriologic Status: Cities of 250,000 or More Population, 1982

CITIES	TOTAL EXTRA-PULMONARY CASES	CASES WITH BACTERIOLOGIC RESULTS								CASES WITH BACTERIOLOGY NOT KNOWN	
		Total		Culture positive		Smear only positive		Negative			
		Number	Percent	Number	Percent	Number	Percent	Number	Percent	Number	Percent
Albuquerque, N.M.	12	9	75.0	4	44.4	2	22.2	3	33.3	3	25.0
Austin, Tex.	3	3	100.0	3	100.0	0	0.0	0	0.0	0	0.0
Baltimore, Md.	50	47	94.0	22	46.8	7	14.9	18	38.3	3	6.0
Birmingham, Ala.	12	12	100.0	12	100.0	0	0.0	0	0.0	0	0.0
Boston, Mass.	34	28	82.4	28	100.0	0	0.0	0	0.0	6	17.6
Buffalo, N.Y.	4	4	100.0	4	100.0	0	0.0	0	0.0	0	0.0
Charlotte, N.C.	10	9	90.0	7	77.8	0	0.0	2	22.2	1	10.0
Chicago, Ill.	139	130	93.5	82	63.1	22	16.9	26	20.0	9	6.5
Cincinnati, Ohio	17	16	94.1	11	68.8	0	0.0	5	31.3	1	5.9
Cleveland, Ohio	19	17	89.5	16	94.1	1	5.9	0	0.0	2	10.5
Columbus, Ohio	12	12	100.0	12	100.0	0	0.0	0	0.0	0	0.0
Dallas, Tex.	28	21	75.0	14	66.7	0	0.0	7	33.3	7	25.0
Denver, Colo.	15	13	86.7	8	61.5	0	0.0	5	38.5	2	13.3
Detroit, Mich.	60	56	93.3	30	53.6	19	33.9	7	12.5	4	6.7
El Paso, Tex.	8	7	87.5	6	85.7	0	0.0	1	14.3	1	12.5
Ft. Worth, Tex.	14	13	92.9	11	84.6	0	0.0	2	15.4	1	7.1
Honolulu, Hawaii	12	12	100.0	5	41.7	2	16.7	5	41.7	0	0.0
Houston, Tex.	81	74	91.4	49	66.2	5	6.8	20	27.0	7	8.6
Indianapolis, Ind.	15	14	93.3	13	92.9	0	0.0	1	7.1	1	6.7
Jacksonville, Fla.	8	8	100.0	4	50.0	3	37.5	1	12.5	0	0.0
Kansas City, Mo.	10	10	100.0	10	100.0	0	0.0	0	0.0	0	0.0
Long Beach, Cal.	11	11	100.0	11	100.0	0	0.0	0	0.0	0	0.0
Los Angeles, Cal.	104	94	90.4	80	85.1	0	0.0	14	14.9	10	9.6
Miami, Fla.	51	50	98.0	47	94.0	2	4.0	1	2.0	1	2.0
Milwaukee, Wisc.	11	10	90.9	7	70.0	0	0.0	3	30.0	1	9.1
Minneapolis, Minn.	7	7	100.0	7	100.0	0	0.0	0	0.0	0	0.0
Newark, N.J.	51	46	90.2	26	56.5	3	6.5	17	37.0	5	9.8
New Orleans, La.	26	17	65.4	16	94.1	0	0.0	1	5.9	9	34.6
New York, N.Y.	306	298	97.4	290	97.3	7	2.3	1	0.3	8	2.6
Norfolk, Va.	5	5	100.0	5	100.0	0	0.0	0	0.0	0	0.0
Oakland, Cal.	6	6	100.0	5	83.3	1	16.7	0	0.0	0	0.0
Oklahoma City, Okla.	5	5	100.0	4	80.0	0	0.0	1	20.0	0	0.0
Omaha, Nebr.	0	0	0.0	0	0.0	0	0.0	0	0.0	0	0.0
Philadelphia, Pa.	61	53	86.9	35	66.0	2	3.8	16	30.2	8	13.1

Table 1–13. (Continued)

CITIES	TOTAL EXTRA-PULMONARY CASES	CASES WITH BACTERIOLOGIC RESULTS								CASES WITH BACTERIOLOGY NOT KNOWN	
		Total		Culture positive		Smear only positive		Negative			
		Number	Percent	Number	Percent	Number	Percent	Number	Percent	Number	Percent
Phoenix, Ariz.	10	10	100.0	7	70.0	1	10.0	2	20.0	0	0.0
Pittsburgh, Pa.	17	16	94.1	13	81.3	0	0.0	3	18.8	1	5.9
Portland, Ore.	12	11	91.7	8	72.7	1	9.1	2	18.2	1	8.3
Sacramento, Cal.	14	14	100.0	13	92.9	1	7.1	0	0.0	0	0.0
St. Louis, Mo.	12	12	100.0	12	100.0	0	0.0	0	0.0	0	0.0
St. Paul, Minn.	1	1	100.0	0	0.0	1	100.0	0	0.0	0	0.0
San Antonio, Tex.	22	21	95.5	21	100.0	0	0.0	0	0.0	1	4.5
San Diego, Cal.	31	30	96.8	18	60.0	1	3.3	11	36.7	1	3.2
San Francisco, Cal.	46	42	91.3	36	85.7	0	0.0	6	14.3	4	8.7
San Jose, Cal.	24	22	91.7	18	81.8	0	0.0	4	18.2	2	8.3
Seattle, Wash.	24	24	100.0	20	83.3	2	8.3	2	8.3	0	0.0
Tampa, Fla.	7	7	100.0	6	85.7	0	0.0	1	14.3	0	0.0
Toledo, Ohio	3	3	100.0	3	100.0	0	0.0	0	0.0	0	0.0
Tucson, Ariz.	10	9	90.0	7	77.8	0	0.0	2	22.2	1	10.0
Tulsa, Okla.	7	5	71.4	3	60.0	1	20.0	1	20.0	2	28.6
Virginia Beach, Va.	4	3	75.0	2	66.7	0	0.0	1	33.3	1	25.0
Washington, D.C.	49	48	98.0	39	81.3	4	8.3	5	10.4	1	2.0
Wichita, Kans.	2	2	100.0	1	50.0	1	50.0	0	0.0	0	0.0
Total: 52 cities	1,502	1,397	93.0	1,111	79.5	89	6.4	197	14.1	105	7.0
San Juan, P.R.	8	8	100.0	6	75.0	0	0.0	2	25.0	0	0.0
Counties[*]											
Atlanta-Fulton Co., Ga.	48	33	68.8	17	51.5	1	3.0	15	45.5	15	31.3
Louisville-Jefferson Co., Ky.	11	10	90.9	6	60.0	2	20.0	2	20.0	1	9.1
Memphis-Shelby Co., Tenn.	9	8	88.9	5	62.5	2	25.0	1	12.5	1	11.1
Nashville-Davidson Co., Tenn.	5	5	100.0	5	100.0	0	0.0	0	0.0	0	0.0
Total: 4 counties	73	56	76.7	33	58.9	5	8.9	18	32.1	17	23.3

[*] Counties which include a principal city of 250,000 or more population, data for principal city were not available separately.
Source: U.S. Dept. of Health and Human Services, Pub. No. (CDC) 84–8249

Fig. 1–10. Tuberculosis: Reported cases (in thousands), by year, United States, 1953–82

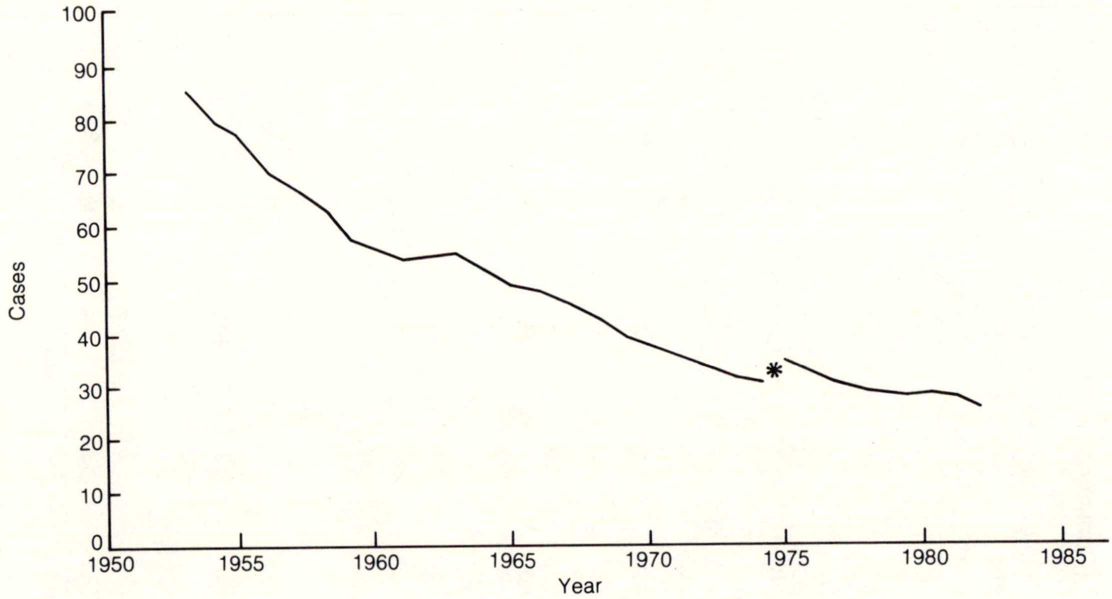

*Case date subsequent to 1974 are not comparable to prior years due to changes in reporting criteria which became effective in 1975.

Source: Morbidity and Mortality Weekly Report, Annual Summary, 1982

it was earlier in this century when it was the second leading cause of death. In 1900, over 80% of the U.S. population was infected with TB before age 20.

There has been a decline in cases from 53 per 100,000 in 1950 to 11 per 100,000 in 1982. The number of cases in thousands and their decline from approximately 85,000 a year in 1950 to about 25,000 in the early 1980s are shown in Fig. 1–10.

Concern arose in the late 1970s when U.S. health professionals noticed the rate of decline in the annual number of reported TB cases per 100,000. The rate of decline between 1978–81 decelerated from a rate of about 6.3% to only 3.2%. This deceleration was attributed to an influx of Asian immigrants who had a higher incidence of tuberculosis than had the indigenous population.

To address this development, Congress appropriated a $5 million annual grant program. The monies were designated for tuberculosis control programs already underway at the Centers for Disease Control. Because of heightened control efforts and slowdowns in Asian immigration, the rate of incidence decline increased to 7.6%

Fig. 1–11. Tuberculosis: Reported cases per 100,000 population, by age, race, and sex, United States, 1982

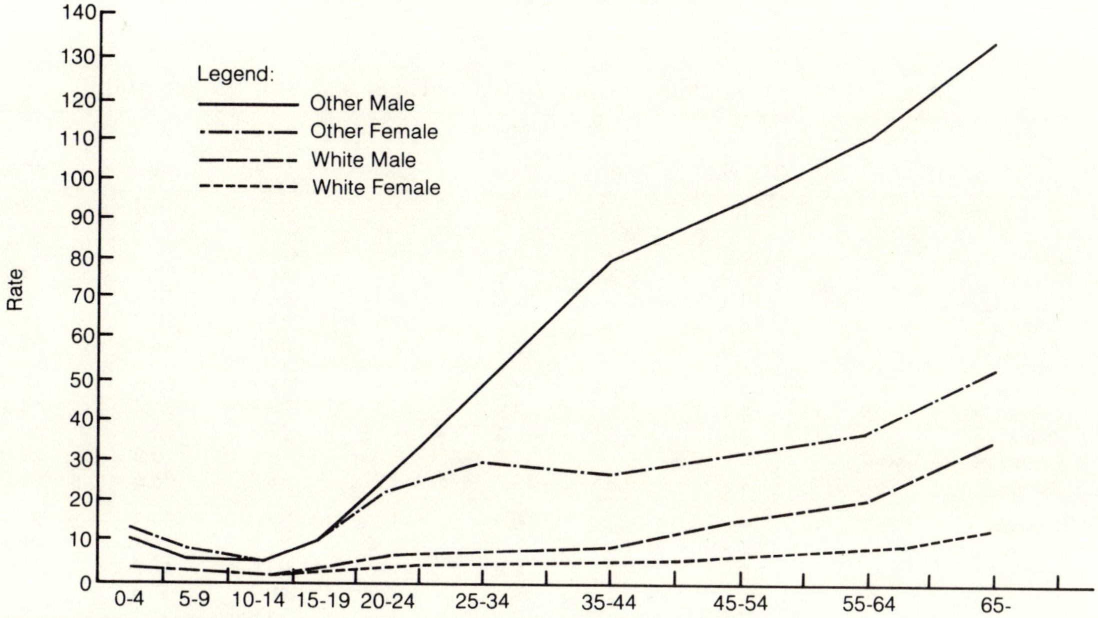

Source: Morbidity and Mortality Weekly Report, Annual Summary 1982

in 1982 over 1981 and 7.3% in 1983 over 1982. The provisional number for 1984 was also encouraging at 9.8 percent.

There is in the mid–1980s, however, renewed concern about a possible upsurge in TB cases due to reactivation of old infections in persons who have developed AIDS. Many of U.S. cases are due to reactivation rather than to a new exposure in a previously uninfected person. Because AIDS impairs the immune system, it weakens the body's defenses against the ever-present bacilli in persons with arrested TB; several cases of reactivation in AIDS patients have been reported.

The number of TB cases reported per 100,000 population in 1982 was greatest for non-white males, whereas the lowest rate persisted for white females (Fig. 1–11). As with many other diseases, the number of TB cases is greater today among white and non-white males than among females, greater among non-whites than whites, and greater among older than younger people. The case rate for 10 to 14 year olds was the lowest of any group for all races.

Non-whites are particularly overrepresented in the number of reported TB cases, possibly because many are immigrants from countries where TB is not under control, as it is in the United States. Cases specified according to race and sex by state for 1982 are shown in Table 1–14. The non-white male rate at 46.5 per 100,000 is much higher than the white male rate of 9.4 and the even lower white female rate of 4.8.

TABLE 1–14. Tuberculosis Case Rates by Race and Sex, States, 1982

STATE	TOTAL	White Total	White Male	White Female	OTHER Total	OTHER Male	OTHER Female
United States	11.0	7.1	9.4	4.8	34.4	46.5	23.4
Alabama	16.0	10.3	15.5	5.4	31.9	48.7	17.4
Alaska	21.9	5.3	5.5	5.1	78.0	76.5	79.6
Arizona	10.5	8.0	11.2	4.9	32.5	40.7	24.5
Arkansas	18.0	14.0	17.2	10.9	37.2	52.2	24.2
California	14.6	10.2	13.1	7.4	39.9	48.1	32.0
Colorado	3.7	2.7	3.2	2.1	19.7	20.0	19.4
Connecticut	4.9	3.2	3.8	2.6	24.3	34.4	15.3
Delaware	9.1	6.6	8.3	5.1	21.2	30.6	12.7
District of Columbia	36.1	5.1	7.3	3.2	48.2	70.8	29.0
Florida	14.1	8.3	12.2	4.7	45.2	65.3	27.0
Georgia	14.7	7.2	9.9	4.6	33.6	47.4	21.3
Hawaii	25.4	4.2	4.7	3.6	37.4	46.7	28.2
Idaho	3.2	2.6	3.8	1.3	28.0	41.7	15.4
Illinois	14.4	7.7	9.4	6.1	48.7	67.6	32.1
Indiana	7.3	5.4	7.1	3.8	29.3	36.1	23.1
Iowa	2.5	1.8	2.5	1.1	39.3	35.7	42.9
Kansas	3.8	2.5	3.3	1.8	21.3	31.7	11.0
Kentucky	16.5	15.0	18.3	11.8	35.0	43.3	27.3
Louisiana	10.8	7.4	11.0	3.8	18.4	26.8	10.8
Maine	5.0	4.7	5.5	4.0	36.4	(50.0)	(20.0)
Maryland	12.7	6.6	8.1	5.1	31.1	44.8	18.7
Massachusetts	8.7	6.2	7.9	4.6	52.7	64.4	42.0
Michigan	9.5	5.8	7.0	4.7	32.5	44.4	21.7
Minnesota	3.8	2.1	2.4	1.7	58.7	79.0	39.1
Mississippi	13.1	8.2	11.4	5.0	21.7	30.1	14.3
Missouri	7.9	7.0	8.8	5.2	15.1	20.7	10.1
Montana	4.6	2.5	2.9	2.1	38.3	52.2	25.0
Nebraska	2.0	1.5	2.0	1.0	13.2	18.2	8.6
Nevada	7.6	6.0	9.3	2.6	19.6	30.0	9.6
New Hampshire	3.5	3.3	5.9	0.8	18.2	(40.0)	—
New Jersey	10.8	6.4	8.0	4.9	36.6	49.1	25.5
New Mexico	9.0	5.1	5.7	4.4	39.4	42.7	36.3
New York	12.8	. .	. .	. .	. .	. .	. .
North Carolina	13.4	6.7	9.9	3.6	34.0	50.5	19.1
North Dakota	2.4	1.4	2.2	0.6	25.9	35.7	15.4
Ohio	5.8	4.0	5.2	2.8	20.8	26.1	16.2
Oklahoma	10.5	7.8	10.8	5.0	27.3	33.3	21.6
Oregon	7.3	5.4	7.5	3.3	52.3	50.9	53.6
Pennsylvania	9.1	6.1	8.9	3.5	37.4	51.7	25.0
Rhode Island	3.5	2.6	2.7	2.5	26.3	33.3	20.0
South Carolina	16.0	7.1	9.8	4.5	35.4	49.2	23.0
South Dakota	5.2	1.6	1.9	1.2	54.2	60.9	48.0

TABLE 1–14. (Continued)

		White			OTHER		
STATE	TOTAL	Total	Male	Female	Total	Male	Female
Tennessee	16.1	14.5	18.5	10.8	23.8	32.4	16.2
Texas	13.4	10.5	14.2	7.0	30.2	41.5	19.6
Utah	3.3	2.3	3.5	1.1	26.6	30.3	22.6
Vermont	2.5	2.5	2.8	2.3	—	—	—
Virginia	12.2	6.7	9.4	4.0	33.3	42.2	25.0
Washington	7.1	4.1	5.4	2.8	46.1	52.6	39.3
West Virginia	8.3	7.7	11.6	4.0	23.3	35.3	12.8
Wisconsin	4.4	3.0	3.7	2.3	29.6	41.7	18.4
Wyoming	2.0	1.4	2.0	0.8	20.0	(25.0)	(14.3)
American Samoa*	12.1	. .	. .	. .	. .	. .	. .
Guam*	46.3	. .	. .	. .	. .	. .	. .
Northern Mariana Is*	443.8	. .	. .	. .	. .	. .	. .
Puerto Rico*	14.8	. .	. .	. .	. .	. .	. .
Trust Terr. Pacific Is*	178.6	. .	. .	. .	. .	. .	. .
U.S. Virgin Is*	—	. .	. .	. .	. .	. .	. .

*Not included in totals.
(—)No cases
(. .)Not available
Notes:
(1) Rates enclosed in parentheses have a population base under 10,000
(2) Cases with race or sex not specified distributed proportionately
(3) Population by race and sex not available for outlying areas of U.S.
Source: U.S. Dept. of Health and Human Services, Publ. No. (CDC) 84–8249

It is interesting to note that Alaska, with a rate of 76.5, the District of Columbia, with a rate of 70.8, Florida, at 65.3, and Minnesota, at 79.0, are not only states with higher overall TB rates but states whose non-white population is more tubercular than the non-white populations of other states. The cases of Florida and Minnesota may be explained in part by the recent arrival of their respective Hispanic and Asian populations, while the District of Columbia's may be explained by the great concentration of non-whites in a small geographic area.

The dispersion of tuberculosis through the United States is shown in Fig. 1–12. The areas of greatest prevalence are those where the concentration of non-white population is the greatest, particularly in the South.

MORTALITY

As recently as 1953, the tuberculosis mortality rate was 12.4 per 100,000. By 1982, the rate had declined to only 0.09 per 100,000, reaching 0.08 by 1984. This victory over death is shown in Table 1–15. The breakdown of deaths by race and type of TB in 1979 is presented in Table 1–16.

Fig. 1–12. Tuberculosis: reported average cases per 100,000 population, by county, United States, 1978–1980

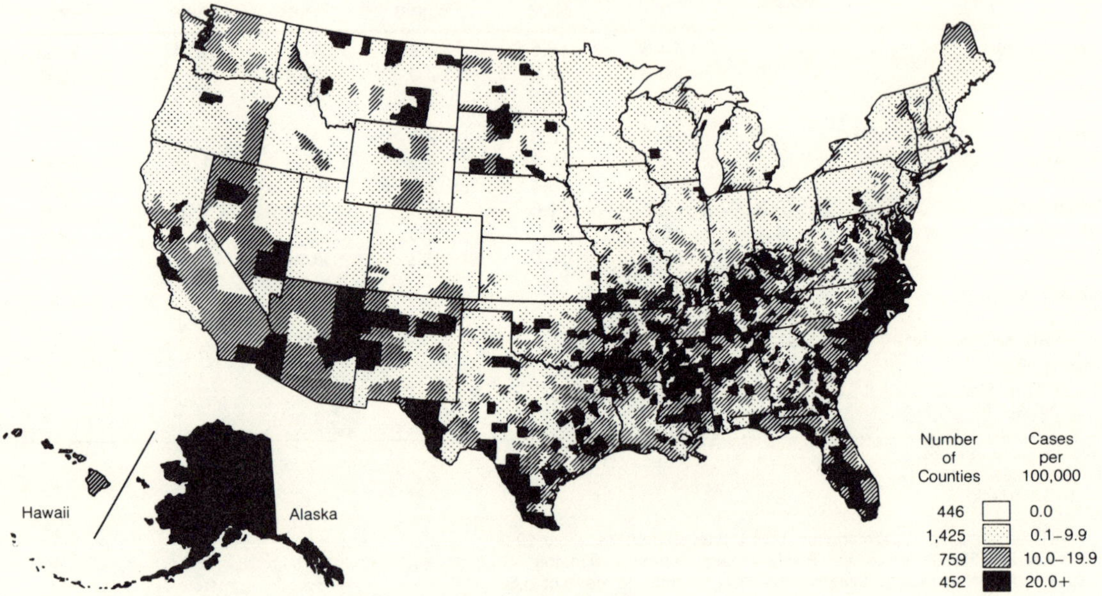

Source: Morbidity and Mortality Weekly Report, Annual Report 1982

TABLE 1–15 Tuberculosis Cases and Case Rates, Deaths and Death Rates, United States, 1953–1982

	TUBERCULOSIS CASES				TUBERCULOSIS DEATHS			
			Percent Change				Percent Change	
YEAR	Number	Rate	Number	Rate	Number	Rate	Number	Rate
1953	84,304	53.0	—	—	19,707	12.4	—	—
1954	79,775	49.3	−5.4	− 7.0	16,527	10.2	−16.1	−17.7
1955	77,368	46.9	−3.0	− 4.9	15,016	9.1	− 9.1	−10.8
1956	69,895	41.6	−9.7	−11.3	14,137	8.4	− 5.9	− 7.7
1957	67,149	39.2	−3.9	− 5.8	13,390	7.8	− 5.3	− 7.1
1958	63,534	36.5	−5.4	− 6.9	12,417	7.1	− 7.3	− 9.0
1959	57,535	32.5	−9.4	−11.0	11,474	6.5	− 7.6	− 8.5
1960	55,494	30.8	−3.5	− 5.2	10,866	6.0	− 5.3	− 7.7
1961	53,726	29.4	−3.2	− 4.5	9,938	5.4	− 8.5	−10.0
1962	53,315	28.7	−0.8	− 2.4	9,506	5.1	− 4.3	− 5.6
1963	54,042	28.7	+1.4	0.0	9,311	4.9	− 2.1	− 3.9
1964	50,874	26.6	−5.9	− 7.3	8,303	4.3	−10.8	−12.2
1965	49,016	25.3	−3.7	− 4.9	7,934	4.1	− 4.4	− 4.7
1966	47,767	24.4	−2.5	− 3.6	7,625	3.9	− 3.9	− 4.9
1967	45,647	23.1	−4.4	− 5.3	6,901	3.5	− 9.5	−10.3
1968	42,623	21.3	−6.6	− 7.8	6,292	3.1	− 8.8	−11.4
1969	39,120	19.4	−8.2	− 8.9	5,567	2.8	−11.5	− 9.7
1970	37,137	18.3	−5.1	− 5.7	5,217	2.6	− 6.3	− 7.1
1971	35,217	17.1	−5.2	− 6.6	4,501	2.2	−13.7	−15.4
1972	32,882	15.8	−6.6	− 7.6	4,376	2.1	− 2.8	− 4.5

	TUBERCULOSIS CASES				TUBERCULOSIS DEATHS			
			Percent Change				Percent Change	
YEAR	Number	Rate	Number	Rate	Number	Rate	Number	Rate
1973	30,998	14.8	−5.7	− 6.3	3,875	1.8	−11.4	−14.3
1974	30,122	14.2	−2.8	− 4.1	3,513	1.7	− 9.3	− 5.6
1975	33,989	15.9	—	—	3,333	1.6	− 5.1	− 5.9
1976	32,105	15.0	−5.5	− 5.7	3,130	1.5	− 6.1	− 6.3
1977	30,145	13.9	−6.1	− 7.3	2,968	1.4	− 5.2	− 6.7
1978	28,521	13.1	−5.4	− 5.8	2,914	1.3	− 1.8	− 7.1
1979	27,669	12.6	−3.0	− 3.8	2,012	0.9	−31.0†	−30.8†
1980	27,749	12.3	+0.3	− 2.4	1,978	0.9	− 1.7	0.0
1981	27,373	11.9	−1.4	− 3.3	1,780*	0.8*	−10.0	−11.1
1982	25,520	11.0	−6.8	− 7.6	1,980*	0.9*	+11.2	+12.5

*Provisional. Deaths for 1981 and 1982 are based on the NCHS 10% sample of death certificates.
†The large decrease in 1979 occurred because late effects of tuberculosis (e.g., bronchiectasis or fibrosis) and pleurisy with effusion (without mention of cause) are no longer included in tuberculosis deaths.
Note: Case date subsequent to 1974 are not comparable to prior years due to changes in counting criteria which became effective in 1975.
Source: U.S. Dept. of Health and Human Services, Pub. No. (CDC) 84–8249.

TABLE 1–16. Tuberculosis Deaths by Race and Form of Disease, States, 1979

STATE	ALL RACES			WHITE			OTHER		
	Total	Respiratory	Other Forms	Total	Respiratory	Other Forms	Total	Respiratory	Other Forms
United States	2,012	1,662	350	1,299	1,111	188	713	551	162
Alabama	53	43	10	29	28	1	24	15	9
Alaska	4	2	2	0	0	0	4	2	2
Arizona	31	25	6	16	14	2	15	11	4
Arkansas	35	32	3	24	22	2	11	10	1
California	178	140	38	134	113	21	44	27	17
Colorado	16	13	3	16	13	3	0	0	0
Connecticut	12	6	6	11	6	5	1	0	1
Delaware	8	7	1	5	5	0	3	2	1
District of Columbia	19	16	3	4	3	1	15	13	2
Florida	126	110	16	65	59	6	61	51	10
Georgia	59	48	11	24	21	3	35	27	8
Hawaii	9	9	0	2	2	0	7	7	0
Idaho	2	1	1	2	1	1	0	0	0
Illinois	108	96	12	58	54	4	50	42	8
Indiana	47	40	7	37	33	4	10	7	3
Iowa	8	6	2	8	6	2	0	0	0
Kansas	13	9	4	11	9	2	2	0	2
Kentucky	61	58	3	55	52	3	6	6	0
Louisiana	59	44	15	26	20	6	33	24	9
Maine	6	6	0	4	4	0	2	2	0
Maryland	29	24	5	15	13	2	14	11	3
Massachusetts	30	20	10	27	18	9	3	2	1
Michigan	61	46	15	36	30	6	25	16	9
Minnesota	12	10	2	12	10	2	0	0	0

TABLE 1–16. (Continued)

STATE	ALL RACES			WHITE			OTHER		
	Total	Respiratory	Other Forms	Total	Respiratory	Other Forms	Total	Respiratory	Other Forms
Mississippi	42	36	6	20	17	3	22	19	3
Missouri	41	36	5	32	30	2	9	6	3
Montana	5	5	0	4	4	0	1	1	0
Nebraska	6	4	2	5	4	1	1	0	1
Nevada	5	3	2	3	2	1	2	1	1
New Hampshire	4	3	1	4	3	1	0	0	0
New Jersey	58	45	13	36	30	6	22	15	7
New Mexico	20	15	5	16	12	4	4	3	1
New York	173	147	26	89	72	17	84	75	9
North Carolina	65	56	9	28	25	3	37	31	6
North Dakota	4	3	1	4	3	1	0	0	0
Ohio	84	74	10	63	55	8	21	19	2
Oklahoma	26	24	2	19	18	1	7	6	1
Oregon	13	13	0	13	13	0	0	0	0
Pennsylvania	115	96	19	90	76	14	25	20	5
Rhode Island	7	6	1	6	6	0	1	0	1
South Carolina	45	37	8	13	13	0	32	24	8
South Dakota	10	6	4	6	5	1	4	1	3
Tennessee	66	53	13	50	41	9	16	12	4
Texas	108	81	27	86	65	21	22	16	6
Utah	2	2	0	2	2	0	0	0	0
Vermont	4	4	0	4	4	0	0	0	0
Virginia	48	38	10	20	19	1	28	19	9
Washington	18	16	2	14	12	2	4	4	0
West Virginia	29	27	2	26	25	1	3	2	1
Wisconsin	28	21	7	25	19	6	3	2	1
Wyoming	0	0	0	0	0	0	0	0	0

Source: U.S. Dept. of Health and Human Services, Pub. No. (CDC) 84-8249

More recently the overall U.S. death rate declined to approximately 1 per 100,000 while a higher death rate of between 1.5 and 2 prevailed in major cities (Table 1–17).

This great advance in disease control is due historically to actions taken by developed countries to isolate and treat active cases in sanitoria and to screen populations for the presence of the disease once the cause and mode of transmission had become known. As early as 1910, researchers, including Koch, began to notice a decline in the incidence of the disease. Striking data from the British Isles confirmed Koch's guess that sanatoria care was the critical factor responsible for abatement of TB incidence and mortality.

The data in Fig. 1–13 indicate the differences in mortality in Ireland contrasted with that of Scotland and England/Wales between 1865 and 1900. In the latter two countries, health insurance

TABLE 1–17. Tuberculosis Deaths and Death Rates: Cities of 250,000 or More Population, 1979 and 1978

CITIES	TUBERCULOSIS DEATHS		DEATH RATE		RANK ACCORDING TO RATE		POPULATION ESTIMATES
	1979	1978	1979	1978	1979	1978	1979
Albuquerque, N.M.	4	3	1.3	1.0	28	50	301,800
Atlanta, Ga.	3	18	0.7	4.1	45	3	430,500
Austin, Tex.	0	4	0.0	1.1	54	46	335,500
Baltimore, Md.	15	33	1.9	4.2	11	2	780,500
Birmingham, Ala.	5	11	1.7	4.1	17	4	286,000
Boston, Mass.	2	6	0.3	1.0	52	51	618,400
Buffalo, N.Y.	7	11	1.9	2.8	12	9	372,500
Charlotte, N.C.	7	4	2.1	1.2	8	40	327,100
Chicago, Ill.	66	105	2.0	3.1	9	6	3,367,000
Cincinnati, Ohio	7	10	1.8	2.5	15	16	396,900
Cleveland, Ohio	8	13	1.3	2.1	30	22	610,200
Columbus, Ohio	8	10	1.5	1.9	22	29	538,800
Dallas, Tex.	12	10	1.2	1.1	34	45	965,900
Denver, Colo.	5	10	1.1	2.1	37	24	461,600
Detroit, Mich.	28	30	2.2	2.2	7	19	1,289,900
El Paso, Tex.	6	7	1.5	1.8	23	30	408,900
Ft. Worth, Tex.	7	6	1.6	1.3	20	39	444,700
Honolulu, Hawaii	4	1	1.1	0.3	36	55	362,200
Houston, Tex.	16	22	1.0	1.2	38	41	1,621,700
Indianapolis, Ind.	7	10	1.0	1.4	39	38	721,900
Jacksonville, Fla.	10	11	1.8	1.9	16	27	569,400
Kansas City, Mo.	6	14	1.3	3.1	31	7	458,600
Long Beach, Cal.	2	3	0.6	0.9	47	52	349,000
Los Angeles, Cal.	37	44	1.3	1.6	29	33	2,801,900
Louisville, Ky.	4	9	1.3	2.8	33	10	319,900
Memphis, Tenn.	10	7	1.5	1.0	24	49	683,500
Miami, Fla.	9	11	2.4	2.9	5	8	374,300
Milwaukee, Wisc.	12	7	2.0	1.1	10	44	613,200
Minneapolis, Minn.	0	4	0.0	1.1	55	43	370,200
Nashville, Tenn.	2	10	0.4	2.2	49	20	453,600
Newark, N.J.	7	9	2.2	2.1	6	21	312,800
New Orleans, La.	29	26	5.1	4.6	1	1	569,100
New York, N.Y.	110	182	1.4	2.4	26	17	7,615,000
Norfolk, Va.	4	6	1.4	2.1	27	23	279,500
Oakland, Cal.	6	4	1.8	1.2	13	42	329,900
Oklahoma City, Okla.	0	4	0.0	1.1	56	47	379,800
Omaha, Nebr.	1	3	0.3	0.8	53	53	379,800
Philadelphia, Pa.	32	50	1.8	2.8	14	11	1,760,200
Phoenix, Ariz.	5	11	0.7	1.5	46	35	758,000
Pittsburgh, Pa.	5	12	1.2	2.7	35	14	432,300
Portland, Ore.	3	10	0.8	2.7	43	12	370,000
Rochester, N.Y.	4	4	1.6	1.6	19	34	251,300
Sacramento, Cal.	4	5	1.5	1.9	21	28	264,700
St. Louis, Mo.	13	14	2.6	2.7	3	13	501,000
St. Paul, Minn.	1	0	0.4	0.0	51	56	270,700

TABLE 1–17. (Continued)

CITIES	TUBERCULOSIS DEATHS		DEATH RATE		RANK ACCORDING TO RATE		POPULATION ESTIMATES
	1979	1978	1979	1978	1979	1978	1979
San Antonio, Tex.	10	11	1.3	1.5	32	36	780,500
San Diego, Cal.	6	11	0.7	1.4	44	37	825,700
San Francisco, Cal.	11	11	1.7	1.7	18	31	657,200
San Jose, Cal.	5	6	0.9	1.0	41	48	586,700
Seattle, Wash.	7	8	1.5	1.6	25	32	479,300
Tampa, Fla.	10	7	3.6	2.4	2	18	277,000
Toledo, Ohio	2	7	0.6	1.9	48	26	363,600
Tucson, Ariz.	3	8	0.9	2.6	40	15	325,000
Tulsa, Okla.	3	7	0.8	2.0	42	25	361,600
Washington, D.C.	16	27	2.4	4.0	4	5	656,000
Wichita, Kans.	1	2	0.4	0.8	50	54	261,000
Total–56 Cities	607	889	1.5	2.1	—	—	41,683,300
All other areas	1,405	2,025	0.8	1.1	—	—	178,415,700
United States	2,012	2,914	0.9	1.3	—	—	220,099,000

Source: U.S. Dept. of Health and Human Services, Pub. No. (CDC) 84–8249

provided for care in private sanatoria but the Irish plan provided a subsidy to TB victims while allowing them to remain at home where they did not receive adequate medical care.

Koch observed the same decline while examining data gathered

Fig. 1–13. Mortality rates for tuberculosis in England, Scotland, and Ireland

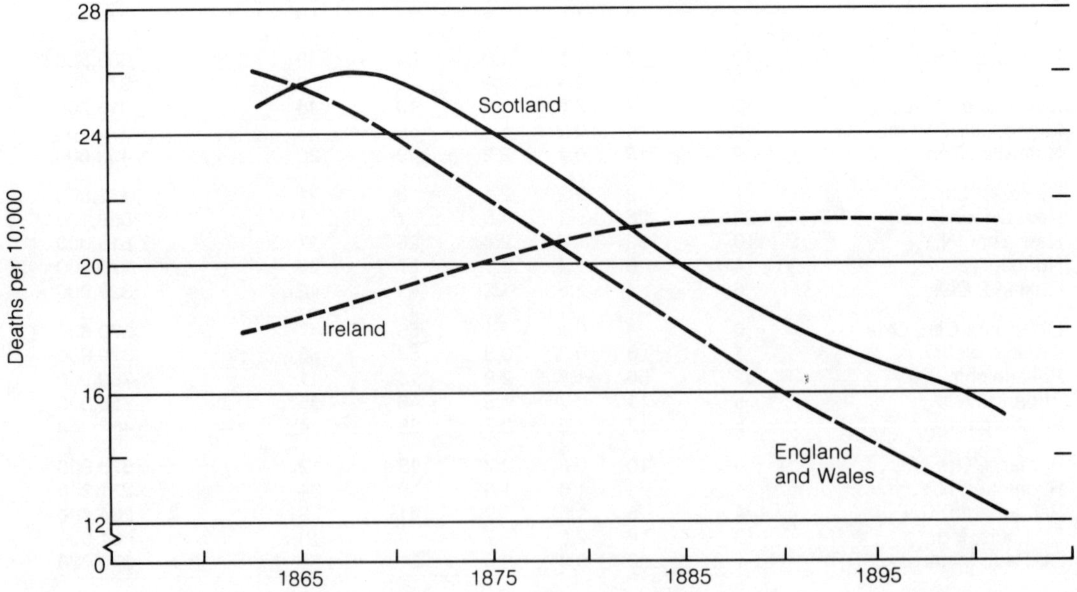

Source: Public Health Reports, Vol. 99, No. 3, 1984.

on TB victims in Manhattan and the Bronx in New York City between 1869 and 1907. The decline was fairly steady, dropping from 43 to 23 deaths per 100,000 between those two years, but then the decline ceased and leveled off (Fig. 1–14). Koch called this leveling off to the attention of New York authorities and recommended that more sanatoria beds be designated for disease victims. This suggestion was implemented by the addition of approximately 5,000 more sanatoria beds and as Koch predicted, TB mortality began to fall once again. Indeed, the drop shown between 1907 and 1920 was slightly steeper than the period before declining from 25 to 10 deaths per 100,000 (Fig. 1–14).

There have been attempts to control TB in underdeveloped countries by administration of the BCG vaccine, which contains an attenuated mycobacterium tuberculosis bacillus. But these efforts have not proven as successful as hoped in that it does not seem to protect children younger than age 5 years, although some protection has been found 5 to 10 years after vaccination in children initially age 0 to 14. These results are better than the famous Chingleput study begun in India in 1968 in which 270,000 people received one of two vaccines or a placebo randomly. After 7½ years, the number of pulmonary TB cases in each group was the same.[b] The deat rates due to tuberculosis in several countries around the world are listed in Table 1–18.

[b]*Morbidity and Mortality Weekly Report* Vol. 32, No. 18

Fig. 1–14. Mortality rates for tuberculosis in New York City

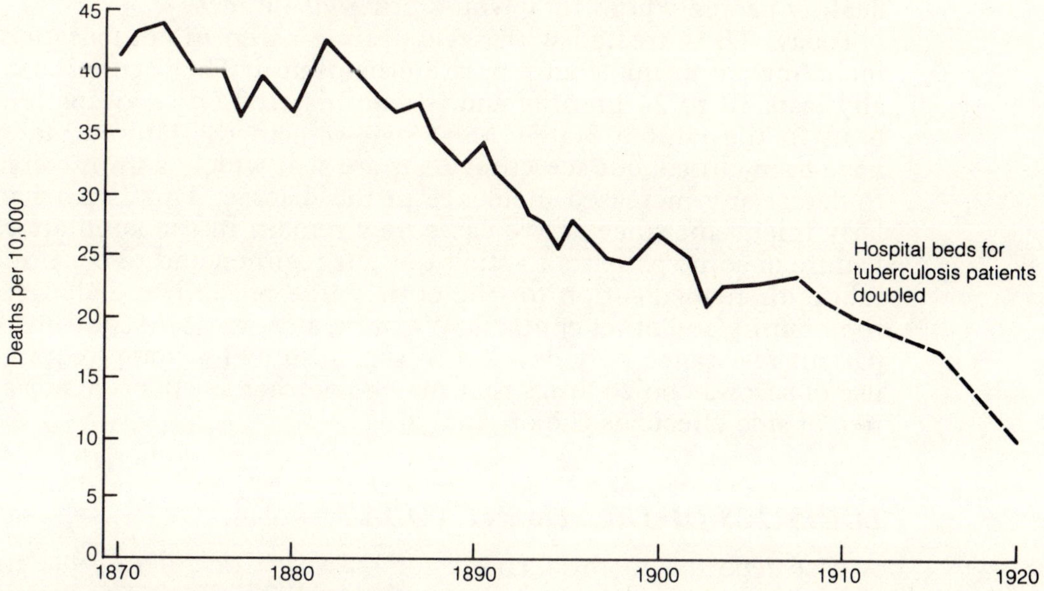

Source: Public Health Reports, Vol. 99, No. 3, 1984.

TABLE 1–18. TB Mortality Rates by Country

COUNTRY	RATE*	YEAR REPORTED
Australia	0.4	80
Austria	4.6	81
Bulgaria	3.7	81
Costa Rica	3.4	81
Chile	12.2	80
France	3.0	80
Hungary	10.8	80
Japan	5.5	80
Kuwait	6.1	79
Poland	0.4	81
United Kingdom†	1.1	81

*Per 100,000
†United Kingdom includes only England and Wales
Source: UN Demographic Yearbook, 1982

The defeat of TB in the United States during the early 20th Century is a particularly interesting epidemiologic story since there was no drug treatment for TB at that time. Treatment in the sanatoria consisted of fresh air, rest, a balanced nutritious diet, and sanitary conditions—factors often missing in the homes of afflicted individuals. Tuberculosis seemed to afflict the poor more than other socioeconomic groups, possibly because they had lowered resistance to disease in general and their close living quarters provided a fertile field for spread of the disease to all members of poor families. At the sanatoria, the routine was a nap after lunch and a walk after dinner, while removing sick individuals from healthy people whom they would otherwise infect.

Today, TB is treated with several drugs often in combination, including isoniazid, rifampin, and ethambutol. The regimen usually lasts 18 to 24 months and is administered on an outpatient basis in the United States. Most sanatoria in the United States have been closed, but screening tests are still widely administered to detect any increased incidence in the disease. This is particularly important since active cases now remain in the population. Failure of some patients to stick to their regimen and to continue taking their medication for the entire time prescribed endangers their family and other contacts. When medication is discontinued, patient resistance may develop so that resumed therapy requires use of second-choice drugs that may be neither as effective nor as free of side effects as the original drug.

LOGISTICS OF TREATMENT TODAY

A case reported to the Centers for Disease Control in 1982 involved a woman who was being treated for TB in Utah. She moved to Montana and discontinued her treatment before finishing her regimen. Because of her contacts with family members, people on the job, people in her community, and relatives in other states, over 700 people in eight states had to be traced and screened for TB. Of these, six cases of active TB were diagnosed, four of them among children younger than age 15 years. Fifty-three other people reacted positively to the TB screening skin test in Utah, Nevada, Montana, and California and were given prophylactic regimens of drug alternatives to isoniazid since the woman's bacilli had become resistant to isoniazid. The alternative drug chosen was rifampin. But controlled trials have not shown rifampin to be effective in preventing TB. Typically, preventive therapy consists of administration of isoniazid at 300 mg per day for 12 months. This outbreak is the largest one in which use of rifampin has been tried prophylactically.

Contacts identified in Illinois, Oklahoma, Washington, and Wyoming luckily showed no positive reaction to TB screening. But the hardship and spread of resistant disease, the tracing, screening, and treatment of large numbers of people could have been avoided completely had the woman completed her treatment as prescribed. The patient's responsibility to follow and complete treatment is important today if patients with active disease are to continue to live among the public at large.[c]

Table 1–19 provides information on the current therapy status of patients living at home in 1981, whether they have completed their drug regimen in that year, were interrupted, stopped or were lost to medical follow-up. As can be seen, there are patients in each region of the United States with a therapy lapse or discontinuance. Public health authorities are becoming concerned about the prevalence of patients remaining under supervision during treatment. Some studies are showing that as many as 20% of outpatients with tuberculosis fail to complete even 6 months of therapy.

[c]*Morbidity and Mortality Weekly Report* Vol. 32, No. 39

TABLE 1–19. Completion of Drug Therapy Started in 1980

REGION AND PROGRAM AREA	Patients Eligible for 24 Months Drugs*	COMPLETED IN 24 MONTHS		DID NOT COMPLETE IN 24 MONTHS		
		Number	Percent	Still On	Stopped	Lost
Region I:						
Connecticut State	138	102	73.9	9	19	8
Maine State	47	45	95.7	0	1	1
Massachusetts State	..	..	..	..	..	..
Massachusetts, Boston	92	65	70.7	14	1	12
New Hampshire State	..	..	..	..	..	..

TABLE 1–19. (Continued)

REGION AND PROGRAM AREA	Patients Eligible for 24 Months Drugs*	COMPLETED IN 24 MONTHS		DID NOT COMPLETE IN 24 MONTHS		
		Number	Percent	Still On	Stopped	Lost
Rhode Island State	. .	. .	. .	. .	. .	. .
Vermont State	17	14	82.4	0	3	0
Total:	294	226	76.9	23	24	21
Region II:						
New Jersey State	. .	. .	. .	. .	. .	. .
New Jersey, Jersey City	. .	. .	. .	. .	. .	. .
New Jersey, Newark	. .	. .	. .	. .	. .	. .
New York State	. .	. .	. .	. .	. .	. .
New York, Buffalo-Erie Co.	. .	. .	. .	. .	. .	. .
New York, New York City	1,168	844	72.3	65	44	215
New York, Rochester-Monroe Co.	. .	. .	. .	. .	. .	. .
Puerto Rico	. .	. .	. .	. .	. .	. .
Puerto Rico, San Juan	. .	. .	. .	. .	. .	. .
Virgin Islands	4	1	25.0	2	0	1
Total:	1,172	845	72.1	67	44	216
Region III:						
Delaware State	. .	. .	. .	. .	. .	. .
District of Columbia	191	154	80.6	19	2	16
Maryland State	. .	. .	. .	. .	. .	. .
Maryland, Baltimore	. .	. .	. .	. .	. .	. .
Pennsylvania State	. .	. .	. .	. .	. .	. .
Pennsylvania, Philadelphia[†]	114	96	84.2	5	7	6
Pennsylvania, Pittsburgh-Allegheny Co.	114	111	97.4	1	0	2
Virginia State	399	379	95.0	2	13	5
Virginia, Norfolk	43	42	97.7	1	0	0
Virginia, Richmond	27	26	96.3	0	0	1
Virginia, Virginia Beach	12	12	100.0	0	0	0
West Virginia State	117	87	74.4	13	11	6
Total:	1,017	907	89.2	41	33	36
Region IV:						
Alabama State	367	352	95.9	9	4	2
Alabama, Birmingham-Jefferson Co.	114	113	99.1	0	0	1
Florida State	. .	. .	. .	. .	. .	
Forida, Jacksonville-Duval Co.	. .	. .	. .	. .	. .	. .
Forida, Miami-Dade Co.	. .	. .	. .	. .	. .	. .
Forida, Tampa-Hillsborough Co.	. .	. .	. .	. .	. .	. .
Georgia State	. .	. .	. .	. .	. .	. .
Georgia, Atlanta-Fulton Co.	. .	. .	. .	. .	. .	. .
Kentucky State	346	324	93.6	2	18	2
Kentucky, Louisville-Jefferson Co.	69	64	92.8	1	1	3
Mississippi State	. .	. .	. .	. .	. .	. .
North Carolina State	. .	. .	. .	. .	. .	. .
North Carolina, Charlotte	. .	. .	. .	. .	. .	. .
South Carolina State	398	371	93.2	14	10	3
Tennessee State	361	344	95.3	6	9	2
Tennessee, Chattanooga-Hamilton Co.	43	39	90.7	1	3	0
Tennessee, Knoxville-Knox Co.	38	35	92.1	0	3	0
Tennessee, Memphis-Shelby Co.	102	87	85.3	5	9	1
Tennessee, Nashville-Davidson Co.	67	61	91.0	2	2	2
Total:	1,905	1,790	94.0	40	59	16

TABLE 1–19. (Continued)

REGION AND PROGRAM AREA	Patients Eligible for 24 Months Drugs*	COMPLETED IN 24 MONTHS		DID NOT COMPLETE IN 24 MONTHS		
		Number	Percent	Still On	Stopped	Lost
Region V:						
Illinois State‡	260	210	80.8	10	22	18
Illinois, Suburban Cook Co.	109	83	76.1	5	15	6
Illinois, Chicago	563	236	41.9	61	15	251
Indiana State	..	..	..	..	..	..
Indiana, Indianapolis-Marion Co.	..	..	..	..	..	..
Michigan State	..	..	..	..	..	..
Michigan, Detroit-Wayne Co.	..	..	..	..	..	..
Minnesota State	77	73	94,8	0	1	3
Minnesota, Minneapolis-Hennepin Co.	60	57	95.0	0	0	3
Minnesota, St. Paul-Ramsey Co.	46	41	89.1	4	0	1
Ohio State	181	134	74.0	30	3	14
Ohio, Akron-Summit Co.	20	15	75.0	3	0	2
Ohio, Cincinnati-Hamilton Co.	65	46	70.8	9	3	7
Ohio, Cleveland-Cuyahoga Co.	140	114	81.4	18	2	6
Ohio, Columbus-Franklin Co.	36	24	66.7	6	0	6
Ohio, Dayton-Montgomery Co.	33	17	51.5	7	4	5
Ohio, Toledo-Lucas Co.	16	12	75.0	2	0	2
Wisconsin State	..	..	..	..	..	..
Wisconsin, Milwaukee	..	..	..	..	..	..
Total:	1,606	1,062	66.1	155	65	324
Region VI:						
Arkansas State	..	..	..	..	..	..
Louisiana State	381	331	86.9	17	0	33
Louisiana, New Orleans	85	49	57.6	6	0	30
New Mexico State	78	76	97.4	1	1	0
New Mexico, Albuquerque-Bernalillo Co.	29	29	100.0	0	0	0
New Mexico, Indian Health Services†	1	1	100.0	0	0	0
Oklahoma State	..	..	..	..	..	..
Oklahoma, Oklahoma City-Co.	..	..	..	..	..	..
Oklahoma, Tulsa City-Co.	..	..	..	..	..	..
Texas State	945	857	90.7	5	45	38
Texas, Austin-Travis Co.	44	42	95.5	0	0	2
Texas, Dallas City-Co.	213	201	94.4	4	3	5
Texas, El Paso City-Co.	106	100	94.3	1	5	0
Texas, Ft. Worth-Tarrant Co.	110	103	93.6	0	2	5
Texas, Houston-Harris Co.	477	389	81.6	22	26	40
Texas, San Antonio-Bexar Co.	145	124	85.5	0	15	6
Total:	2,614	2,302	88.1	56	97	159
Region VII:						
Iowa State	71	60	84.5	0	3	8
Kansas State	64	60	93.8	2	2	0
Kansas, Wichita-Sedgwick Co.	19	15	78.9	0	1	3
Missouri State†	111	92	82.9	0	12	7
Missouri, St. Louis Co.	53	48	90.6	3	1	1
Missouri, Kansas City	35	23	65.7	5	3	4
Missouri, St. Louis-City	59	46	78.0	6	2	5
Nebraska State	..	..	..	..	..	..
Nebraska, Omaha-Douglas Co.	..	..	..	..	..	..
Total:	412	344	83.5	16	24	28

TABLE 1–19. (Continued)

REGION AND PROGRAM AREA	Patients Eligible for 24 Months Drugs*	COMPLETED IN 24 MONTHS		DID NOT COMPLETE IN 24 MONTHS		
		Number	Percent	Still On	Stopped	Lost
Region VIII:						
Colorado State	. .	. .	. .	. .	. .	. .
Colorado, Denver	63	57	90.5	2	1	3
Montana State	21	13	61.9	3	2	3
North Dakota State	34	29	85.3	3	0	2
South Dakota State	32	27	84.4	1	1	3
Utah State	36	27	75.0	3	1	5
Wyoming State	. .	. .	. .	. .	. .	. .
Total:	186	153	82.3	12	5	16

*Excludes patients who died or moved during the 24 months.
†Data are for 6 months of 1980.
‡Includes 93 agencies out of 101.
‖Excludes Puerto Rico, U.S. Virgin Islands, and Guam.
(. .)Not available.
Note: Programs listed under State are excluded from State totals.
Source: U.S. Dept. of Health and Human Services, Pub. No. (CDC) 84–8249

When contacts of unarrested cases were traced back to various localities, a number of other TB cases were found (Table 1–20). A process was used that was similar to the one in the case of the woman from Utah in 1982.

TABLE 1–20. Tuberculosis Cases Found among Contacts, 1982

REGION AND PROGRAM AREA	CONTACTS EXAMINED		TUBERCULOSIS CASES FOUND AMONG CONTACTS			
			Close		Other	
	Close	Other	Number	Rate*	Number	Rate*
Region I:						
Connecticut State	740	467	5	7	0	0
Maine State	71	271	1	14	1	4
Massachusetts State	. .	. .	. .	. .	. .	. .
Massachusetts, Boston	515	0	9	17	0	0
New Hampshire State	. .	. .	. .	. .	. .	. .
Rhode Island State	134	111	1	7	0	0
Vermont State	32	256	0	0	1	4
Total:	1,492	1,105	16	11	2	2
Region II:						
New Jersey State	1,297	0	11	8	0	0
New Jersey, Jersey City	134	0	1	7	0	0
New Jersey, Newark	235	0	3	13	0	0
New York State†	147	91	3	20	0	0
New York, Buffalo-Erie Co.	. .	. .	. .	. .	. .	. .
New York, New York City‡	1,478	260	23	16	1	4
New York, Rochester-Monroe Co.	. .	. .	. .	. .	. .	. .
Puerto Rico	596	250	11	18	1	4

TABLE 1–20. (Continued)

REGION AND PROGRAM AREA	CONTACTS EXAMINED		TUBERCULOSIS CASES FOUND AMONG CONTACTS			
			Close		Other	
	Close	Other	Number	Rate*	Number	Rate*
Virgin Islands	0	0	0	0	0	0
Total:	3,887	601	52	13	2	3
Region III:						
Delaware State	125	225	0	0	0	0
District of Columbia	554	227	7	13	7	31
Maryland State	1,067	2,172	8	7	2	1
Maryland, Baltimore	949	42	29	31	0	0
Pennsylvania State	1,630	1,313	9	6	0	0
Pennsylvania, Philadelphia	672	383	12	18	0	0
Pennsylvania, Pittsburgh-Allegheny Co.	222	314	2	9	1	3
Virginia State	2,616	4,680	37	14	8	2
Virginia, Norfolk	201	160	0	0	0	0
Virginia, Richmond	345	402	3	9	2	5
Virginia, Virginia Beach	119	229	2	17	0	0
West Virginia State	352	506	4	11	0	0
Total:	8,852	10,653	113	13	20	2
Region IV:						
Alabama State	1,584	3,326	20	13	3	1
Alabama, Birmingham-Jefferson Co.	735	522	4	5	0	0
Florida State	2,335	2,501	10	4	2	1
Florida, Jacksonville-Duval Co.	333	477	2	6	0	0
Florida, Miami-Dade Co.	650	860	1	2	3	3
Florida, Tampa-Hillsborough Co.	267	1,201	2	7	1	1
Georgia State	2,490	2,233	47	19	9	4
Georgia, Atlanta-Fulton Co.	457	126	4	9	0	0
Kentucky State	2,022	4,611	18	9	8	2
Kentucky, Louisville-Jefferson Co.	249	313	5	20	0	0
Mississippi State	..	..	..	..	..	..
North Carolina State	..	..	..	..	..	..
North Carolina, Charlotte	..	..	..	..	..	..
South Carolina State	4,962	0	35	7	0	0
Tennessee State	2,288	0	8	3	0	0
Tennessee, Chattanooga-Hamilton Co.	250	0	1	4	0	0
Tennessee, Knoxville-Knox Co.	233	0	0	0	0	0
Tennessee, Memphis-Shelby Co.	587	0	4	7	0	0
Tennessee, Nashville-Davidson Co.	556	0	0	0	0	0
Totals	19,998	16,170	161	8	26	2
Region V:						
Illinois State‖	1,211	805	6	5	5	6
Illinois, Suburban Cook Co.	..	..	..	..	..	..
Illinois, Chicago	..	..	..	..	..	..
Indiana State	..	..	..	..	..	..
Indiana, Indianapolis-Marion Co.	388	390	4	10	0	0
Michigan State	1,899	14,714	19	10	1	0
Michigan, Detroit-Wayne Co.	661	1,718	11	17	6	3
Minnesota State	481	329	0	0	0	0
Minnesota, Minneapolis-Hennepin Co.	213	66	0	0	0	0
Minnesota, St. Paul-Ramsey Co.	68	49	2	29	0	0

TABLE 1–20. (Continued)

REGION AND PROGRAM AREA	CONTACTS EXAMINED		TUBERCULOSIS CASES FOUND AMONG CONTACTS			
			Close		Other	
	Close	Other	Number	Rate*	Number	Rate*
Ohio State	917	525	17	19	15	29
Ohio, Akron-Summit Co.	31	52	0	0	0	0
Ohio, Cincinnati-Hamilton Co.	90	67	2	22	2	30
Ohio, Cleveland-Cuyahoga Co.	477	329	6	13	2	6
Ohio, Columbus-Franklin Co.	149	61	0	0	0	0
Ohio, Dayton, Mongtomery Co.	62	43	0	0	0	0
Ohio, Toledo-Lucas Co.	65	45	6	92	4	89
Wisconsin State +	162	58	7	43	0	0
Wisconsin, Milwaukee	206	39	0	0	0	0
Total:	7,080	19,290	80	11	35	2
Region VI:						
Arkansas State	..	..	..	..	..	..
Louisiana State	2,059	0	38	18	0	0
Louisiana, New Orleans	160	0	9	56	0	0
New Mexico State	238	729	2	8	0	0
New Mexico, Albuquerque-Bernalillo Co.	45	50	0	0	0	0
New Mexico, Indian Health Services	309	102	2	6	0	0
Oklahoma State	922	1,206	25	27	4	3
Texas State	3,421	1,684	48	14	6	4
Texas, Austin-Travis Co.	101	221	2	20	0	0
Texas, Dallas City-Co.	594	50	8	13	0	0
Texas, El Paso City-Co.	411	165	4	10	0	0
Texas, Ft. Worth-Tarrant Co.	399	17	6	15	0	0
Texas, Houston-Harris Co.	2,932	103	56	19	0	0
Texas, San Antonio-Bexar Co.	574	216	3	5	2	9
Total:	12,165	4,543	203	17	12	3
Region VII:						
Iowa State	214	223	2	9	0	0
Kansas State	216	455	1	5	0	0
Kansas, Wichita-Sedgwick Co.	91	39	3	33	0	0
Missouri State	2,142	505	10	5	1	2
Missouri, St. Louis Co.	747	0	5	7	0	0
Missouri, Kansas City	62	176	1	16	0	0
Missouri, St. Louis City	178	247	0	0	0	0
Nebraska State	42	40	0	0	0	0
Nebraska, Omaha-Douglas Co.	30	13	0	0	0	0
Total:	3,722	1,698	22	6	1	1
Region VIII:						
Colorado State	243	79	1	4	0	0
Colorado, Denver	233	263	6	26	0	0
Montana State‡	22	34	0	0	0	0
North Dakota State	24	135	1	42	0	0
South Dakota State	192	734	3	16	0	0
Utah State	129	496	1	8	1	2
Wyoming State	..	..	..	..	..	..
Total:	843	1,741	12	14	1	1

TABLE 1–20. (Continued)

REGION AND PROGRAM AREA	CONTACTS EXAMINED		TUBERCULOSIS CASES FOUND AMONG CONTACTS			
			Close		Other	
	Close	Other	Number	Rate*	Number	Rate*
Region IX:						
Arizona State‡	108	18	0	0	0	0
Arizona, Phoenix-Maricopa Co.‡	164	86	0	0	0	0
Arizona, Tucson-Pima Co.‡	14	47	0	0	0	0
Arizona, Indian Health Services‡	176	98	0	0	0	0
California State	..	..	..	..	..	..
California, Long Beach	..	..	..	..	..	..
California, Los Angeles	..	..	..	..	..	..
California, Oakland-Alameda Co.	..	..	..	..	..	..
California, Sacramento City-Co.	..	..	..	..	..	..
California, San Diego City-Co.	..	..	..	..	..	..
California, San Francisco City-Co.	652	1,006	23	35	3	3
California, San Jose-Santa Clara Co.	..	..	..	..	..	..
Hawaii State	280	78	4	14	0	0
Hawaii, Honolulu	294	46	1	3	0	0
Nevada State	122	160	2	16	0	0
Nevada, Clark Co.	45	162	0	0	1	6
Guam	..	..	..	..	..	..
Total:	1,855	1,701	30	16	4	2
Region X:						
Alaska State	224	171	11	49	3	18
Idaho State	..	..	..	..	..	..
Oregon State	..	..	..	..	..	..
Oregon, Portland-Multnomah Co.	..	..	..	..	..	..
Washington State	558	507	20	36	1	2
Washington, Seattle-King Co.	263	812	13	49	0	0
Total	1,045	1,490	44	42	4	3
Total all areas	60,939	58,992	733	12	107	2
U.S. Total‖	60,343	58,742	722	12	106	2

* Rate per 1,000 contacts examined.
† Data are for 6 of 62 counties for 6 months of 1982.
‡ Data are for 6 months of 1982.
** Includes 95 agencies out of 101.
+ Data are for 2 months of 1982.
‖ Excludes Puerto Rico, U.S. Virgin Islands, and Guam.
(. .) Not available.
Note: Program listed under State are excluded from State totals.
Source: U.S. Dept. of Health and Human Services pub. No. (CDC)84–8249

To combat the lack of supervision of clinic outpatients, outreach programs have been developed in which workers, often of the same ethnic background as the patients, visit them in their homes and administer medication to them. One such program in New York City lasting 24 months assigned workers to 98 patients who had stopped therapy. At the end of the period, 80% of these patients were either cured or on their medication. Shorter regimens of treatment have also been introduced and are undergoing study for their efficacy. One regimen under study since October 1981 requires patients to be seen twice monthly instead of once a month, receiving their medication for 6 months instead of the much longer typical schedule of up to 24 months. Patient supervision is tighter on this schedule and the shortened length of treatment could allow annual savings in drugs and services of up to $10 million.

As discussed, discontinuation of one's drug therapy before its prescribed course can lead to a tubercular relapse, often in a drug-resistant form, and the transmission of this drug-resistant disease to healthy, never-infected individuals. People so infected are said to have primary, drug-resistant, disease which can be more difficult to treat than nonresistant forms.

To determine the extent of this problem, the Centers for Disease Control analyzed 12,118 mycobacterial cultures from 20 city and state laboratories between 1975 and 1982. Organisms resistant to one or more antitubercular drugs were found in 6.9% of the samples. Resistance to isoniazid and streptomycin was greatest. Ninety-two percent of patients resistant to a TB drug were resistant to one or both of these drugs (Fig. 1–15).

Fig. 1–15. Percentages of tuberculosis patients with primary drug resistance, by race/ethnic group—United States, 1975–1982

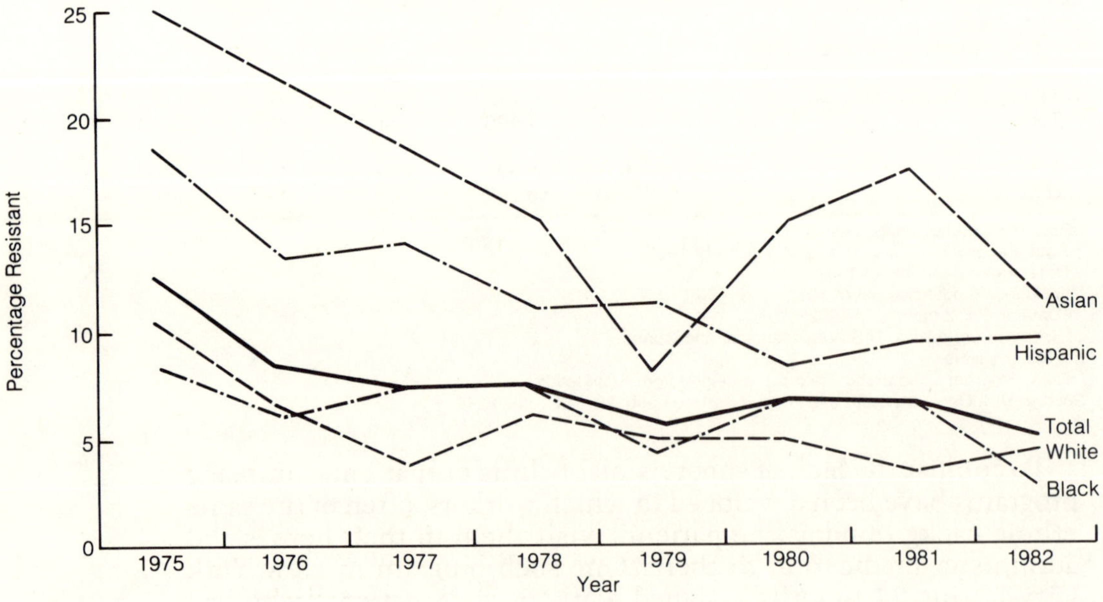

Source: Morbidity and Mortality Weekly Report, Annual Summary 1983

During the course of the survey, the percentage of primary drug-resistant cultures declined with the greatest remaining prevalence in Asian and Hispanic populations (Fig. 1–16).

Fig. 1–16. Tuberculosis: primary drug resistance rates, United States, 1975–1982

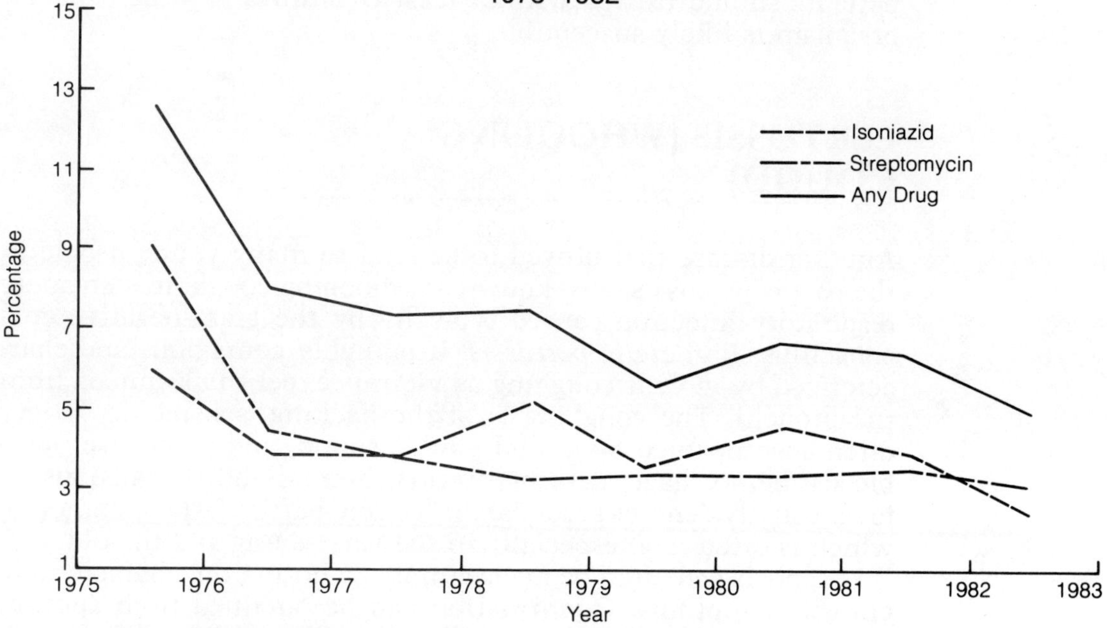

Source: Morbidity and Mortality Weekly Report, Vol. 32, No. 40, October 14, 1983

The reason for the decline in primary, drug-resistant TB is unknown, but the centers suspect that changing patterns of anti-TB therapy may be partly responsible. Use of rifampin and isoniazid in combination has resulted in less drug resistance during therapy, and this combination is being used more often now than in the 1970s. The resistance found during the survey was 4% for isoniazid, 3.8% for streptomycin, and 1.1% for thionamide. Other drugs, such as rifampin, ethambutol, kanamycin, capreomycin, and cycloserine were less than 1%.

Drug resistance was highest among Asians and Hispanics, but it is not known whether they acquired their infections in the United States or in another country from which they came. Developing countries in Asia and Latin America are known to have higher rates of primary resistant disease than the United States. One reason is that people in these countries can obtain antitubercular drugs over the counter and treat themselves since resources for treating these populations and monitoring them are inadequate.

In light of these findings, the Centers for Disease Control recommend that several kinds of patients be tested for drug-resistant TB, including Asians and Hispanics, persons previously treated with anti-TB drugs, persons who do not become culture negative by the fourth month of therapy, and persons who have been exposed to drug-resistant TB. Until sensitivity is known, high-risk patients should treated with at least two drugs to which the TB organism is likely susceptible.

PERTUSSIS (WHOOPING COUGH)

Another disease that proved to be fatal to many young people in the past is pertussis, also known as whooping cough. It is an acute respiratory infection caused typically by the gram-negative coccobacillus, *Bordetella pertussis*. It is highly contagious and characterized by violent coughing as victims expel thick mucus from the bronchi. The coughing is of the hacking, spasmodic variety often accompanied by a loud whoop sound, and can cause nosebleeds, hemorrhage, detached retina, hernia, and convulsions. A fever usually denotes secondary infection, particularly pneumonia, which is often fatal especially in the very young and the old.

Diagnosis can often be made simply by noting the characteristic clinical symptoms. Confirmation can be obtained from sputum culture in the early stage and fluorescent antibody screening of smears during later stages when the bacterium is no longer detectable on culture.

Treatment consists of medication to minimize cough and fluid buildup and administration of antibiotics to prevent secondary infection. Antibiotics are also used to lessen the contagious stage of the disease, although the decline in pertussis that has occurred during the last several decades is due largely to the development and widespread use of a pertussis vaccine. Controversy has developed over administration of the pertussis vaccine in recent years as central nervous system (CNS) disorders—including convulsions and brain damage leading to death—have been reported in children, particularly infants, after they had received the vaccine. The media have publicized cases of severely damaged children reported to have suffered their affliction within 48 to 72 hours after administration of the vaccine and have raised questions about the benefit of using the vaccine since it is thought that very few cases of pertussis occur today in the United States. However, the fact that there are very few cases compared to the number once reported is associated with the widespread use of the pertussis vaccine, which is mandated for children entering school in 44 states.

When controversy flared in the United Kingdom in 1974, vaccinations for pertussis decreased markedly. This was followed by two outbreaks of pertussis, one in 1977–1979 with more than 100,000 cases and 36 deaths, and one in 1982 with 65,000 cases and 14 reported deaths.

Authorities in the United States have also noted that the number of pertussis cases reported in the National Hospital Discharge Survey are higher than that reported by the states to the Atlanta Centers for Disease Control, which keeps the national count. It is also surmised that many pertussis cases may fail to be diagnosed or hospitalized and that the official count is considerably less than the actual. Since most American children have been vaccinated, this observation has led some researchers to question the effectiveness of the vaccine as a further complication to the debate about its use.

In evaluating the evidence for and against the vaccine, researchers point to the lack of any rigorous study of reported cases of vaccine-related side effects. They make the additional observation that infants comprise a population in which the side effects following administration of the vaccine, such as convulsions and sudden death, are thought to occur at low percentages irrespective of the vaccine, i.e., in babies not vaccinated.

Concerned critics of the vaccine remain unconvinced by such arguments. The effects of negative publicity about the vaccine may be materializing, since 79 pertussis cases in Maryland were reported to the Atlanta Centers for Disease Control in 1982. This was a sharp increase from the 10 to 18 cases reported annually for the 10 years previous. The largest proportion of patients were younger than age 1 year and residing in Baltimore. Of the infants exposed, 20 were in infants who had not received three doses of the pertussis vaccine; 26 had not been vaccinated in compliance with the age-recommended schedule. Fifty-seven percent of all the cases were hospitalized, the average length of stay being 8.6 days. Twelve patients developed pneumonia, two seizures, and one an encephalopathy.

This increase in Maryland cases was confirmed by reviews of hospital admissions and laboratory specimen submissions for 1981 and 1982. The pertussis cases and deaths reported in the United States between 1920 and 1981 are shown in Fig. 1–17. An increase in both is noticeable beginning in 1976.

In light of these considerations, most medical authorities still feel that the benefits of vaccine administration outweigh the risk. The Centers for Disease Control recommend three doses of the vaccine before age 6 months, a fourth dose at 1 year, and a booster

Fig. 1–17. Pertussis (whooping cough): reported cases and deaths per 100,000 population, by year, United States, 1922–82

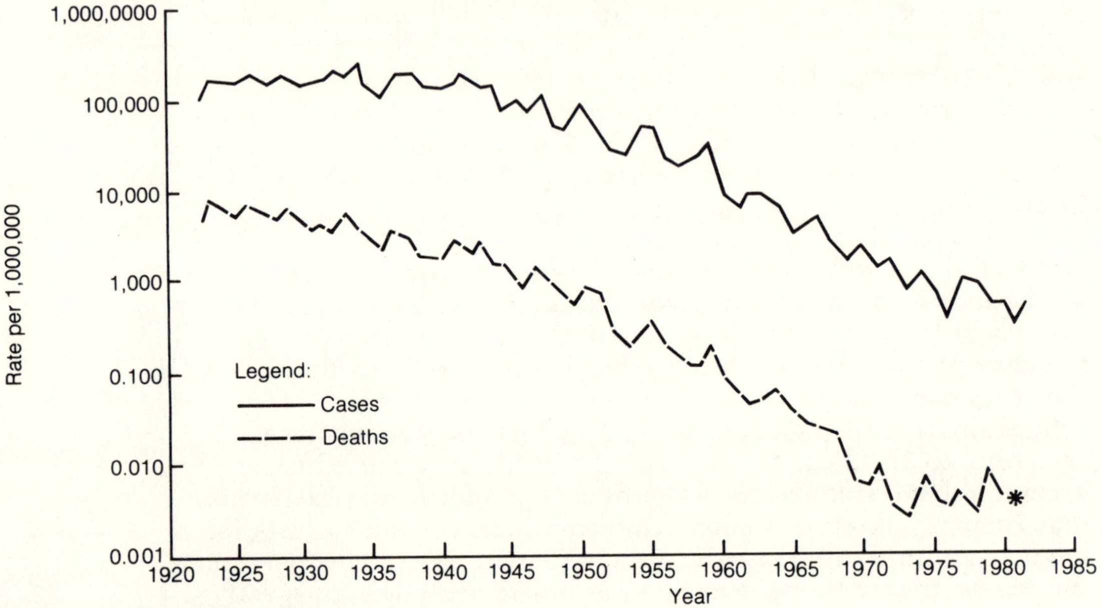

*Data not available for 1981 and 1982.

Source: Morbidity and Mortality Weekly *Report, Annual Summary* 1982

between ages 4 and 6 years.

Nevertheless, there are vaccination risk estimates from the Netherlands, a country that like the United States uses a combination diphtheria, tetanus, and pertussis vaccine. Both use an inactivated whole-cell virus. Dose schedules differ, however, in that the Netherlands does not vaccinate any child older than 14 months, whereas American children are given DPT until age 7 years. Both countries have experienced a steep decline in pertussis.

Estimates from the Netherlands of vaccine-related side effects include the occurrence of permanent brain damage in 1 of every 350,000 children, shock or convulsions in 1 per 2,500. The rate for the latter determined by one U.S. study was 1 per 1750.[d]

These estimates have led the Netherlands to adopt a vaccine with a lower pertussis antigen concentration. Reports uncovered by the media in the United States indicate that a split virus vaccine was developed by Eli Lilly Company several years ago, which might well be safer than the present whole-virus product. But Lilly discontinued manufacturing the vaccine in the early 1980s. Efforts

[d]Cody CL et al: Nature and rates of adverse reactions associated with DPT and DT immunization in infants and children. *Pediatrics* 68:650–660, 1981.

will no doubt be made to perfect a better vaccine in the United States due to parental if not governmental or medical pressure.

DIPHTHERIA

As already noted, in the United States, vaccine for pertussis is usually delivered with vaccine for diphtheria. Administration of diphtheria vaccine has made this acute respiratory disease rare in the United States. When common, diphtheria typically struck children younger than age 15 years and had a mortality rate of 10%.

The infection, caused by a gram-positive rod, affects the tonsils, nasopharynx, and larynx in its classic form with transmission of the rods through airborne exhalation droplets. Within a week of contact, a thick mucous membrane forms over the affected tissues, which bleeds if attempts are made to remove it. Failure to remove it, however, can occasionally lead to suffocation. A cough and

Fig. 1–18. Diphtheria: reported cases per 100,000 population, by year, United States, 1955–83

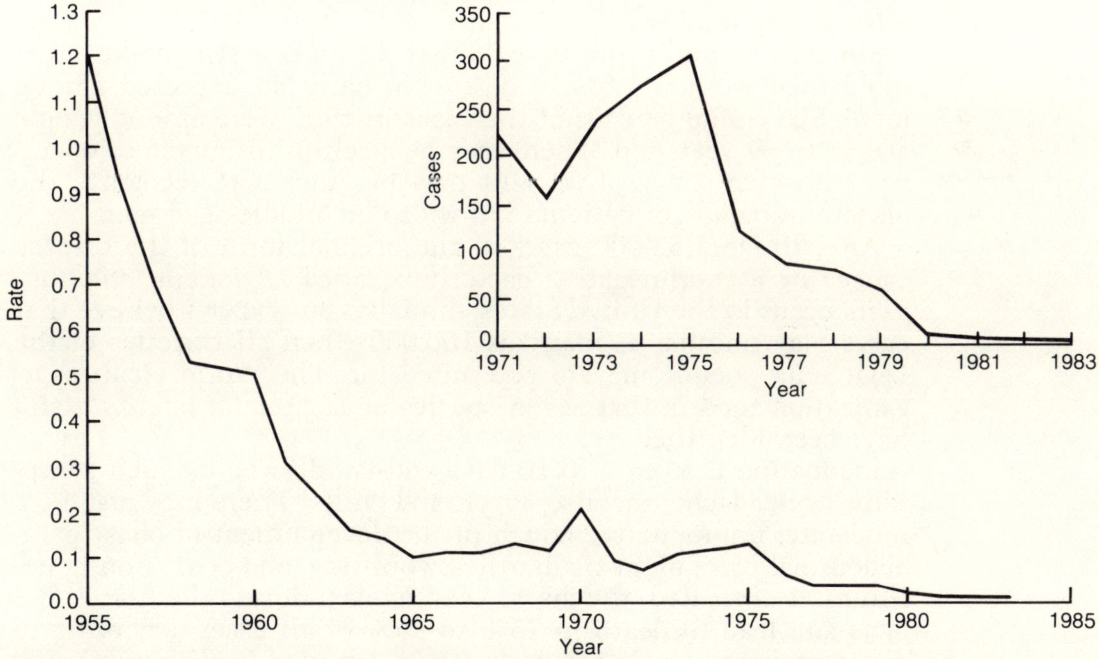

Source: Morbidity and Mortality Weekly Report, Annual Summary 1983

symptoms similar to whooping cough also accompany the characteristic membrane symptom.

Treatment involves the administration of antibiotics, diphtheria antitoxin and supportive care. The patient is usually isolated and monitored for signs of suffocation, shock, and transient neuritis, which can develop as long as 2 or 3 months after disease onset.

As Fig. 1–18 shows, the incidence of diphtheria has decreased markedly since 1955, although there was an increase in the number of cases between 1965 and 1970. Again, between 1972 and 1975, a slight upsurge of cases occurred in Washington state. These cases were not of the respiratory variety but involved cutaneous sites. This is the prevalent form today in the United States especially in the Northwest and Southwest. However, between 1983 and 1985, all reported cases were noncutaneous respiratory cases.

LEGIONNAIRES' DISEASE

Researchers have recently named a newly recognized illness, Legionnaires' disease, after American legion members who became mysteriously ill while meeting in Philadelphia in 1976. This acute respiratory infection had an affinity for middle-aged men who were often heavy smokers.

Since 1976 monitoring reveals that the disease still strikes men more than women (68% of diagnosed cases are reported among men). Sixty-nine percent of the cases in 1981 were among people age 50 to 69 years old. There may be a self-fulfilling effect operative, however, since physicians may be quicker to recognize the disease in paradigm patients known to be middle-aged men.

An estimated 52,000 cases of the original form of the disease caused by a gram-negative bacterium called *Legionella pneumophila* occur in the United States annually. But experts believe that cases may number as many as 100,000 when all varieties of the Legionella pneumonia are accounted for. The World Health Organization reports that seven species of *Legionella pneumophila* have been identified.

Incubation is from 2 to 10 days and is followed by such symptoms as headache, malaise, fever, and chills. There may also be a moderate, unproductive cough or the development of chest pain, abdominal pain, pleuritic diarrhea, vomiting, and confusion or delirium. If untreated, the disease can worsen during the first 4 to 6 days and lead to death in 15% to 25% of all cases according to different estimates. In the early 1980s, reported fatality was lower at about 10% to 12.5%. The patient may develop rales or ronchi without consolidation and patchy localized infiltrates that move to multilobar involvement; consolidation may be reflected on serial radiographs.

Unfortunately, tissue gram stains show little evidence of the bacterium, and diagnosis is confirmed by a fourfold increase in antibody titer that is measured by an indirect immunofluorescent test that takes 6 to 8 weeks to perform. Thus, prompt needed treatment of 500 mg of erythromycin every 6 hours for 14 to 21 days must be initiated through clinical recognition of the symptoms. Other therapy, such as oxygen administration, is supportive.

The source of the *Legionella pneumophila* is thought to be water in contaminated cooling systems and contaminated potable water. Spread of the disease from person to person has not been definitively established, although airborne transmission is suspected from source to host. Identification of this disease has answered questions surrounding mysterious outbreaks of severe febrile respiratory disease before 1976, and Legionnaires' disease has been recognized since 1976 in outbreaks in the United States and Europe.

ITS PATTERN

A seasonal pattern has been noted through monitoring. Of all reported cases, 44% have developed between July and September. Figure 1–19 shows the number of reported cases in the United States between 1978 and 1983.

In 1983, there were 852 reported cases of legionellosis in the United States. They occurred primarily in the north central and north mountain states (Fig. 1–20).

The age distribution of 455 sporadic cases reported nationally to the Atlanta Centers for Disease Control is shown in Table 1–21. Fifty percent of the cases were in patients 50–69 years old while the male-female ratio was 1.7 : 1.

Risk factors identified worldwide for contracting this disease include a history of cigarette smoking, alcohol consumption, location (either residential or work) near a construction site, recent travel (holiday or business), and stay in a hotel or hospital. Clusters of cases have been reported for specific hotels both in the United States and abroad and for hospitals where the infection is suspected to be endemic. The nosocomial incidence of legionellosis was first noticed in a hospital study in 1977.

Fig. 1–19. Legionellosis: reported sporadic cases, by month of onset, United States, 1978–82

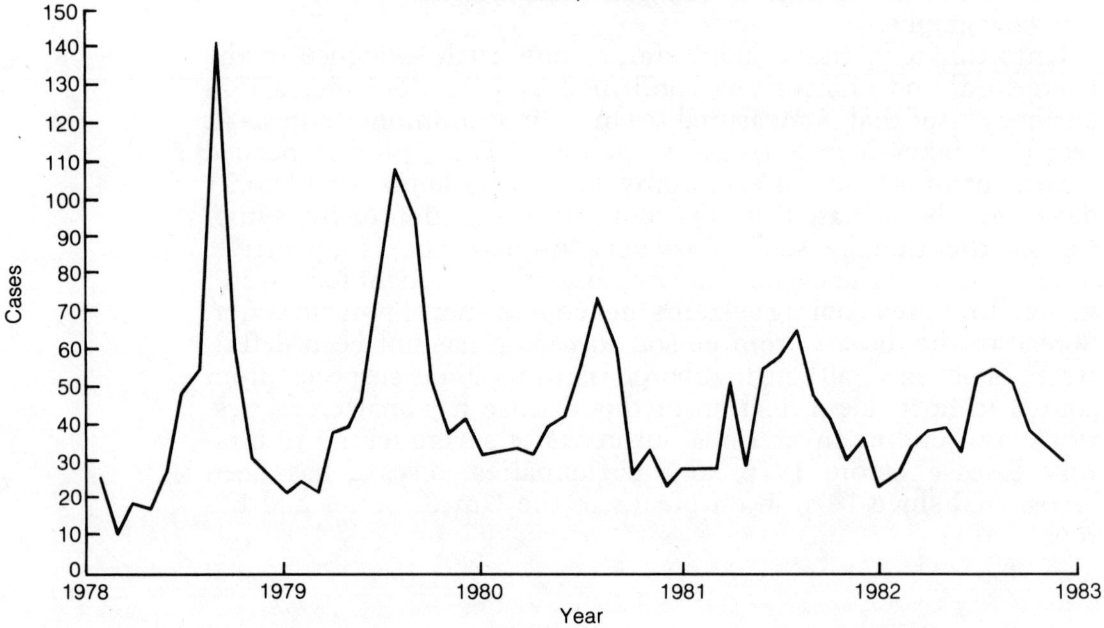

Source: Morbidity and Mortality Weekly Report, Annual Summary 1983

TABLE 1–21. Legionellosis: Age Distribution of Sporadic Cases, United States, 1982

AGE GROUP	NUMBER OF CASES	(%) TOTAL CASES
0–9	5	1
10–19	8	2
20–29	22	5
30–39	48	11
40–49	56	12
50–59	92	20
60–69	127	28
70–79	62	14
80+	33	7
Unk.	2	
Total	455	100

Source: Morbidity and Mortality Weekly Report, Annual Summary, 1982

Fig. 1–20. Legionellosis: reported cases per 100,000 population, by state, United States, 1983

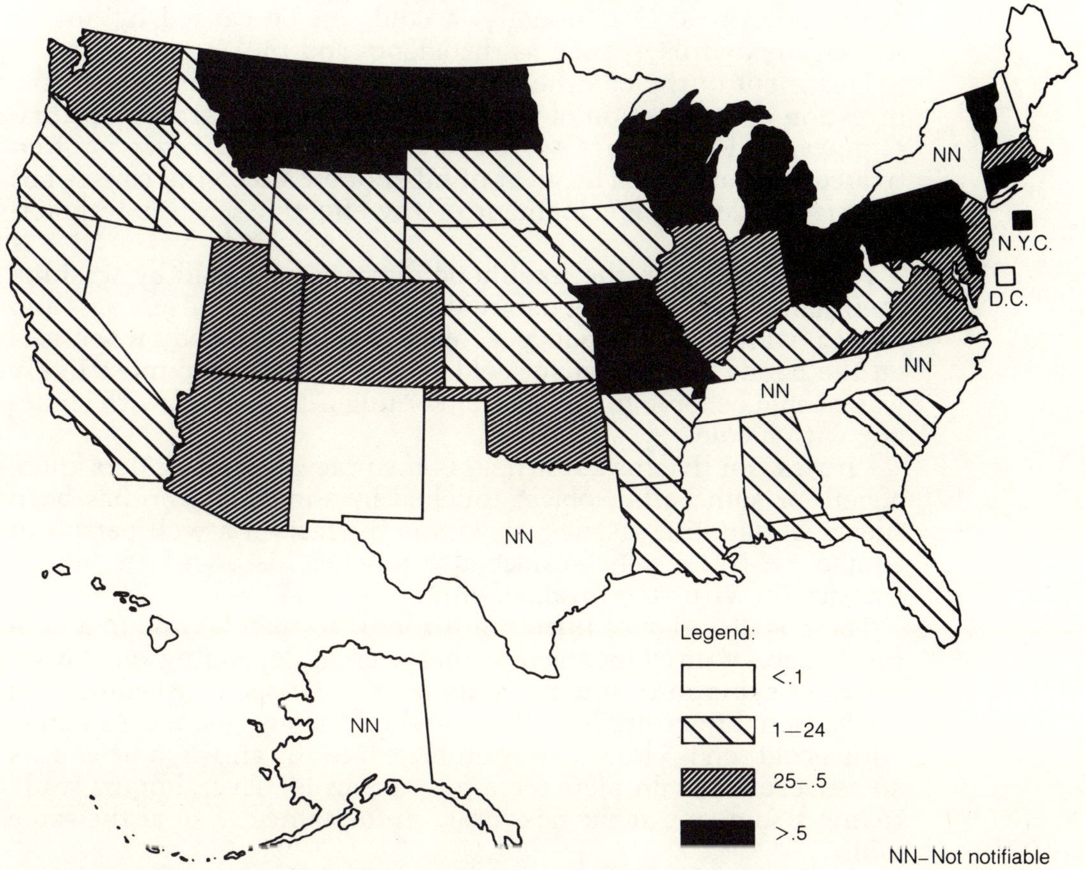

Source: Morbidity and Mortality Weekly Report, Annual Summary 1983

THE COMMON COLD

An acute respiratory illness that seldom if ever by itself causes mortality but that accounts for major morbidity in otherwise healthy individuals is the common cold. Outbreaks occur typically from September through April, the greatest incidence occurring in winter.

Symptoms include headache, stuffy nose, sore throat, fatigue, and temperature mildly above normal. It can persist from 2 to 14 days. Caused by more than 100 different viruses, fewer than 60% of cases are related to a specific virus. The rhinoviruses cause between 25% and 30% of all adult colds. Another 15% are attributed to coronaviruses discovered in England in 1960. There are at last count at least 32 strains of coronaviruses and over 100 different rhinoviruses. Occasionally, a cold can be caused by any of several myxoviruses, such as the adeno- and the enteroviruses.

Treatment of the common cold remains symptomatic with the ingestion or application of nasal and chest decongestants, antihistamines, and analgesics to lessen headache pain. Fever is often treated with aspirin. The great number of possible viral causes has thus far made the development of any effective vaccine impractical.

People can lessen the likelihood of catching a cold by washing their hands and avoiding habitual touching of the nose, eyes, and mouth, which can introduce a cold virus into the body when it is on the hands. This mode of cold transmission is the most likely way people become infected after coming into contact with someone with a cold.

Viruses can live for a few hours on surfaces such as a doorknob, pencil, or some other object touched by someone who has been sneezing, handling tissues, or wiping his face. If a well person in contact with the same surface also touches his own face, he can transfer the virus to portals of entry.

There is also risk of infection if someone spends time in a confined space with someone who has a cold, depending on the severity of symptoms and the amount of time spent. According to the National Institute for Allergy and Infectious Disease, someone with a cold sends virus-bearing droplets into the air when he coughs and sneezes. The droplets remain in the air for several hours ready to infect someone at the next desk, in the same car, or at the same table.

So far, the work and claims of Nobel Prize winner Linus Pauling that large doses of vitamin C can prevent the common cold are controversial although there is some sentiment in the scientific community that ingestion of vitamin C may minimize the severity of a cold once it develops.

Each year an estimated 400 million colds strike the U.S. population. They account for 21% of all acute illness. Children younger than age 4 years average eight colds annually, while adults average two. One Michigan study found that young boys have more colds than girls. But women tend to have more colds later in life. Since the greatest incidence of colds is in children, women who traditionally have been in contact with children more than men would be expected to have more colds than their husbands who may be away from a sick child most of the time.

The common cold results in 297 million days of restricted activity including 38 million school days and 34 million work days with an estimated cost to individuals of $550 million a year just for cold remedies alone.

The most promising and perhaps only prophylactic measure developed to protect against cold viruses is an interferon nasal spray tested in 1986 at the University of Virginia School of Medicine and Australia's University of Adelaide. The spray prevented cold development in 80% of the patients exposed to the spray before exposure to rhinoviruses, which cause 50% of all colds. If approved by the FDA, Schering-Plough will market the spray. Although many respiratory infections like the common cold are not serious, their sheer volume poses an enormous burden on health resources. The National Ambulatory Care Survey gathered data on the extent of utilization for acute respiratory conditions in the mid-1970s.

THE BURDEN OF ACUTE RESPIRATORY DISEASES

The number and percentage distribution of doctor office visits by diagnosis for acute respiratory conditions made during the mid-1970s is shown in Table 1–22. More than one-half of all visits, almost 93 million visits of 163 million due to respiratory problems, were for acute upper respiratory disorders not counting influenza illness. Twenty-eight percent of all respiratory-related visits were for chronic conditions, and another 10% were for influenza and pneumonia.

TABLE 1–22. Number and Percentage Distribution of Office Visits for Acute and Chronic Diseases of the Respiratory System, by Diagnosis: United States, 1975–76

DIAGNOSIS AND ICDA CODE*		VISITS (IN THOUSANDS)	PERCENT DISTRIBUTION
All respiratory disease diagnoses	460–519	163,401	100.0
Acute upper respiratory infections, except influenza	460–466,490	92,705	56.7
Acute nasopharyngitis (common cold)	460	4,445	2.7
Acute sinusitis	461	2,598	1.6
Acute pharyngitis	462	17,414	10.7
Acute tonsilitis	463	12,573	7.7
Acute laryngitis and tracheitis	464	2,982	1.8
Acute upper respiratory infection of multiple or unspecified sites	465	33,248	20.3
Acute bronchitis and bronchiolitis, and bronchitis unqualified	466,490	19,446	11.9
Influenza	470–474	10,312	6.3
Pneumonia	480–486	5,194	3.2

* Based on the Eighth Revision International Classification of Diseases, Adapted for Use in the United States (ICDA).
Source: Vital and Health Statistics, Series 13, No. 42

TABLE 1–23. Number of Office Visits for Selected Acute Diseases of the Respiratory System and for All Other Morbidity-related Groups by Diagnostic or Therapeutic Services Ordered or Provided, by Diagnosis: United States, 1975–76

PROCEDURE	DIAGNOSIS AND ICDA CODE*								
Diagnostic or therapeutic service	Acute nasopharyngitis and acute upper respiratory infection of multiple or unspecified sites (460,465)	Acute sinusitis (461)	Acute pharyngitis (462)	Acute tonsillitis (463)	Acute laryngisits and tracheitis (464)	Acute bronchitis and bronchiolitis, and bronchitis unqualified (466,490)	Influenza (470–474)	Pneumonia (480–486)	All other morbidity-related ICDA† groups (000–458, 520–629, 680–738, 780–796)
All visits	37,693	2,598	17,414	12,573	2,982	19,446	10,312	5,194	667,261
					Percent‡				
Limited history and/or examination	66.0	82.2	68.8	65.4	68.8	66.2	54.5	64.7	67.7
General history and/or examination	12.8	6.8	9.7	11.5	10.4	13.1	9.9	17.8	18.8
Clinical laboratory test	14.3	9.4	30.8	24.9	14.8	13.9	14.0	19.3	27.0
X-ray	3.0	7.4	1.3	1.3	*2.1	12.6	4.7	34.8	8.0
Blood pressure check	25.1	20.6	18.8	10.0	16.3	30.5	26.3	27.2	42.4
Drug prescribed**	81.8	90.5	77.4	79.0	77.0	76.9	79.8	63.6	65.5
Injection	26.7	34.0	24.9	31.5	25.2	29.2	45.0	21.9	19.1
Medical counseling	7.8	3.4	5.6	7.9	*8.9	9.3	7.7	10.3	16.6
Other diagnostic and therapeutic services¶	4.9	13.2	3.5	2.8	*3.8	8.2	4.9	6.1	36.0

* Based on the *Eighth Revision International Classification of Diseases. Adapted for Use in the United States* (ICDA).

† For this report excludes categories relating to special conditions and examinations without sickness, complications of pregnancy, childbirth, and the puerperium; congenital anomalies; certain causes of perinatal morbidity and mortality; accidents, poisoning, and violence; diagnosis "none" and "unknown."

‡ Percents will not add to 100.0 because more than one service may have been provided.

** Includes prescription and nonprescription drugs.

¶ Includes electrocardiogram, hearing test, vision test, endoscopy, immunization, office surgery, physiotherapy, psychotheray and therapeutic listening, and other diagnostic or therapeutic services.

Source: Vital and Health Statistics, Series 13, No. 42

Information about the diagnostic or therapeutic services ordered or provided according to acute respiratory diagnosis is summarized in Table 1–23. The most common services rendered were a limited physical examination, history review, and prescription for a medication.

The physician specialty visited by those with acute respiratory problems seeking treatment by way of physician office visit is shown in Table 1–24. Not surprisingly, the type of physician most often visited by acute respiratory patients was the general family practice physician and the pediatrician.

TABLE 1–24. Number of Office Visits for Acute Pharyngitis or Acute Laryngitis and Tracheitis, Number and Percentage of Drug Visits, Number of Drug Mentions, Drug Mention Rate, and Drug Intensity Rate, by Selected Characteristics: United States, 1980

SELECTED CHARACTERISTIC	OFFICE VISITS: All visits	OFFICE VISITS: Drug visits*		DRUG MENTIONS	DRUG MENTION RATE†	DRUG INTENSITY RATE†
	Number in thousands	Number in thousands	Percent	Number in thousands	Rate per visit	
Sex						
Both sexes	10,277**	9,020	87.8	16,139	1.57	1.79
Female	5,669	4,916	86.7	8,949	1.58	1.82
Male	4,608	4,104	89.1	7,190	1.56	1.75
Age (years)						
Under 15	5,229	4,428	84.7	7,901	1.51	1.78
15–24	1,646	1,483	90.1	2,392	1.45	1.61
25–44	2,113	1,906	90.2	3,286	1.56	1.72
45 and over	1,288	1,203	93.4	2,560	1.99	2.13
Race						
White	9,524	8,418	88.4	14,980	1.57	1.78
Black	625	486	77.7	972	1.56	2.00
Problem status						
New problem	6,756	5,945	88.0	10,089	1.49	1.70
Old problem	3,521	3,075	87.3	6,050	1.72	1.97
Major reason for visit						
Acute problem	9,345	8,237	88.2	14,620	1.56	1.77
Chronic problem, routine	269	*237	88.2	*488	1.81	2.06
Chronic problem, flareup	509	427	83.8	831	1.63	1.95
Non-illness care	153	*118	*77.5	*200	1.31	1.69

* A visit in which one or more drugs were ordered or provided.
† Drug mentions divided by number of visits.
‡ Drug mentions divided by number of drug visits.
** Includes races other than white and black not shown as separate categories.
Source: Vital and Health Statistics, Series 13, No. 42

Table 1–25 shows the drug recommendation or utilization rate for patients according to their age, sex, and race who present with acute pharyngitis or acute laryngitis and tracheitis. One-half of the 10 million visits for people with this symptom were made by children under age 15. Only 13% of such visits were made by people

TABLE 1–25. Number of Office Visits for Selected Acute Diseases of the Respiratory System and Percentage Distribution of Visits by Physician Specialty, According to Diagnosis: United States, 1975–76

DIAGNOSIS AND ICDA CODE*		VISITS (IN THOUSANDS)	PHYSICIAN SPECIALTY						
			Total	General and family practice	Internal medicine	Pediatrics	General surgery	Otolaryngology	All other specialties
			Percent distribution						
Acute nasopharyngitis and acute upper respiratory infection of multiple or unspecified sites	460,465	37,693	100.0	60.4	8.2	21.6	3.5	2.0	4.5
Acute sinusitis	461	2,598	100.0	70.1	7.5	7.3	1.0	7.5	6.6
Acute pharyngitis	462	17,414	100.0	53.6	7.4	28.4	2.6	3.9	4.1
Acute tonsillitis	463	12,573	100.0	57.2	2.4	28.2	2.4	4.0	5.8
Acute laryngitis and tracheitis	464	2,982	100.0	36.3	6.2	40.9	2.3	9.1	5.2
Acute bronchitis and bronchiolitis, and bronchitis unqualified	466,490	19,446	100.0	57.3	13.6	20.3	2.8	0.3	5.7
Influenza	470-474	10,312	100.0	78.5	7.3	8.8	2.0	0.3	3.1
Pneumonia	480-486	5,194	100.0	50.5	14.9	27.0	3.3	0.0	4.3

*Based on the *Eighth Revision International Classification of Diseases, Adapted for Use in the United States* (ICDA).
Source: Vital and Health Statistics, Series 13, No. 71

over age 45, but the drug mention rate for the older group was higher than that of the younger. While almost everyone has experienced the annoyance and debilitation of an acute respiratory infection several times in their lives, chronic respiratory infections involving only a portion of the general population are also becoming more widespread. As cigarette smoking has become popular, pollution become more pervasive and many new chemical agents become available for general use, chronic respiratory conditions such as emphysema, bronchitis and asthma have become more common as discussed in the next chapter.

Chronic Lung Disease 2

In addition to the previously discussed acute infections of the respiratory system, there are various chronic disorders that seem to be growing in prevalence. Such diseases include chronic obstructive pulmonary disease (COPD), which is a disease classification that can include chronic bronchitis and/or emphysema. Other chronic lung disorders are asthma, respiratory allergies, and several occupational diseases, such as black lung and silicosis.

CHANGES IN DISEASE CLASSIFICATION

Since the 1950s, the discernment of morbidity and mortality trends for some of these diseases and for respiratory disease as a whole is complicated by several factors. One problem is the disease classification changes that have occurred in the International Classification of Diseases between the sixth and seventh revisions and between the seventh and eighth.

The ratio of deaths attributed to unqualified and chronic bronchitis in the sixth classification of diseases compared to the seventh is 1.07 to 1.00. Some criteria in the sixth revision, which called for a syndrome to be considered bronchitis, were missing in the seventh or specifically ruled out. The same thing occurred between the seventh and eighth revisions, which had a comparability ratio of 1.06. Although the number of deaths attributed to

Fig. 2–1. Revisions of the *International Classification of Diseases*

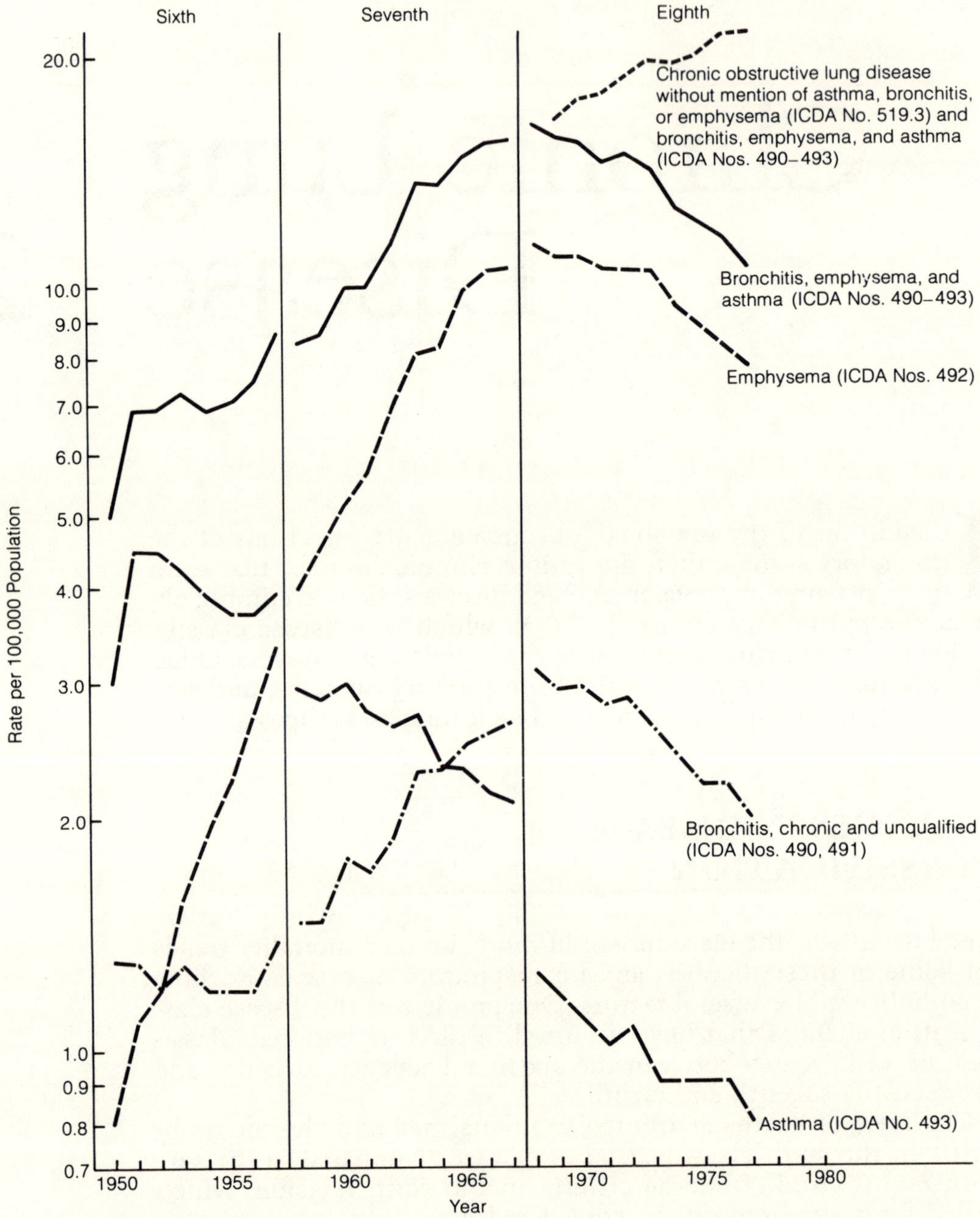

Death rates for bronchitis, emphysema, asthma **and other chronic obstructive lung diseases: United States, 1950–1977**

Source: Vital and Health Statistics, Series 20, No. 17

unqualified and chronic bronchitis increased over this entire period from 1,953 in 1950 to 4,313 in 1977, the lack of comparability between bronchitis criteria in each revision, if not recognized, would lead one to think that the increase was less than it actually was. Without the classification changes of each revision, the increase would have been larger than the numbers just stated.

The breaks or discontinuities due to different designation ratios between different revisions of the International Classification of Diseases can be seen in Fig. 2–1, which supposedly shows the general trend in mortality for some chronic respiratory diseases.

Although drastic trend changes appear to have occurred between 1968 and 1977 (third portion of Fig. 2–1), they probably did not occur because another complication entered the picture, obscuring what was happening with these diseases.

During the latter part of the 1960s, physicians who had generally recorded the cause of death on certificates specifically as emphysema or bronchitis began using the more general nonspecific referent of COPD, which often included one or both of these syndromes. In addition, COPD is not an International Classification designation but one introduced by the National Center for Health Statistics for the United States.

Before this shift in physician practice, COPD was mentioned in medical textbooks as a general title embracing various respiratory disorders in which there is a hindrance to the patient's air flow. Patients with asthma, emphysema, and bronchitis all fell into this loose classification, but it was not used commonly to designate the cause of death on death certificates.

As can be seen in Fig. 2–1, after the late 1960s, mortality from emphysema, asthma, and bronchitis appears to be declining while the new dotted line at the top designating COPD deaths shows a higher mortality than all the other lines as well as an upward trend.

THE TRUE TREND

In light of the change in recording the cause of death, researchers have decided that the data for emphysema and chronic obstructive lung disease, ICDA 492 and 519.3, for 1969–77 show a truer mortality curve for emphysema deaths than emphysema data alone. Measured in this way, the age-adjusted death rate due to emphysema did not decline between 1968 and 1977 but increased 31.3% from 9.6 to 12.6 per 100,000. This was 18 times the rate for 1950.

The number of deaths attributed to these several diseases alone and in the combination just described are shown in Table 2–1. If

TABLE 2–1. Number of Deaths from Specified Diseases of Respiratory System, by Race and Sex: United States, 1968–82 (Numbers after causes of death are category numbers of the *Eighth Revision International Classification of Diseases, Adapted for Use in the United States*, 1965 (ICDA). The asterisk before category number 519.3 indicates that the title to which this number corresponds was not included in ICDA but was introduced by the National Center for Health Statistics.)

CAUSE OF DEATH, RACE, AND SEX	1982	1977*	1976*	1975*	1974*	1973*	1972*,†	1971*	1970*	1969	1968
Bronchitis, emphysema, and asthma and Chronic obstructive lung disease without mention of asthma, bronchitis or emphysema (490-493 and *519.3)‡											
Total	59,869**	43,325	45,882	43,061	41,179	41,042	38,978	36,605	35,333	33,848	. . .
White, male	36,970**	31,802	31,851	30,374	29,281	29,542	28,172	26,695	25,921	25,096	. . .
White, female	18,417**	11,575	11,122	9,986	9,320	8,833	8,156	7,398	6,886	6,343	. . .
All other, male	6,363**	2,209	2,196	1,989	1,961	2,003	1,984	1,828	1,857	1,766	. . .
All other, female	2,392**	739	713	712	617	664	666	684	669	643	. . .
Chronic obstructive lung disease without mention of asthma, bronchitis, or emphysema (519.3)‡											
Total	NA	23,962	21,472	17,593	14,299	11,334	8,210	6,321	4,444	2,704	. . .
White, male		16,718	15,184	12,573	10,315	8,177	5,944	4,647	3,271	2,000	. . .
White, female		5,736	4,937	3,956	3,049	2,369	1,592	1,164	785	473	. . .
All other, male		1,186	1,079	838	757	628	566	405	330	192	. . .
All other, female		322	272	226	178	160	108	105	58	39	. . .
Bronchitis, emphysema, and asthma (490–493)											
Total	19,442	22,363	24,410	25,468	26,880	29,708	30,768	30,284	30,889	31,144	33,078
White, male	11,526	15,084	16,667	17,801	18,966	21,365	22,228	22,048	22,650	23,096	24,536
White, female	6,390	5,839	6,185	6,030	6,271	6,464	6,564	6,234	6,101	5,870	6,153
All other, male	1,808	1,023	1,117	1,151	1,204	1,375	1,418	1,423	1,527	1,574	1,726
All other, female	1,107	417	441	486	439	504	558	579	611	604	663
Bronchitis, unqualified (490)											
Total	3,495	704	744	696	680	768	778	710	832	799	843
White, male	2,010	268	319	326	301	326	352	309	365	361	359
White, female	1,301	358	340	292	281	333	294	294	318	311	342
All other, male	116	43	48	49	67	73	68	61	88	76	88
All other, female	68	35	37	29	31	36	64	46	61	51	54
Chronic bronchitis (491)											
Total		3,609	3,895	4,016	4,417	4,779	5,084	4,881	5,014	5,044	5,362
White, male		2,344	2,595	2,744	3,026	3,332	3,582	3,507	3,632	3,699	3,908
White, female		1,087	1,110	1,087	1,164	1,212	1,222	1,114	1,140	1,075	1,147
All other, male		130	152	141	167	180	212	188	197	214	239
All other, female		48	38	44	60	55	68	72	45	56	68
Emphysema (492)											
Total	12,793	16,376	17,796	18,795	19,907	22,249	22,580	22,539	22,721	22,939	24,185
White, male	8,533	11,911	13,128	14,092	15,011	17,100	17,528	17,553	17,919	18,243	19,361
White, female	3,622	3,646	3,808	3,775	3,979	4,069	3,982	3,858	3,640	3,522	3,568
All other, male	504	683	722	757	783	910	900	949	982	1,001	1,073
All other, female	134	136	138	171	134	170	170	179	180	173	183
Asthma (493)											
Total	3,154	1,674	1,975	1,961	1,876	1,912	2,326	2,154	2,322	2,362	2,688
White, male	983	561	625	639	628	607	766	679	734	793	908
White, female	1,467	748	927	876	847	850	1,066	968	1,003	962	1,096

TABLE 2–1. (Continued)

CAUSE OF DEATH, RACE, AND SEX	1982	1977*	1976*	1975*	1974*	1973*	1972*,†	1971*	1970*	1969	1968
All other, male	351	167	195	204	187	212	238	225	260	283	326
All other, female	373	198	228	242	214	243	256	282	325	324	358

*Excludes deaths of nonresidents of the United States.
†Based on a 50-percent sample of deaths.
‡The subcategory ICDA No. 519.3 was first introduced for data year 1969. Beginning with data year 1972 the subtitle for 519.3 was modified by the addition of "without mention of asthma, bronchitis, or emphysema."
**ICDA 492, 494-496 does not use 519.3
Source: Vital and Health Statistics, Series 20, No. 17

one looks at the number of deaths for 1969, one can see the changes that have taken place in classifying emphysema, bronchitis, and COPD. The total number of respiratory deaths in 1969 was 33,848, COPD without mention of any other condition constituted 7% of total deaths at 2,704, while chronic bronchitis at 5,044 deaths that year amounted to 15% of the total and emphysema at 22,939 deaths composed 67% of the total number of deaths.

Looking at the 1977 entries, one sees that the situation has become reversed, with COPD constituting 51% of the total 46,325 deaths, chronic bronchitis at 3,609 only 7%, and emphysema at 16,376 only 35% instead of its former 67% share of the whole. But rather than really decreasing its share of the death toll, emphysema has been picked up as COPD as has bronchitis to a lesser extent. Thus, COPD has correspondingly come to account for a larger proportion of respiratory deaths.

Table 2–2 presents the death rates reported in various countries for chronic bronchitis, emphysema, and asthma combined.

Table 2–2. Death Rates For Chronic Bronchitis, Emphysema, and Asthma in Several Countries by Latest Reported Year*

COUNTRY	RATE	YEAR
Australia	15.4	80
Austria	26.3	81
Bulgaria	27.8	81
Chile	8.1	80
El Salvadore	21.5	80
France	12.8	80
Greece	20.3	81
Hungary	65.8	80
Japan	10.9	80
Kuwait	4.8	79
Poland	28.4	80
United Kingdom†	38.6	81

*per 100,00
†United Kingdom includes only England and Wales
Source: UN Demographic Yearbook, 1982

CHRONIC BRONCHITIS

Chronic bronchitis is often a long-standing disease in which the ill suffer with a persistent cough, mucopurulent expectoration, and difficulty in breathing on exertion. There is enlargement of the tracheobronchial mucous glands and enlargement or inflammation of peripheral airways that contain excess mucus.

Clinically, chronic bronchitis has been defined as the production of at least two tablespoons of sputum per day for 3 consecutive months occurring in at least 2 consecutive years. Chest sounds and wheezing may be heard. Laboratory tests may show increased hematocrit and increased bronchovascular markings and enlarged pulmonary arteries on chest films.

Medical researchers believe that chronic bronchitis in adults is almost always caused by smoking. Patients usually present with symptoms between ages 40 and 60 years. The disease is often accompanied by emphysema and if the patient seeks help when symptomatic as when FEV (forced expiratory volume of air) is less than 1.5 liters, the 5-year survival rate is judged to be about 50%.

DEATH RATE

Alone, chronic bronchitis is not usually fatal but coupled with other disease, particularly other respiratory diseases such as pneumonia or emphysema, it often leads to death. Mortality is low because chronic bronchitis is commonly listed in Part II of a death certificate as a contributory cause of death.

The age-adjusted death rate for chronic bronchitis and unqualified bronchitis (not designated as chronic) together was 1.1 per 100,000 for both 1950 and 1957, increasing from 1.2 to 2.1 between 1958 and 1967 and decreasing from 2.3 to 1.5 between 1968 and 1982 when reported deaths from both chronic and unqualified bronchitis declined from 6,205 to 3,495 (Table 2–1). Note that the latter decline may be due to changed recording practices as just described.

Those with the greatest death rate due to this disease from 1950 through 1982 were white males. By 1977, they had 2.3 times the rate of white females, 1.6 times the rate for all non-white males, and 4.2 times the non-white female rate. The death rate, which went up according to age, is shown for each age, race, and sex group between 1960 and 1982 in Table 2–3.

TABLE 2–3. Death Rates for Chronic and Unqualified Bronchitis, by Age, Race, and Sex; and Corresponding Age-adjusted Rates: United States, 1960–82 (For 1968–77 rates are based on deaths assigned to category numbers 490, 491 of the *Eighth Revision International Classification of Diseases, Adapted for Use in the United States*, 1965 (ICDA), for 1960–67 rates are based on deaths assigned to category numbers 501, 502 of the Seventh Revision adopted in 1955. For method of age adjustment, see appendix I)

RACE, SEX, AND YEAR	ALL AGES	25–34 Years	35–44 Years	45–54 Years	55–64 Years	65–74 Years	75–84 Years	85 Years and Over	Age-adjusted Rate
Both sexes				Rate per 100,000 population					
1982	1.5	0.0	0.1	0.6	2.1	6.5	13.4	24.6	—
1977*	2.0	0.1	0.2	0.9	3.6	9.6	17.8	25.9	1.4
1976*	2.2	0.1	0.2	1.1	4.0	10.2	19.4	30.3	1.5
1975*	2.2	0.1	0.3	1.0	4.5	10.8	19.9	26.7	1.6
1974*	2.4	0.1	0.3	1.3	4.7	12.0	22.7	29.0	1.7
1973*	2.6	0.1	0.4	1.3	5.2	13.1	24.7	37.6	1.9
1972*,†	2.8	0.2	0.5	1.7	5.6	15.1	24.0	33.7	2.1
1971*	2.7	0.1	0.4	1.5	5.8	14.0	24.3	33.8	2.0
1970*	2.9	0.1	0.4	1.8	6.3	14.4	25.7	31.8	2.1
1969	2.9	0.1	0.4	1.9	6.1	14.9	25.4	40.2	2.2
1968	3.1	0.1	0.4	1.8	7.0	16.0	27.4	43.2	2.3
1967	2.7	0.1	0.4	1.7	6.0	13.8	23.8	33.6	2.1
1966	2.6	0.1	0.4	1.8	5.9	13.9	23.1	34.0	2.1
1965	2.5	0.1	0.4	1.6	5.5	13.0	20.7	31.6	1.9
1964	2.3	0.1	0.4	1.5	5.0	12.1	19.2	32.8	1.8
1963	2.3	0.1	0.4	1.4	4.7	12.1	19.2	35.0	1.8
1962	1.9	0.1	0.3	1.2	4.1	9.6	15.6	27.9	1.5
1961	1.7	0.1	0.3	1.0	3.6	8.2	13.1	21.9	1.3
1960	1.8	0.1	0.3	1.1	3.6	8.8	13.5	25.4	1.4
White, male									
1982	2.1	—	—	—	—	—	—	—	
1977*	2.9	0.1	0.1	1.2	4.9	16.5	33.5	43.7	2.1
1976*	3.2	0.1	0.2	1.2	5.8	18.0	37.5	58.1	2.4
1975*	3.4	0.1	0.2	1.3	6.6	19.2	39.6	57.0	2.6
1974*	3.7	0.1	0.2	1.6	6.7	21.9	45.0	57.1	2.9
1973*	4.1	0.1	0.3	1.4	8.0	23.9	49.3	71.0	3.2
1972*,†	4.4	0.2	0.5	2.1	9.0	27.3	49.0	62.5	3.5
1971*	4.3	0.1	0.4	1.8	9.4	26.3	48.6	63.9	3.4
1970*	4.6	0.1	0.5	2.2	10.1	27.4	52.4	56.5	3.7
1969	4.7	0.1	0.6	2.5	10.1	28.9	50.0	70.6	3.8
1968	5.0	0.1	0.4	2.4	11.4	30.2	54.0	78.2	4.0
1967	4.4	0.1	0.4	2.4	10.1	26.6	47.5	60.5	3.6
1966	4.4	0.1	0.4	2.5	9.9	27.2	46.5	66.0	3.6
1965	4.1	0.1	0.5	2.2	9.6	25.4	39.3	58.4	3.3
1964	3.8	0.1	0.4	2.3	8.8	23.7	35.4	57.5	3.1
1963†	3.7	0.1	0.4	2.0	8.9	23.4	34.7	53.6	3.1
1962†	3.0	0.1	0.3	1.7	7.4	18.3	26.9	42.5	2.5
1961	2.6	0.1	0.3	1.5	6.1	15.1	23.2	33.0	2.1
1960	2.7	0.1	0.3	1.7	6.0	16.1	23.5	36.3	2.2
White, female									
1982	1.3	—	—	—	—	—	—	—	—

TABLE 2–3. (Continued)

RACE, SEX, AND YEAR	ALL AGES	25–34 Years	35–44 Years	45–54 Years	55–64 Years	65–74 Years	75–84 Years	85 Years and Over	Age-adjusted Rate
1977*	1.5	0.1	0.2	0.8	2.6	5.3	9.7	20.4	0.9
1976*	1.5	0.1	0.2	0.9	2.6	5.2	10.2	21.1	0.9
1975*	1.5	0.0	0.2	0.9	2.9	5.4	9.7	14.7	0.9
1974*	1.5	0.1	0.3	1.0	3.1	5.3	10.8	18.0	1.0
1973*	1.7	0.1	0.3	1.0	3.0	6.3	11.1	23.9	1.0
1972*	1.6	0.1	0.4	1.1	2.8	6.9	10.2	20.7	1.0
1971*	1.5	0.1	0.3	1.1	3.0	5.7	10.3	20.5	1.0
1970*	1.6	0.1	0.3	1.5	3.1	5.8	10.1	20.8	1.1
1969	1.5	0.1	0.3	1.2	2.7	5.3	10.5	27.5	1.0
1968	1.7	0.1	0.3	1.1	3.3	6.2	11.2	27.3	1.1
1967	1.3	0.1	0.3	1.0	2.5	4.7	8.9	21.9	0.9
1966	1.3	0.1	0.3	1.1	2.6	4.4	8.6	20.0	0.9
1965	1.2	0.1	0.3	1.0	2.1	4.0	9.0	18.4	0.8
1964	1.1	0.1	0.3	0.9	1.7	3.6	8.8	20.7	0.8
1963‡	1.1	0.1	0.3	0.8	1.3	3.4	9.0	26.0	0.8
1962‡	0.9	0.1	0.3	0.7	1.4	2.7	7.7	19.3	0.7
1961	0.8	0.1	0.2	0.5	1.4	2.6	6.4	15.2	0.6
1960	0.9	0.0	0.2	0.6	1.3	2.9	6.7	19.6	0.7
All other, male				Rate per 100,000 population					
1982	4.7	—	—	—	—	—	—	—	—
1977*	1.3	—	0.5	1.1	3.8	7.0	15.4	19.4	1.3
1976*	1.5	0.1	0.5	2.5	4.9	9.3	14.5	13.2	1.6
1975*	1.4	0.3	0.5	1.1	5.0	9.3	13.8	17.2	1.5
1974*	1.8	0.1	0.9	1.7	6.0	13.1	14.8	24.6	1.9
1973*	2.0	0.4	1.0	2.2	6.7	8.7	23.9	34.0	2.1
1972*,†	2.2	—	1.1	3.5	7.9	14.2	19.1	35.3	2.5
1971*	2.0	0.5	1.4	2.3	6.9	10.6	21.3	26.5	2.2
1970*	2.3	0.3	0.6	3.1	8.9	11.7	21.2	27.1	2.5
1969	2.5	0.3	0.7	3.7	8.6	13.2	26.1	27.3	2.7
1968	2.8	0.4	1.3	4.0	10.0	15.4	24.2	39.0	3.1
1967	2.3	0.2	1.2	3.5	7.4	14.4	22.8	17.9	2.6
1966	2.1	0.4	1.3	3.0	6.6	13.2	15.1	8.3	2.3
1965	2.2	0.2	0.8	2.6	6.1	12.8	18.8	29.4	2.3
1964	1.9	0.1	1.3	2.1	6.2	10.9	16.9	18.8	2.0
1963‡	2.2	0.2	1.0	2.3	6.4	16.0	10.9	34.5	2.3
1962‡	2.0	0.3	0.4	2.5	4.0	11.5	16.1	27.6	2.0
1961	1.8	0.3	0.5	2.1	5.0	11.4	8.8	13.3	1.8
1960	1.8	0.2	0.3	2.4	5.8	10.9	10.0	19.1	1.8
All other, female									
1982	0.4	—	—	—	—	—	—	—	—
1977*	0.5	0.1	0.2	0.6	1.1	2.8	3.7	4.5	0.5
1976*	0.5	0.0	0.1	0.6	2.0	2.3	3.4	3.3	0.5
1975*	0.5	0.3	0.3	0.4	1.1	2.1	3.2	6.4	0.5
1974*	0.6	0.1	0.5	0.4	1.8	3.4	5.0	2.1	0.7
1973*	0.7	0.1	0.5	1.3	2.0	1.9	4.5	8.0	0.7
1972*,†	1.0	0.2	0.5	1.1	1.7	4.3	2.8	17.1	0.9
1971*	0.9	0.2	0.7	1.1	1.9	3.6	4.8	13.2	0.9

TABLE 2–3. (Continued)

RACE, SEX, AND YEAR	ALL AGES	25–34 Years	35–44 Years	45–54 Years	55–64 Years	65–74 Years	75–84 Years	85 Years and Over	Age-adjusted Rate
1970*	0.8	—	0.7	0.9	2.9	2.1	4.7	6.4	0.8
1969	0.8	0.4	0.1	1.3	1.7	2.9	4.0	7.7	0.8
1968	1.0	0.3	1.0	1.3	2.4	2.6	5.9	9.8	1.0
1967	0.8	0.3	0.6	0.5	1.6	3.4	3.9	7.0	0.8
1966	0.7	0.1	0.6	1.0	1.2	2.2	3.2	3.8	0.7
1965	0.8	0.4	0.6	0.4	1.5	2.1	0.9	6.1	0.7
1964	0.9	0.2	0.9	1.0	1.8	1.6	2.9	11.1	0.8
1963‡	0.9	0.3	0.6	0.4	0.9	2.9	4.2	19.0	0.8
1962‡	0.9	0.2	0.5	0.6	1.4	3.0	4.3	7.5	0.8
1961	0.7	0.1	0.5	0.3	1.4	1.2	3.9	25.0	0.6
1960	0.9	0.1	0.2	0.4	0.8	2.2	4.8	17.4	0.7

*Excludes deaths of nonresidents of the United States.
†Based on a 50% sample of deaths.
‡Figures by race exclude data for residents of New Jersey because this State did not require reporting of the item for these years.
Source: Vital and Health Statistics, Series 20, No. 17

PREVALENCE

When the actual prevalence of chronic bronchitis was assessed as a morbidity measure by the government in 1970, the number of cases for persons of different ages, at different income levels, and living in different circumstances were as shown in Table 2–4.

Interestingly, prevalence was much greater among persons living in nonfarm areas, but there was no indication that city pollution might be a causative agent except for people older than age 65. People in this age category living in central city areas had a higher prevalence of chronic bronchitis than those living outside central cities. This differential did not show up among younger people, but this may reflect the cumulative insult to the lungs that eventually leads to disease when one reaches advanced age.

On the other hand, it is not known whether the old living in central cities have lived there all their lives and whether or not they are or have been at the same socioeconomic level as those who do not have chronic bronchitis in advanced age.

The prevalence rate of this disease in older people with low incomes does appear to be higher than in those with higher incomes.

But children younger than age 17 years in 1970 showed a reverse pattern. Children from middle income homes, those with incomes between $10,000 and $15,000 a year (equivalent to a

TABLE 2–4. Prevalence of Chronic Bronchitis Reported in Health Interviews, by Age, Family Income, and Place of Residence: United States, 1970

FAMILY INCOME AND PLACE OF RESIDENCE	ALL AGES	UNDER 17 YEARS	17–44 YEARs	45–64 YEARS	65 YEARS AND OVER
	Rate per 1,000 persons				
Total	32.7	38.9	23.2	35.4	41.2
Family income					
Less than $3,000	39.5	30.0	28.3	54.6	46.3
$3,000–$4,999	35.0	36.2	28.4	34.3	43.8
$5,000–$6,999	31.0	36.4	17.6	43.4	39.0
$7,000–$9,999	32.3	37.9	25.3	35.3	34.8
$10,000–$14,999	32.6	46.9	21.8	29.0	
$15,000 or more	30.8	38.8	23.7	30.3	
Place of residence					
SMSA	33.0	39.8	24.0	34.3	42.0
Central city	31.9	35.4	24.0	33.9	45.5
Not central city	33.8	43.1	24.0	34.5	38.2
Outside SMSA:					
Nonfarm	33.0	38.5	22.2	39.0	40.8
Farm	24.9	26.0		28.2	

Source: National Center for Health Statistics: Prevalence of selected chronic respiratory conditions: United States, 1970. *Vital and Health Statistics*. Series 10-No. 84. DHEW Pub. No. (HRA) 74-1511. Health Resources Administration. Washington. U.S. Government Printing Office. Sept. 1973.

1986 salary of $30,000 to $45,000) had a higher reported prevalence of chronic bronchitis than those with incomes less than $10,000. This may reflect a greater tendency for economically advantaged children to be counted because of more accurate parent recall or more medical attention.

On the assumption that children from both middle income and high income families (incomes over $15,000 in 1970) obtained more medical treatment and attended more to their illnesses, both should show about the same reported prevalence. This would be true even when both sets of economically advantaged children had fewer bouts of bronchitis in reality than poorer children. Yet, as Table 2–4 shows, the two advantaged groups differ. Upper income children reported more illnesses than low income children but substantially less than middle income children.

One might speculate that upper income children were less sick due to greater economic advantages than middle income children. But this hypothesis is unlikely since both middle and upper income children live in circumstances better than those in which disease would be common. What may explain the difference is a possibly greater sophistication of the high income families in knowing how to care for a child with bronchitis without consulting a physician. This would be especially true if the high income parents were themselves physicians.

The course of drug therapy for acute bronchitis patients according to several patient characteristics is shown in Table 2–5. More visits for this problem were made by females who also had a higher medication recommendation rate.

TABLE 2–5. Number of Office Vists for Bronchitis, Acute; or Not Specified as Acute or Chronic, Number and Percentage of Drug Visits, Number of Drug Mentions, Drug Mention Rate, and Drug Intensity Rate, by Selected Characteristics: United States, 1980.

SELECTED CHARACTERISTIC	OFFICE VISITS: All visits	OFFICE VISITS: Drug visits*		DRUG MENTIONS	DRUG MENTION RATES†	DRUG INTENSITY RATE‡
	Number (in thousands)	Number (in thousands)	Percentage	Number (in thousands)	Rate per visit	
Sex						
Both sexes	8,323**	7,855	94.4	16,349	1.96	2.08
Female	4,382	4,237	96.7	9,179	2.09	2.17
Male	3,940	3,618	91.8	7,170	1.82	1.98
Age (years)						
Under 15	3,101	2,911	93.9	5,328	1.72	1.83
15–24	818	763	93.2	1,559	1.91	2.04
25–44	1,312	1,293	98.5	2,682	2.04	2.07
45–64	1,875	1,787	95.3	3,797	2.03	2.12
65 and over	1,210	1,102	90.7	2,983	2.45	2.71
Race						
White	7,246	6,909	95.3	14,103	1.95	2.04
Black	916	850	92.8	2,086	2.28	2.45
Problem status						
New problem	5,012	4,837	96.5	9,850	1.97	2.04
Old problem	3,311	3,018	91.2	6,499	1.96	2.15
Major reason for visit						
Acute problem	7,203	6,941	96.4	14,094	1.96	2.03
Chronic problem, routine	587	447	76.1	1,277	2.18	2.86
Chronic problem, flareup	413	364	88.0	771	1.87	2.12
Post surgery/post injury	12	12	100.0	24	2.00	2.00
Non-illness care	108	91	84.9	183	1.69	2.01

*A visit in which one or more drugs were ordered or provided
†Drug mentions divided by number of visits
‡Drug mentions divided by number of drug visits
**Includes races other than white and black not shown as separate categories
Source: Vital and Health Statistics, Series 13, No. 71

EMPHYSEMA

Older individuals with bronchitis often suffer from emphysema as well. Unlike chronic bronchitis sufferers, those who have only emphysema do not always present with a cough or expectoration of mucus. But they experience weight loss, progressive difficulty in breathing on exertion, and distant chest sounds. They can show a normal hematocrit and on X-ray large central pulmonary arteries and hyperinflated lungs. Pulmonary alveoli become distended or ruptured.

Again, it most often occurs in men ages 45 to 65 who have smoked heavily, lived in a cold, damp or urban environment, or had a dusty work history. The crude death rate in 1982 was 22.9 deaths per 100,000 and the age-adjusted death rate for emphysema and chronic obstructive pulmonary disease considered as one disease classification because of reasons cited earlier in this discussion reached an all-time high in the late 1970s at 12.6 per 100,000.

There were 40,338 deaths due to this disease in 1977. From 1969 when emphysema was considered alone to 1977 when it was combined with COPD the age-adjusted death rate rose 31.3%.

MORTALITY

Although the increase in death due to this disease has been continuous, the tide for males has been rising at a decreasing rate. This may be a hint of a future flattening and eventual decline of the emphysema/COPD death curve as the campaign against cigarette smoking continues to take hold over the next few decades. If today's 20-year-olds smoke less, they will likely show a lowered death rate from this slowly developing disease in 25 years.

It is more than coincidental that the three respiratory diseases which have taken an increasingly larger death toll since 1950 are emphysema, lung-bronchus-trachea cancer, and cancer of the larynx. Each of these diseases has been linked to cigarette smoking, and it is unfortunate that these diseases caused in part by avoidable conditions have offset the gains in respiratory health and survival in other diseases, such as tuberculosis and P&I.

The age, sex, and race breakdown of the death rate for emphysema/COPD is shown in Table 2–6. As can be seen, the death rate increases for each succeeding age group from 25 through 84 years. The percentage increases for white and non-white females were larger than they were for white males, while white males started showing a rate decrease by 1982. Thus, women are catching up with men in their death toll for this disease just as they are for

TABLE 2–6. Death Rates for Emphysema and Chronic Obstructive Lung Disease Without Mention of Asthma, Bronchitis, or Emphysema, by Age, Race, and Sex, and Corresponding Age Adjusted Rates United States, 1960–82. [For 1969–70, rates are based on deaths assigned to category numbers 492, *519.3 used with the *Eighth Revision International Classification of Diseases, Adapted for Use in the United States*, 1965 (ICDA); for 1968 on deaths assigned to category number 492 of the Eighth Revision; and for 1960–67 rates are based on deaths assigned to category number 527.1 of the Seventh Revision adopted in 1955. The asterisk before category number 519.3 indicates that the title to which this number corresponds was not included in ICDA but was introduced by the National Center for Health Statistics (NCHS).]

RACE, SEX, AND YEAR	ALL AGES	25–34 YEARS	35–44 YEARS	45–54 YEARS	55–64 YEARS	65–74 YEARS	75–84 YEARS	85 YEARS AND OVER	AGE-ADJUSTED RATE
Both sexes	Rate per 100,000 population								
1982[**]	22.9	0.1	0.8	7.4	36.9	49.8	215.4	243.8	—
1977[*]	18.7	0.1	1.1	7.8	35.9	102.2	181.8	169.2	12.6
1976[*]	18.3	0.2	1.2	8.1	36.9	101.6	174.7	169.5	12.5
1975[*]	17.1	0.2	1.2	7.9	36.3	97.3	161.4	143.5	11.9
1974[*]	16.2	0.1	1.1	7.9	35.4	94.5	151.6	134.3	11.5
1973[*]	16.0	0.1	1.2	8.1	36.7	94.0	147.1	138.4	11.6
1972[*†]	14.7	0.1	1.2	7.6	34.4	88.3	135.9	122.3	10.9
1971[*]	14.0	0.1	1.4	8.2	33.1	83.3	125.5	116.9	10.4
1970[*]	13.4	0.2	1.4	7.6	33.0	82.0	116.5	99.8	10.1
1969	12.7	0.2	1.5	7.5	31.7	77.1	110.6	107.9	9.6
1968	12.1	0.2	1.4	7.1	30.7	74.0	105.8	103.5	9.2
1967	10.6	0.2	1.1	6.3	27.2	65.1	91.5	92.2	8.1
1966	10.4	0.1	1.2	6.3	27.1	63.9	90.1	87.8	8.0
1965	9.6	0.1	1.1	6.3	25.2	60.5	82.6	83.9	7.6
1964	8.3	0.1	1.0	5.7	22.6	51.2	68.9	68.3	6.5
1963	8.0	0.2	0.9	5.7	22.2	50.8	64.0	70.8	6.4
1962	6.7	0.1	1.0	4.6	18.7	42.2	53.0	55.4	5.3
1961	5.6	0.1	0.8	3.7	16.5	35.4	43.8	46.8	4.5
1960	5.2	0.1	0.8	4.0	15.5	32.6	38.6	38.4	4.2
White, male									
1982[**]	25.1	—	—	—	—	—	—	—	—
1977[*]	31.3	0.1	1.4	10.2	55.2	189.6	398.0	415.8	23.1
1976[*]	31.1	0.2	1.2	11.0	58.2	192.7	382.2	424.8	23.3
1975[*]	29.5	0.2	1.3	10.6	58.1	188.4	360.1	345.7	22.4
1974[*]	28.2	0.1	1.2	11.2	58.1	182.9	335.4	322.7	21.8
1973[*]	28.2	0.1	1.4	11.3	61.9	186.2	329.1	322.5	22.1
1972[*†]	26.4	0.2	1.2	10.9	58.7	177.5	302.4	292.3	20.9
1971[*]	25.2	0.1	1.7	11.7	58.0	169.3	278.8	270.7	20.1
1970[*]	24.5	0.1	1.7	11.4	58.0	169.1	259.1	224.3	19.5
1969	23.5	0.2	1.8	11.4	57.4	160.6	244.3	234.5	18.9
1968	22.6	0.2	1.7	10.7	56.0	156.5	232.5	229.6	18.3
1967	20.1	0.1	1.5	10.0	51.1	138.2	201.1	203.4	16.3
1966	19.7	0.2	1.6	9.9	52.0	134.7	198.3	192.5	16.1
1965	18.4	0.1	1.5	10.2	48.2	128.2	177.3	177.1	15.1
1964	15.7	0.2	1.3	9.8	43.0	107.9	146.5	144.8	13.0
1963[‡]	15.5	0.2	1.3	9.7	43.4	107.8	134.9	149.1	12.8

TABLE 2–6. (Continued)

RACE, SEX, AND YEAR	ALL AGES	25–34 YEARS	35–44 YEARS	45–54 YEARS	55–64 YEARS	65–74 YEARS	75–84 YEARS	85 YEARS AND OVER	AGE-ADJUSTED RATE
1962‡	12.8	0.1	1.4	7.9	36.8	88.9	109.8	112.3	10.6
1961	10.7	0.1	1.1	6.1	32.6	72.8	88.6	89.2	8.8
1960	9.8	0.1	1.1	6.9	30.1	66.8	78.3	74.9	8.2
White, female									
1982**	15.9	—	—	—	—	—	—	—	—
1977*	9.8	0.0	0.6	5.2	20.1	44.6	64.9	70.7	5.8
1976*	9.2	0.1	0.9	5.3	19.6	41.6	61.9	65.0	5.6
1975*	8.2	0.1	1.0	5.1	19.0	36.8	51.5	59.3	5.1
1974*	7.4	0.1	0.8	5.1	17.2	34.5	48.6	52.2	4.7
1973*	6.8	0.0	0.9	4.8	16.0	31.5	43.7	56.8	4.4
1972*†	6.0	0.1	1.0	4.4	14.4	27.8	38.1	45.1	3.9
1971*	5.5	0.1	0.8	4.6	12.7	24.2	35.7	46.4	3.6
1970*	4.9	0.1	0.9	4.2	12.2	22.1	29.8	38.3	3.3
1969	4.4	0.1	0.8	3.8	10.6	19.0	28.8	47.0	3.0
1968	4.0	0.1	0.8	3.4	10.0	16.6	26.8	43.4	2.7
1967	3.2	0.1	0.5	2.8	7.7	13.3	22.5	36.1	2.2
1966	3.0	0.1	0.7	2.6	6.7	13.7	21.2	34.1	2.1
1965	2.8	0.1	0.7	2.4	5.9	12.0	20.8	35.4	1.9
1964	2.3	0.1	0.6	2.0	5.2	9.7	18.0	28.6	1.6
1963‡	2.2	0.1	0.4	2.1	4.8	9.1	17.7	28.1	1.5
1962‡	1.8	0.1	0.5	1.7	3.8	7.5	15.7	25.4	1.3
1961	1.5	0.1	0.3	1.2	3.0	6.6	12.4	22.7	1.1
1960	1.3	0.1	0.4	1.1	2.9	5.5	11.3	16.9	1.0
All other, male									
1982**	14.2	—	—	—	—	—	—	—	—
1977*	13.5	0.6	2.5	14.3	48.5	101.6	184.2	184.7	14.7
1976*	13.3	0.4	2.8	14.2	47.2	99.7	184.6	183.8	14.4
1975*	12.0	0.2	3.4	13.9	43.9	86.8	171.4	139.1	13.3
1974*	11.8	0.2	3.8	12.1	44.5	100.4	140.7	145.6	13.3
1973*	12.0	0.4	2.6	14.5	47.6	94.7	147.4	154.7	13.5
1972*†	11.5	0.8	2.6	15.4	46.0	84.8	160.8	117.7	13.3
1971*	11.0	0.8	3.7	15.0	43.7	84.2	120.8	128.6	12.5
1970*	10.8	0.5	4.0	12.1	45.7	79.8	131.0	104.7	12.2
1969	10.1	0.2	3.6	15.1	39.6	78.1	107.4	118.2	11.6
1968	9.2	0.7	3.6	16.1	35.1	66.1	106.5	75.6	10.6
1967	7.8	0.8	2.5	11.6	29.5	60.7	82.1	110.3	8.9
1966	7.5	0.4	3.4	13.2	28.9	55.1	70.9	102.8	8.7
1965	7.1	0.2	2.1	12.9	28.7	49.0	75.0	102.9	8.1
1964	6.2	0.2	2.7	8.7	28.5	47.9	54.1	50.0	7.2
1963‡	6.3	0.2	2.7	10.3	25.4	46.4	57.6	96.6	7.2
1962‡	4.9	0.5	2.0	6.5	21.6	42.6	34.2	41.4	5.7
1961	4.6	0.4	2.4	7.3	18.0	31.6	40.9	53.3	5.2
1960	4.2	0.3	2.4	7.3	18.2	31.7	26.7	47.8	4.9
All other, female									
1982**	4.6	—	—	—	—	—	—	—	—

TABLE 2–6. (Continued)

RACE, SEX, AND YEAR	ALL AGES	25–34 YEARS	35–44 YEARS	45–54 YEARS	55–64 YEARS	65–74 YEARS	75–84 YEARS	85 YEARS AND OVER	AGE-ADJUSTED RATE
1977*	3.0	0.0	0.9	4.4	10.6	14.6	31.6	35.6	2.8
1976*	2.7	0.1	0.9	4.1	10.3	14.8	23.5	27.3	2.7
1975*	2.8	0.3	1.4	4.6	8.5	15.2	25.3	20.0	2.7
1974*	2.1	0.3	0.6	3.2	7.6	13.7	18.1	23.7	2.2
1973*	2.3	0.2	1.0	4.1	9.3	11.9	22.3	19.3	2.4
1972*†	2.0	—	1.8	2.6	7.2	9.2	20.6	29.3	2.0
1971*	2.1	0.1	1.2	4.8	7.3	11.7	15.6	13.1	2.2
1970*	1.8	0.3	1.1	3.0	5.7	9.5	15.3	20.3	1.9
1969	1.6	0.4	1.3	3.1	5.0	6.7	14.9	26.2	1.7
1968	1.4	—	1.2	2.5	5.6	6.1	10.5	26.2	1.5
1967	1.2	0.3	1.2	1.8	3.5	6.2	9.1	15.8	1.2
1966	1.2	—	1.0	1.8	4.1	6.4	7.7	15.1	1.2
1965	1.0	0.3	0.6	2.3	3.2	4.4	8.5	10.2	1.1
1964	0.8	0.1	0.6	2.3	2.2	2.0	5.4	13.3	0.8
1963‡	1.1	0.1	0.7	1.9	3.9	5.4	6.3	23.8	1.1
1962‡	0.9	0.2	1.0	1.1	2.9	3.0	10.3	15.0	1.0
1961	0.7	0.1	0.3	0.9	1.6	4.3	8.9	12.5	0.7
1960	0.7	0.1	0.7	1.4	2.0	2.9	2.4	12.4	0.7

*Excludes deaths of nonresidents of the United States.
†Based on a 50% sample of deaths.
‡Figures by race exclude data for residents of New Jersey because this State did not require reporting of the item for these years.
**Does not use 519.3 but ICDA codes 492, 494–496
Source: Vital and Health Statistics, Series 20 No. 17

respiratory cancer. Epidemiologists suspect women's equal right to smoke as causative in the increasing equalization in their emphysema death rate. On the brighter side, female increases, although larger than those of men, have like the men's shown a pattern of increasing at a declining rate between 1950 and 1977.

PREVALENCE

The prevalence of emphysema determined through survey in 1970 is shown in Table 2–7. Treatment of those afflicted with COPD and/or emphysema involves bronchodilator therapy, use of antimicrobials for respiratory infection, and sometimes oxygen administration. Patients also need to be educated about the effects of smoking and lifestyle factors on their conditions.

ASTHMA

Descriptions of asthma attacks go back to the second century A.D.

TABLE 2–7. Prevalence of Emphysema Reported on the Basis of Physicians' Diagnosis in Health Interviews, by Age, Family Income, and Place of Residence: United States, 1970

FAMILY INCOME AND PLACE OF RESIDENCE	ALL AGES	UNDER 45 YEARS	45–64 YEARS	65 YEARS AND OVER
	Rate per 1,000 persons			
Total	6.6	1.0	13.9	31.7
Family income				
Less than $3,000	14.5	*	28.0	27.0
$3,000–$4,999	12.0	*	18.9	40.4
$5,000–$6,999	7.5	*	17.1	43.1
$7,000–$9,999	5.1	*	12.9	38.3
$10,000–$14,999	3.4	*	10.6	*
$15,000 or more	3.4	*	8.5	*
Place of residence				
SMSA	5.4	0.7	11.4	28.0
Central city	6.1	*	12.8	26.5
Not central city	4.9	*	10.3	29.3
Outside SMSA:				
Nonfarm	8.8	1.5	19.4	38.7
Farm	7.7	*	*	*

Source: National Center for Health Statistics: Prevalence of selected chronic respiratory conditions: United States, 1970. *Vital and Health Statistics*. Series 10-No. 84. DHEW Pub. No. (HRA) 74–1511. Health Resources Administration. Washington. U.S. Government Printing Office, Sept. 1973.

but as of the 1980s there still is not definitive understanding of the mechanism or varying causes of this disease. What is known, contrary to past opinion, is that asthma is not always due to a psychological disorder, inferior genes, or allergies. Nor is it an inconsequential medical disorder.

Asthma is a disease in which bronchial airways are narrowed because of spasm of the bronchial tubes or swelling of their mucous membranes. This becomes acute during attacks when an asthmatic suffers shortness of breath and wheezing. Autopsy findings in those who have died during an attack reveal hyperdistended lungs with thick tenacious, mucous-plugging, bronchioles, and mucosal and basement membrane thickening. Eosinophils (a type of white blood cell important in modulating immune reactions) are widely present.

TRIGGERS OF ATTACK

Triggers of asthma attacks can be extrinsic, such as allergens like dust, mold, animal dander, or drugs. There may be a true allergy to a drug or in cases where aspirin triggers an attack, asthmatics may find that other anti-inflammatory medications, including phenylbutazone and indomethacin, will elicit a similar attack. Other agents known to precipitate asthma attacks are yellow food dye #5, tartrazine yellow, and sulfur dioxide (a food preservative often used to keep vegetable greens such as lettuce from turning brown). This agent is also present in some beers, wines, and other foods.

Attacks also follow exercise, although many asthmatics exercise without provoking an attack. Other triggers can be reflexes and respiratory infections. Asthma often begins when a child suffers from a respiratory infection. Several viruses including syncytial virus, influenza type A, and adenovirus have been associated with the onset of asthma.

Researchers have observed that bronchial smooth muscle exhibits a 100-fold increased response to histamine in persons infected with a weakened live virus. Investigators conjecture that viruses may damage the airways' protective lining, exposing histamine-reactive receptors. Histamines seem to play a role in asthma even though antihistamine drugs so effective for other kinds of allergic reactions have proved largely ineffective in treating asthma. Indeed, it may be that other receptors are also exposed, which are sensitive to powerful bronchoconstrictors released by mast cells. Mast cells have been implicated for some time in allergic reactions.

Extrinsically caused, allergy-related asthma is thought to characterize most childhood asthma cases. Unless present before age 2 years, childhood asthma typically has a better prognosis than adult-onset asthma, which occurs in people older than age 40. Often childhood asthma disappears by early adulthood, although this is not always true. The profile of children prone to developing asthma is one in which there is a family history of allergy and a pattern of allergic eczema in infancy.

It is now believed that four of five childhood asthmatics have an allergic component in their disease. The predisposing allergy may be to certain common foods— particularly eggs, wheat, milk, and corn or to inhaled allergens, such as household dust. Parents' smoking may increase the risk of respiratory ailments. According to the National Institute for Allergy and Infectious Disease at least one study has found that tobacco smoke aggravated asthma in 67% of those whose parents smoked.

It is estimated that 8.9 million Americans suffer from asthma. Indeed, asthma and other allergies are the leading chronic disease complex among children younger than age 17. The rank of asthma among chronic diseases causing limitation of activity among the general population is shown in Table 2–8.

The number of asthma cases per 1,000 population between 1969 and 1984 is shown in Table 2–9.

TABLE 2–8. Prevalence of the Leading Chronic Conditions Causing Limitation of Activity, U.S., 1979

RANK	CONDITION	PREVALENCE (IN THOUSANDS)
1	Deformities or orthopedic impairments	5,620
2	Arthritis*	5,372
3	Heart conditions	5,305
4	Hypertension*	3,203
5	Diabetes	1,593
6	Visual impairments	1,486
7	Asthma	1,274
8	Displacement of intervertebral disc	1,207
9	Emphysema	1,118
10	Hearing impairments	776
11	Paralysis	753
12	Hernia of abdominal cavity	703
13	Diseases of the urinary system	640
14	Arteriosclerosis*	615
15	Cerebrovascular disease	614

* Not elsewhere classified.
Source: Health Interview Survey NCHS

TABLE 2–9. Asthma Cases* Between 1969 and 1984

ASTHMA YEAR	CASES
1969	8.1
1971	9.1
1972	8.7
1973	9.9
1974	11.6
1975	11.7
1980	11.0*
1981	14.0
1982	14.0
1983	15.0
1984	15.0

*Rates have been rounded through conversion from a per 100,000 to a per 1,000 ratio.
Source: National Institute of Allergy and Infectious Disease

The number of disability days associated with asthma by sex and age in the United States in 1975 is estimated in millions in Tables 2–10. The benefit allowed by Social Security in just 1 year to workers disabled by asthma and other chronic respiratory diseases totalled $90.5 million in the late 1970s.

The disposition of medication therapy for asthmatic sufferers by various patient characteristics is shown in Table 2–11. The tendency not to recommend drug usage for children as much as for

TABLE 2–10. Disability Days Associated with Asthma by Sex and Age: United States, 1975 Estimates (*in millions*)*

SEX AND AGE (YEARS)	RESTRICTED ACTIVITY DAYS	BED DAYS	WORK LOSS DAYS	SCHOOL LOSS DAYS
Both sexes				
All ages	94	36	5	6
Under 17	28	11		
17–44	23	8		
45–64	23	7		
65+	21	10		
Male				
All ages	49	18	4	4
Under 17	17	6		
17–44	9	3		
45–64	10	2		
65+	13	6		
Female				
All ages	45	18	2	2
Under 17	11	5		
17–44	14	5		
45–64	13	5		
65+	7	3		

*Figures may not add because of rounding.
Data are based on household interviews of the civilian, noninstitutional population.
Source: Derived from unpublished data from the Health Interview Survey 1970, National Center for Health Statistics. Adjusted by age and sex with 1975 Census Estimates. Prepared by Epidemiology and Biometry Branch, MIDP, NIAID.

adults is reflected in asthma data since so many asthmatics are children.

ALLERGIC RHINITIS (HAY FEVER)

Millions of people suffer from a runny or congested nose, tearing eyes, and sneezing fits either seasonally from the end of summer into early fall if they are allergic to ragweed pollen, or all year round if they are allergic to allergens continually in the environment, such as dust and mold spores.

Originally, people thought the syndrome, which was most noticeable at the end of the summer, was caused by hay and thus the misnomer "hay fever" has come into general use to refer to this particular allergic rhinitis problem. The medical term "rhinitis" literally means inflammation of the nose.

Rhinitis has an extrinsic and intrinsic form. Extrinsic rhinitis is caused by external environmental factors, such as the ragweed

TABLE 2–11. Office Visits for Asthma, Number and Percentage of Drug Visits, Number of Drug Mentions, Drug Mention Rate, and Drug Intensity Rate, by Selected Characteristics: United States, 1980

SELECTED CHARACTERISTIC	OFFICE VISITS: All visits	OFFICE VISITS: Drug visits*		DRUG MENTIONS	DRUG MENTION RATE†	DRUG INTENSITY RATE‡
	Number (in thousands)	Number (in thousands)	Percent	Number (in thousands)	Rate per visit	
Sex						
Both sexes	5,921**	5,477	92.5	11,655	1.97	2.13
Female	3,262	2,999	91.9	6,738	2.07	2.25
Male	2,659	2,478	93.2	4,917	1.85	1.98
Age (years)						
Under 15	2,335	2,126	91.0	3,495	1.50	1.64
15–24	737	716	97.2	1,262	1.71	1.76
25–44	1,106	1,031	93.2	2,271	2.05	2.20
45–64	1,065	989	92.8	2,876	2.70	2.91
65 and over	678	616	90.8	1,750	2.58	2.84
Race						
White	5,234	4,830	92.3	10,441	1.99	2.16
Black	648	607	93.8	1,134	1.75	1.87
Problem status						
New problem	1,204	1,148	95.3	2,616	2.17	2.28
Old problem	4,717	4,329	91.8	9,039	1.92	2.09
Major reason for visit						
Acute problem	1,653	1,518	91.9	3,243	1.96	2.14
Chronic problem, routine	2,812	2,561	91.1	5,036	1.79	1.97
Chronic problem, flareup	1,214	1,169	96.3	2,976	2.45	2.55
Non-illness care	241	228	94.6	401	1.66	1.76

*A visit in which one or more drugs were ordered or provided
†Drug mentions divided by number of visits
‡Drug mentions divided by number of drug visits
**Includes races other than white and black not shown as separate categories
Source: Vital and Health Statistics, Series 13, No. 71

pollen, pollens from other plants, grasses, trees and dust, molds and foods. Overuse of nasal sprays can also induce greater nasal congestion by a rebound effect and people have had nasal side effects from drugs like reserpine and propranolol.

Intrinsic rhinitis, on the other hand, seems to be unrelated to inhalation or digestion of these agents and may be related to nose function or physiology. One form of intrinsic rhinitis occurs during pregnancy due to hormonal conditions. A deviated septum and nasal polyps can also lead to chronic rhinitis. Moreover, rhinitis can be induced in some by exposure to cold temperatures. This is often referred to as vasomotor rhinitis. It is categorized with intrinsic rhinitis disorders since its etiology is not clearly understood. The National Institute of Allergy and Infectious Disease (NIAID) estimates that approximately 60% to 70% of chronic rhinitis cases are of undetermined origin. Researchers suspect that an imbalance in the nervous system of the nose may be responsible for many of these cases.

The nose is a complex organ controlling the humidity and temperature of breathed-in air; removing foreign bodies, such as pollens and dust from the respiratory system; and initiating an immune response to foreign bodies, such as viruses that invade the body through inhalation.

TREATMENT

By studying nasal tissue and allergens outside of the body, scientists have been able to determine the dynamics of allergic rhinitis as one in which sensitized mast cells in contact with allergens release substances, called mediators, that cause surrounding tissue to swell and itch. A well-known mediator in the swelling and itching of tissue during allergic reactions is histamine. With the development of antihistamine drugs in the 1940s, allergic rhinitis sufferers were able to find effective relief from their symptoms. Before that time, the only recourse for sufferers was sensitivity testing and allergy shots, an expensive and time-consuming treatment that doesn't always suppress rhinitis reactions. Many people still seek therapy in an attempt to arrest the mechanism of their disease in a more pervasive way than the symptomatic relief available through antihistamine drug usage. One reason is that some of these drugs have side effects ranging from dry mouth to drowsiness to psychological reactions in the form of anxiety attacks. Nevertheless, many people do take such drugs on a daily basis without any noticeable adverse effect and gain symptomatic relief.

Others seek immunotherapy in the hope that treatment of their allergy will prevent the onset of asthma. Investigators now believe that allergic rhinitis sufferers' fear of asthma has been exaggerated and that only 7% of such persons go on to develop asthma. Past estimates of this risk, which have contributed to excessive anxiety, were as high as 35%.

Determination of the substances one is allergic to has traditionally been done through skin testing. In this procedure, sera containing various allergens are injected into the patient or applied through skin scratches on the back or arm. If a patient is allergic to the substance, a red flare and swelling develop around the site of the scratch to varying degrees, depending on the severity of the allergic reaction. This usually happens within 15 minutes as IgE antibodies specific to the allergen gather at the site of its introduction. If there is no reaction, the assumption is that there are no IgE antibodies for the particular allergen and the patient is not allergic to the introduced substance.

In recent years, laboratory blood tests have been developed to determine the sensitivity of a patient to various antigens. Two tests—the Histamine Release Test and the RAST test—are being used, but they are not considered to be as diagnostically accurate as skin testing.

GENES

The genetic component in allergies is well established. In one study, 48% of allergy sufferers had an immediate family history of allergic disease. Only 12% of nonallergic persons had such a background. Clearly, there are also cases of allergic children whose parents are allergy free, but this is not the norm.

Theory concerning the role of IgE antibodies supposes that this kind of antibody developed to fight parasitic infections and that its presence in persons not afflicted with parasites harmful to the body is vestigial. The fetus in utero produces IgE antibodies at 22 weeks' gestation and they have been found in the sera of some umbilical cords although it is not generally thought that IgE antibodies cross the placental barrier between mother and child. Still, infants have reacted allergically to substances to which they have not previously been exposed. This suggests that they are exhibiting an allergic response passed on through their mother. There have been reports of babies fed exclusively through nursing who exhibit an allergy to cow's milk, sensitized it would seem, by antibodies to cow's milk in their mother's milk. Thus, nursing may be another avenue of immune transference between mother and child.

This is a particularly interesting point of speculation since early studies in the 1950s seem to show that more than one-half of allergy high-risk infants fed cow's milk developed allergies whereas only 14% of similar infants that did not drink cow's milk developed allergy problems. This finding led to the manufacture of soy and other cow's milk substitutes for infant formula. But a 1973 survey of more than 400 children found no difference in allergy development among children fed cow's, mother's, or soy milk, except that those fed soy milk may have had a somewhat more severe allergic response when allergic. In light of these findings, study of the question of immune transference goes on.

PREVALENCE

There are more than 5 million children who have allergic rhinitis.

In children younger than 10 years it seems to develop more often in boys. After age 10 it develops more often in girls. The number of hay fever sufferers, not counting those with non-hay fever rhinitis per 1,000 population between 1969 and 1975, is shown in Table 2–12.

TABLE 2–12. Hay Fever Sufferers Between 1969 and 1975*

HAYFEVER YEAR	RATE PER 1,000 POPULATION
1969	4.1
1971	3.5
1972	3.7
1973	4.1
1974	4.7
1975	5.0

*These data represent the chronic conditions obtained through questions pertaining to 2-week disability days, doctor visits, limitation of activity and hospitalization and do not reflect the prevalence of chronic conditions for that year.
Source: Unpublished data from the Health Interview Survey, National Center for Health Statistics. Data are based on household inteviews. Prepared by Epidemiology and Biometry Branch, MIDP, NIAID, Report of the Task Force on Asthma and the Other Allergic Diseases. National Institute of Allergy and Infectious Disease, March 1980.

Fig. 2–2. Ragweed density in the United States

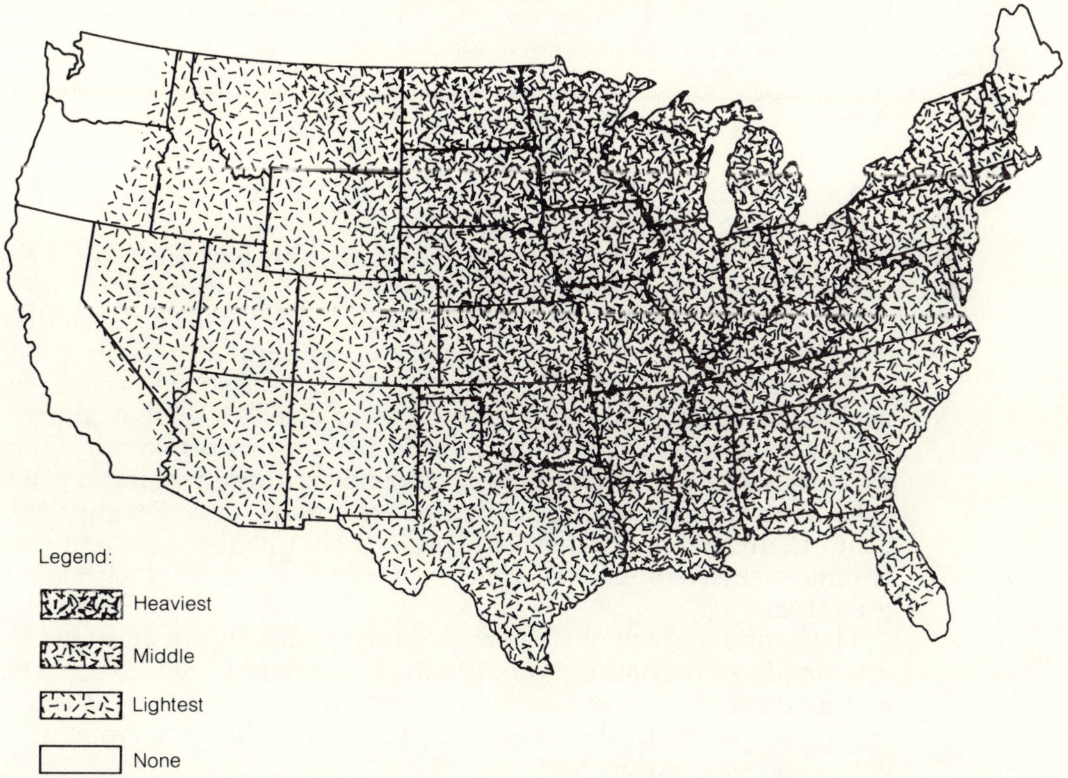

Source: Report of the Task Force on Asthma and the Other Allergic Diseases, National Institute of Allergy and Infectious Disease, March 1980.

TABLE 2–13. Disability Days Associated with Hay Fever by Sex and Age: United States, 1975 Estimates (*in millions*)*

SEX AND AGE	RESTRICTED ACTIVITY DAYS	BED DAYS	WORK LOSS DAYS	SCHOOL LOSS DAYS
Both sexes				
All ages (years)	28	6	3	2
Under 17	6	2	—	
17–44	10	2	1	
45–64	8	2	1	
65+	3	1	1	
Male				
All ages (years)	8	2	1	1
Under 17	3	1	—	
17–44	2	1	—	
45–64	2	—	—	
65+	2	—	1	
Female				
All ages (years)	19	4	2	1
Under 17	3	1	—	
17–44	8	1	1	
45–64	7	1	1	
65+	2	1	—	

*Figures may not add because of rounding.
Data are based on household interviews of the civilian, noninstitutional populations.
Source: Derived from unpublished data from the Health Interview Survey 1970 National Center for Health Statistics. Adjusted by age and sex with 1975 Census Estimates. Prepared by Epidemiology and Biometry Branch, MIDP, NIAID, National Institute for Allergy and Infectious Disease

Areas of the United States where rhinitis-producing pollen is prevalent are illustrated in Fig. 2–2.

In all, there are approximately 14.9 million hay fever sufferers in the United States. In 1975, they lost 3.5 million work-days, which cost them more than $154 million in wages. The disability days associated with allergic rhinitis are presented in Table 2–13.

The number and percentage distribution of office visits made by people suffering from chronic respiratory disease, such as allergic rhinitis and others is shown in Table 2–14. The proportion of women patients seeking medical help for various chronic respiratory diseases is greater for each type except for emphysema. Seventy percent of emphysema patients are men. It should also be noted that chronic disease sufferers are older typically than patients with acute infections.

The seriousness of chronic respiratory problems encountered by private physicians during office visits is shown in Table 2–15. The complaint judged most serious was emphysema although at times any of the several other problems, such as asthma or bronchitis, could become acutely serious.

The diagnostic or treatment modalities given to chronically ill

TABLE 2–14. Number, Percentage Distribution, and Average Annual Rate of Office Visits for Selected Chronic Diseases of the Respiratory System and Percentage Distribution for All Other Morbidity-related Groups, by Selected Patient Characteristics: United States, 1975–76

SELECTED PATIENT CHARACTERISTICS	DIAGNOSIS AND ICDA CODE						
	Chronic bronchitis (491)	Emphysema (492)	Asthma (493)	Chronic Pharyngitis and naso-pharyngitis (502)	Chronic sinusitis (503)	Hay fever (507)	All other morbidity-related ICDA groups (000–458, 520–629, 680–738, 780–796)
	Visits (in thousands)						
All visits	1,646	5,223	10,951	2,486	8,284	17,012	667,261
	Percent distribution						
	100.0	100.0	100.0	100.0	100.0	100.0	100.0
Sex							
Female	50.6	29.6	54.9	58.2	58.8	56.3	61.5
Male	49.4	70.4	45.1	41.9	41.2	43.7	38.5
Race							
White	92.4	91.9	87.3	94.8	89.9	94.4	90.3
Black and all other	*7.7	*8.1	12.7	*5.2	10.1	5.6	9.7
Age (years)							
Under 15	*1.5	*1.1	32.9	25.5	10.3	29.2	11.7
15–24	*6.3	*0.1	10.9	*13.1	14.8	16.6	12.1
25–44	*19.3	*4.8	18.1	30.8	35.7	30.9	24.4
45–64	45.3	44.9	28.1	*18.8	27.4	17.7	30.2
65 and over	*27.7	49.0	10.1	*11.9	11.7	5.6	21.7
Median visit age in years	57.4	64.7	32.0	33.0	37.8	27.3	. . .
Standard error of median visit age in years	3.0	2.2	4.4	5.8	2.7	2.2	. . .
	Visit rate per 1,000 population						
All visits	4.0	12.5	26.2	6.0	19.9	40.8	. . .
Sex							
Female	3.9	7.2	27.8	6.7	22.6	44.4	. . .
Male	4.0	18.3	24.6	5.2	17.0	36.9	. . .
Race							
White	4.2	13.2	26.4	6.5	20.5	44.3	. . .
Black and all other	*2.3	*7.7	25.4	*2.4	15.3	17.3	. . .

*May be an unreliable estimate
Source: Vital and Health Statistics, Series 13, No. 42

respiratory patients during office visits are shown in Table 2–16. As with acutely ill patients, chronic patients usually have a limited physical exam and/or history review and drug medication. But chronic bronchitis and emphysema patients additionally have their blood pressure taken either because of their age or the nature of their pulmonary condition which often impacts on heart function.

TABLE 2–15. Office Visits for Selected Chronic Diseases of the Respiratory System and Percentage Distribution of Visits by Problem Status and by Problem Seriousness, According to Diagnosis: United States, 1975–76

DIAGNOSIS AND ICDA CODE*		VISITS (IN THOUSANDS)	TOTAL	PROBLEM STATUS: New problem	PROBLEM STATUS: Continuing problem	PROBLEM SERIOUSNESS: Not serious	PROBLEM SERIOUSNESS: Slightly serious	PROBLEM SERIOUSNESS: Serious or very serious
			Percentage distribution					
Chronic bronchitis	491	1,646	100.0	27.0	73.0	39.6	40.6	19.7
Emphysema	492	5,223	100.0	13.1	86.9	10.0	31.8	58.2
Asthma	493	10,951	100.0	9.5	90.6	21.6	46.3	32.1
Chronic pharyngitis and nasopharynigitis	502	2,486	100.0	38.7	61.3	57.3	33.7	9.0
Chronic sinusitis	503	8,284	100.0	50.7	49.3	54.6	36.3	9.0
Hay fever	507	17.012	100.0	16.7	83.3	57.0	36.8	6.2

*Based on the *Eighth Revision International Classification of Disease, Adapted for Use in the United States* (ICDA).
Source: Vital and Health Statistics, Series 13, No. 42

The physician specialty sought out by patients with chronic respiratory disease for office based care is presented in Table 2–17. Chronically ill patients, as indicated, were seen by general practitioners, internists, pediatricians, and allergists.

OCCUPATIONAL LUNG DISEASE

As has been discussed, many lung diseases are caused by environmental agents in combination with constitutional factors that vary from person to person. Pollen antigens in the environment can cause allergic rhinitis in allergy-prone individuals with high circulation of IgE antibodies in their system. But pollen inhaled by other nonallergic individuals will produce no external allergic reaction.

Cigarette smoking will cause lung diseases, such as emphysema or lung cancer in large numbers of average individuals. Statistically, the odds are against the average person who smokes. Some people, on the other hand, are genetically more resistant to lung disease and can smoke all their lives without developing serious lung disease. Others are constitutionally weaker and develop lung cancer without ever having smoked.

Similarly, there are other stimuli for disease development in the work environment that affect large numbers of workers of average or less-than-average health. The National Institute for Occupational Safety and Health (NIOSH) estimates that 100,000 persons die yearly from occupationally related respiratory disease; 400,000

Table 2–16. Office Visits for Selected Chronic Diseases of the Respiratory System and for All Other Morbidity-related Groups by Diagnostic or Therapeutic Services Ordered or Provided, by Diagnosis: United States, 1975–76

DIAGNOSTIC OR THERAPEUTIC SERVICE	DIAGNOSIS AND ICDA CODE*						
	Chronic bronchitis (491)	Emphysema (492)	Asthma (493)	Chronic pharyngitis and naso-pharyngitis (502)	Chronic sinusitis (503)	Hay fever (507)	All other morbidity-related ICDA† groups (000–458, 520–629, 680–738, 780–796)
	Visits (in thousands)						
All visits	1,646	5,223	10,951	2,486	8,284	17,012	667,261
	Percent of visits‡						
Limited history and/or examination	53.6	71.7	53.0	57.2	68.5	38.2	67.7
General history and/or examination	25.8	12.5	10.1	14.9	7.0	6.9	18.8
Clinical laboratory test	32.3	17.2	6.0	7.5	10.3	4.8	27.0
X-ray	24.1	13.4	5.8	5.7	6.7	2.1	8.0
Blood pressure check	53.3	62.7	19.9	20.0	35.9	9.2	42.4
Electrocardiogram	14.9	9.7	1.3	0.0	1.2	0.7	4.6
Drug prescribed**	59.4	63.1	49.4	67.6	79.0	31.9	65.5
Injection	27.5	22.8	26.4	14.9	29.5	22.6	19.1
Immunization	3.2	4.2	40.7	14.5	1.1	52.7	1.6
Medical counseling	17.8	16.7	11.5	*8.4	9.5	10.3	16.6
Other diagnostic and therapeutic services¶	*8.6	11.4	7.7	11.6	16.1	10.7	29.9

*Based on the *Eighth Revision International Classification of Diseases, Adapted for Use in the United States* (ICDA).
†For this report excludes categories relating to special conditions and examinations without sickness; complications of pregnancy, childbirth and the puerperium: congenital anomalies; certain causes of perinatal morbidity and mortality; accidents, poisonings, and violence; diagnosis "none" and "unknown."
‡Percents will not add to 100.0 because more than one service may have been provided.
**Includes prescription and nonprescription drugs.
¶Includes hearing test, vision test, endoscopy, office surgery, physiotherapy, psychotherapy or therapeutic listening, and other diagnostic or therapeutic services.
Source: Vital and Health Statistics, Series 13, No. 42

new cases develop annually. The most common diseases of this sort are dust related. Those who inhale silica dust in the stone, glass, and blasting industries suffer from silicosis. Those who inhale carbon and silica dust during coal mining often suffer from black lung disease. Pneumoconiosis, silicosis, and anthracosilicosis are sometimes used interchangeably when speaking about either of these similar dust-induced lung conditions.

BLACK LUNG

Most of the pioneering work done to investigate and identify Black Lung disease occurred in England and continental countries during

TABLE 2–17. Office Visits for Selected Chronic Diseases of the Respiratory System and Percentage Distribution of Visits by Physician Specialty, According to Diagnosis: United States, 1975–76

			PHYSICIAN SPECIALTY						
DIAGNOSIS AND ICDA CODE*		VISITS (IN THOUSANDS)	Total	General and family practice	Internal medicine	Pediatrics	Otolaryngology	Allergy	All other specialties (residual)
			Percentage distribution						
Chronic bronchitis	491	1,646	100.0	52.9	25.8	0.3	1.2	0.6	19.2
Emphysema	492	5,223	100.0	52.4	30.3	0.6	0.0	3.1	13.6
Asthma	493	10,951	100.0	29.5	10.6	21.9	0.7	32.3	5.0
Chronic pharyngitis and nasopharyngitis	502	2,486	100.0	30.3	4.2	14.9	34.3	11.9	4.4
Chronic sinusitis	503	8,284	100.0	60.5	10.2	5.6	13.5	* 0.8	9.4
Hay fever	507	17,012	100.0	25.3	9.9	17.8	9.6	30.6	5.8

*Based on the Eighth Revision International Classification of Diseases, Adapted for Use in the United States (ICDA).
Source: Vital and Health Statistics, Series 13, No. 42

the 19th Century. Frequent warnings began to appear in the medical literature about an "unusual chest disease" among bituminous coal miners. By 1936, the Medical Research Council of Great Britain undertook intensive study of the etiology and pathology of the disease. In the United States, study of anthracite coal miners was begun in the late 1920s, but until the late 1940s it was generally assumed that bituminous coal workers were not afflicted by the disease.

When an initial study of anthracite coal workers was conducted among 2,711 Pennsylvania miners and 135 disabled miners in 1928, 23% had evidence of anthracosilicosis or anthracite pneumoconiosis, a disease that results from breathing anthracite coal dust. Mortality from lung disease was much higher among the miners than among males in the general population.

It was not until 1941 that a link between pneumoconiosis and bituminous coal mining was suspected. Because bituminous mining exposes coal miners to silica, their disease is also referred to as silicosis. By 1950, it was established that coal miners' pneumoconiosis was a serious problem among anthracite (hard coal) and bituminous (soft coal) miners.

LUNG CHANGES

Clinically, the disease is one of progressively greater and greater difficulty in breathing caused by the inhalation of carbon and silica dust. Fibrosis develops in the lung with nodules that conglomerate in the advanced stage. In the early stage the disease is often referred to as anthracosilicosis; the term *'pneumoconiosis'* is applied to the advanced stage in which there is distention of both the bronchi and other thoracic structures.

Physically, there may be little evidence of lung damage until a pulmonary infection occurs or pulmonary circulation is impaired. Early tissue change appears on chest films after 10 or more years of exposure to coal dust at a stage when an affected individual may have symptoms of chronic bronchitis. At this stage, pulmonary function values may still be normal. After 20 to 25 years, the person may be experiencing emphysema symptoms and lung tissue is massively fibrotic. Mixed in this fibrotic tissue are black areas consisting of dust particles in small clusters, the residue of dust-laden phagocytes.

Complicated pneumoconiosis occurs more quickly in the upper and central lobes of the lung where extensive areas of dead tissue containing coal dust form tumor-like masses in one or both lungs.

TABLE 2–18. Prevalence Among Coal Miners: History of Specified Chest Conditions by Age (by percent positive replies).

MEDICAL HISTORY	AGE					
	Less than 35	35–44	45–54	55–64	65 or more	Total
Working miners:						
Pneumonia	20.5	22.7	25.2	26.0	*[a]	24.0
Asthma	3.9	5.1	5.8	8.8	*	5.9
Pleurisy	8.1	7.4	11.3	15.1	2	10.5
Bronchitis	6.5	4.8	7.6	8.9	*	6.9
Tuberculosis	0	.4	.9	1.2	*	.7
Dust on the lungs	1.3	4.9	8.7	14.1	*	7.8
Heart trouble	2.9	3.3	6.1	9.7	*	5.6
Other chest trouble	6.9	4.7	5.7	5.6	*	5.6
Nonworking miners:						
Pneumonia	*	26.3	30.0	31.5	19.4	30.6
Asthma	*	3.9	12.6	15.7	8.3	14.2
Pleurisy	*	18.4	12.6	14.7	8.3	14.4
Bronchitis	*	9.2	17.8	14.5	5.6	14.4
Tuberculosis	*	0	3.3	2.3	5.6	2.4
Dust on the lungs	*	11.8	40.5	34.3	27.8	33.5
Heart trouble	*	7.9	18.9	27.7	19.4	24.7
Other chest trouble	*	17.1	11.0	13.1	19.4	13.3

[a]Less than 10 persons in age group
Source: Pneumoconiosis in Appalachian Bituminous Coal Miners, HEW, Bureau of Occupational Safety and Health 1969

EARLY U.S. STUDY

Between 1963 and 1965, a detailed investigation of coal miners' lung disease was conducted among bituminous coal miners in Appalachia.[a] Over 2,500 working miners and 1,191 nonworking miners were studied. Inclusion of nonworking or no–longer–working miners was important to the study design because no–longer–working miners are often sick miners: the very population that is of greatest interest in this type of study. The miners were asked an array of questions about their personal health history, whether they had ever experienced lung disease symptoms or had ever been diagnosed as having a lung disease. The miners replied yes or no. The results are shown in Table 2–18.

The high percentage of men in each age range listed who had a history of pneumonia is noteworthy. It is also true to expectation that the percentage of nonworking miners who reported dust on the lungs, asthma, pleurisy, and bronchitis was higher than it was for working miners, particularly among men in older brackets.

In addition to the problems just cited, 10% of the working miners reported a persistent, productive cough, while 28% of the non-

[a]Lainhart WS: *Prevalence of Coal Miners' Pneumoconiosis* in *Appalachian Bituminous Coal Miners,* HEW 1969.

TABLE 2–19. Prevalence Among Coal Miners: History of Dyspnea

DEGREE OF DYSPNEA	WORKING MINERS		NONWORKING MINERS	
	Number	Percent	Number	Percent
None	1,209	47.6	174	15.4
Slight	1,001	39.4	336	29.7
Moderate	239	9.4	208	18.4
Marked	62	2.5	138	12.2
Severe	28	1.1	275	24.3
Total	2,539	100.0	1,131	100.0
Disabled or unknown dyspnea history	10		30[a]	
Total	2,549		1,161	

[a]Of nonworking miners, 44 disabled due to noncardiopulmonary causes
Source: Pneumoconiosis in Appalachian Bituminous Coal Miners, HEW, Bureau of Occupational Health and Safety, 1969

Fig. 2–3. Prevalence of persistent productive cough by years underground and cigarette-smoking habits among working and nonworking miners

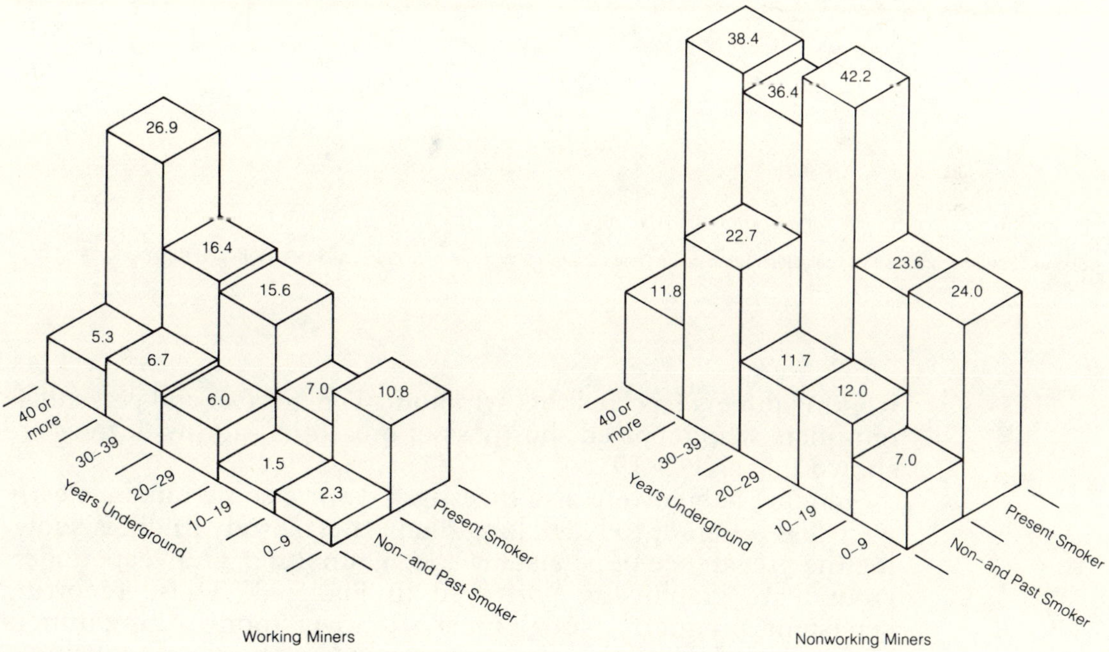

Source: Pnuemoconiosis In Appalachian Bituminous Coal Miners, HEW, Bureau of Occupational Health and Safety, 1969

Fig. 2–4. Prevalence of marked and severe dyspnea by years underground and cigarette-smoking habits among working and nonworking miners

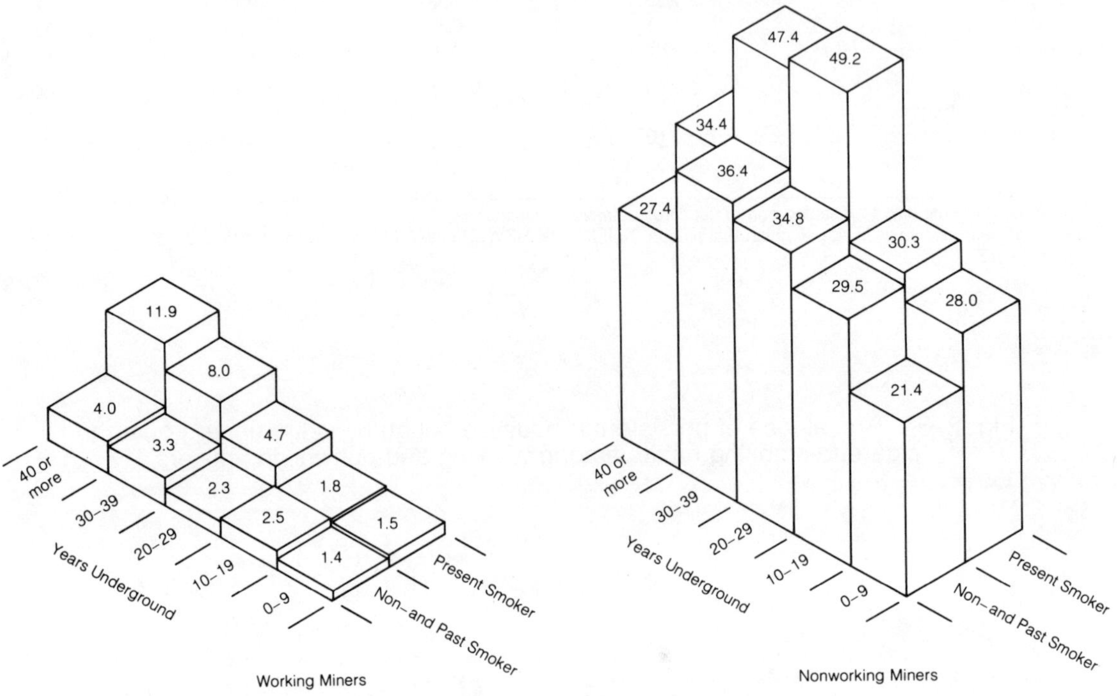

Source: Pneumoconiosis In Appalachian Bituminous Coal Miners, HEW, Bureau of Occupational Health and Safety, 1969.

working miners reported this symptom. The number and percentage of miners who reported shortness of breath in varying degrees are shown in Table 2–19.

Smoking habits were also investigated since some miners clearly were less resistant to black lung than others. Study findings showing the prevalence of persistent cough, smoking, and years underground are graphically portrayed in Fig. 2–3. Those reporting persistent, productive cough most often were nonworking miners who had worked many years underground and were current smokers. Slightly more than 38% of those underground longest reported persistent cough compared to only 2.3% reporting this symptom among relatively new nonsmoking workers.

Similarly, smokers underground longest who were no longer working as miners reported more dyspnea (shortness of breath) than any other group except those underground 30 to 39 years who presumably were so sick that they stopped working earlier than those underground for 40 or more years (Fig. 2–4).

Pneumoconiosis diagnosed through chest films and various clinical symptoms among different kinds of miners is depicted in Fig. 2–5. As indicated, the highest percentage of pneumoconiosis was among nonworking miners, and chronic cough was clinically related to pathologic findings more than dyspnea.

THE DISEASE TODAY

Estimates of the prevalence today of black lung disease range from 5% to 15% of the coal workforce. Four thousand deaths are attributed to it annually. The prevalence of 5% was determined by a recently completed NIOSH study that has been criticized for inconsistencies in its chest film readings and its limited period of study. The results of the study are summarized in Table 2–20.

Fig. 2–5. Prevalence of cough and dyspnea by degree of pneumoconiosis among working and nonworking miners.

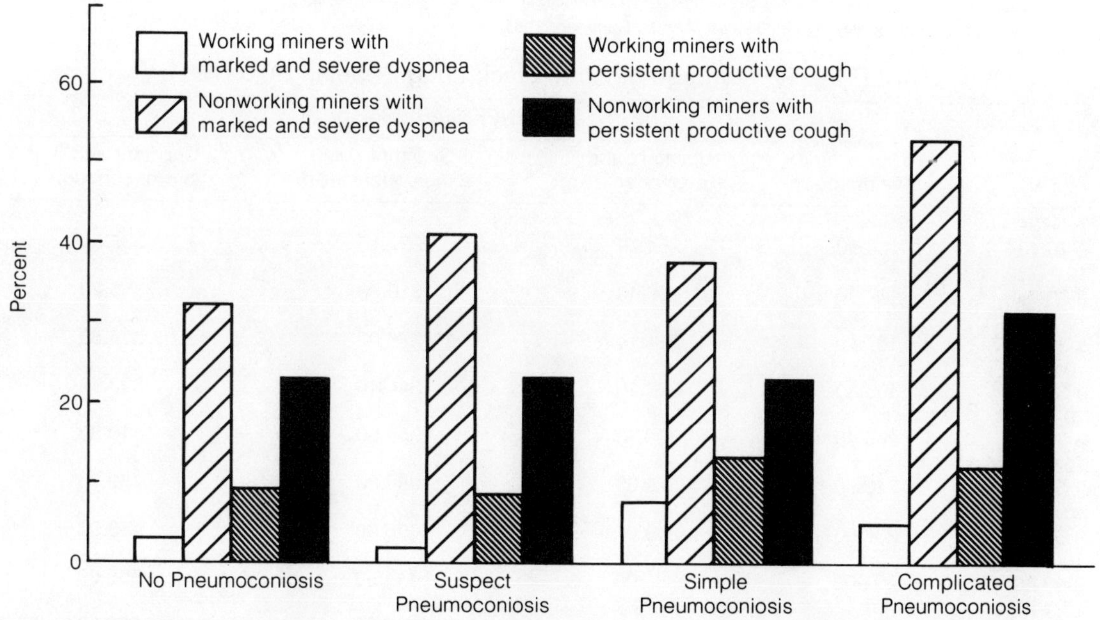

Source: Pneumoconiosis in Appalachian Bituminous Coal Miners, HEW, Bureau of Occupational Health and Safety, 1969

In 1969, funds were made available to miners disabled by black lung disease by the passage of the Federal Coal Mine Health and Safety Act. Benefits were liberalized in 1977 under the Black Lung Benefits Revenue Act. The monthly disability benefit granted to qualifying miners between 1973 and 1981 is shown in Table 2–21.

TABLE 2–20. Pneumoconiosis: Coal Workers' Pneumoconiosis, Round Three, NIOSH National Coal Study, October 1, 1978–December 15, 1980

YEARS MINING	CATEGORY* 0	1	2	3	PMF	TOTAL
0–9	39,050	416	14	1	2	39,483
	98.90%	1.05%	0.04%	0.00%	0.00%	
10–19	6,167	424	32	1	4	6.618
	93.19%	6.41%	0.33%	0.02%	0.08%	
20–29	2,228	410	52	5	9	2,704
	82.40%	15.16%	1.92%	0.19%	0.33%	
30–39	2,094	628	130	9	58	2,919
	71.74%	21.51%	4.45%	0.31%	1.99%	
40+	369	135	32	4	14	554
	66.61%	24.37%	5.78%	0.72%	2.53%	
Total	49,908	2,013	250	20	87	52,278
	95.47%	3.85%	0.48%	0.04%	0.17%	

*0, Absence of small opacities
1, Small opacities definitely present, but normal lung marking still visible
2, Numerous opacities, but normal lung marking still visible
3, Numerous opacities and normal lung marking partially or totally obscured
Progressive massive fibrosis
Source: Morbidity and Mortality Weekly Report, Annual Summary 1981

TABLE 2–21. Average Monthly Black Lung Benefit, 1973–1981

YEAR	BENEFICIARIES Claimant	Claimant and 1 dependent ($)	Claimant and 2 dependents ($)	Claimant and 3 or more dependents ($)
7-1-73–9-30-73	169.80	254.70	297.10	339.50
10-1-73–9-30-74	177.60	266.40	310.80	355.20
10-1-74–9-30-75	187.40	281.10	328.00	374.80
10-1-75–9-30-76	196.80	295.20	344.40	393.50
10-1-76–9-30-77	205.40	308.10	359.50	410.80
10-1-77–9-30-78	219.90	329.80	384.80	439.70
10-1-78–9-30-79	232.00	348.00	405.90	463.90
10-1-79–9-30-80	254.00	381.00	444.50	508.00
10-1-80–9-30-81	279.80	419.60	489.60	559.50

Source: Black Lung Benefit Act, Annual Report; US Department of Labor 1982

The number of active and terminated-plus-active claims for each state in 1979 and 1980 reported in thousands are listed in Table 2–22. The greatest number of claims have been in Alabama, Illinois, Kentucky, Ohio, Pennsylvania, and West Virginia—the coal mining states. The total expenditure in 1980 was $1.5 billion.

Various measures are used to reduce the amount of dust in the air that miners breathe, including water sprays in the mines and respirators for the miners. The maximum exposure to dust particles allowable in the United States is the standard set forth in the United Kingdom namely, 2 mg/meter.

Preventive measures, such as adherence to federal dust standards and the education of employers and workers, can do much to reduce the incidence of these occupational diseases. In similar fashion, much can be done to avoid the food-borne diseases, which are described in the next chapter. Prevention plays a greater role in reducing the incidence and suffering of many respiratory and infectious diseases than does treatment.

TABLE 2–22. Distribution of Black Lung Funds by State, July 1, 1973–December 31, 1980 (in thousands)

STATE	ACTIVE CLAIMS		ALL CLAIMS*
	As of December 31, 1979	As of December 31, 1980	AS OF DECEMBER 31, 1980
United States	784,206	1,343,274	1,545,110
Alabama	32,166	51,224	58,930
Alaska	352	563	648
Arizona	3,089	5,157	5,974
Arkansas	5,286	8,948	10,254
California	11,353	18,166	21,318
Colorado	12,297	19,715	22,636
Connecticut	2,432	3,865	4,375
Delaware	1,412	2,671	2,996
District of Columbia	492	811	982
Florida	15,611	26,110	29,707
Georgia	1,389	2,630	2,976
Hawaii	33	105	105
Idaho	399	612	652
Illinois	46,825	75,665	89,045
Indiana	24,945	41,756	48,900
Iowa	8,333	13,443	16,128
Kansas	4,148	7,293	8,426
Kentucky	64,911	109,561	124,872
Louisiana	586	783	950
Maine	64	161	177
Maryland	11,960	19,338	22,786
Massachusetts	354	740	823
Michigan	15,840	25,789	29,621
Minnesota	186	425	549
Mississippi	382	705	870
Missouri	7,522	12,234	14,382

1980 (in thousands)

STATE	ACTIVE CLAIMS As of December 31, 1979	ACTIVE CLAIMS As of December 31, 1980	ALL CLAIMS* AS OF DECEMBER 31, 1980
Montana	1,503	2,290	2,697
Nebraska	145	233	285
Nevada	584	928	1,173
New Hampshire	37	91	104
New Jersey	8,286	14,253	16,776
New Mexico	3,302	5,254	5,925
New York	6,572	11,850	13,835
North Carolina	2,933	4,829	5,345
North Dakota	221	302	354
Ohio	77,248	134,153	156,798
Oklahoma	5,057	9,128	10,368
Oregon	1,176	1,793	2,132
Pennsylvania	196,364	357,931	410,839
Rhode Island	38	93	117
South Carolina	512	1,162	1,287
South Dakota	143	185	209
Tennessee	19,237	30,174	34,840
Texas	2,124	3,306	3,836
Utah	4,674	8,381	9,435
Vermont	374	556	674
Virginia	44,163	75,243	84,778
Washington	2,908	5,475	6,217
West Virginia	125,594	212,411	240,960
Wisconsin	593	945	1,136
Wyoming	4,021	7,635	8,478
All other	4,030	6,203	7,430

*Active and terminated claims

Source: Black Lung Benefits Act, Annual Report; US Department of Labor 1982

Enteric Infections 3

TYPES OF INFECTION

Unlike respiratory infections, which are usually airborne, enteric infections are often transmitted to a healthy host through water or food containing a disease agent, usually a bacterium, parasite, or virus. Enteric infections typically affect the gastrointestinal tract. Symptoms include nausea, vomiting, severe diarrhea, and stomach cramps. Travelers often develop these symptoms after drinking water in a foreign locale. The water contains viruses for which the traveler has no immunity, viruses not found in home water. The disease agent causing these self-limiting episodes is usually unidentified. These and other passing enteric infections caused by some unidentified agent are often referred to simply as gastroenteritis.

Other life-threatening enteric infections can occur in anyone, native and visitor alike, who ingests food or water contaminated by certain bacteria. The bacteria produce toxins that cause the loss of water and electrolytes from the small intestine in severe diarrhea, which quickly leads to dehydration. Others such as *E. coli*, salmonella, and shigella attack the mucosa of the colon, causing ulceration, bleeding, and secretion of water.

SALMONELLOSIS

Salmonellosis is an enteric infection caused by gram-negative bacilli. They may cause bacteremia, enterocolitis (gastroenteritis), or typhoid. The typhoid variety *S. typhi* is the most lethal form, causing a mortality of about 3% to 10%. Other forms are less severe and usually cause mild-to-moderate illness. Ten serotypes of salmonella cause most of the salmonellosis outbreaks in the United

States. These serotypes can live in food, water, ice, and sewage. Most of them cause gastroenteritis designated as Salmonella enteritidis followed by a serotype.

In adults, infection is usually transmitted by improperly cooked or processed foods, although persons have contacted nontyphoid types of salmonellosis from powdered milk, candy bars, pharmaceuticals, and exposure to infected persons. A healthy carrier working as a food handler is often the source of typhoid infection. Five percent of infected persons become carriers. Children may become infected through fecal-oral spread. In rural areas, typhoid is typically transmitted through drinking water contaminated with fecal excretion from a carrier.

The symptoms of salmonellosis infections include fever and abdominal pain, delirium, and stupor. Enterocolitis involves severe diarrhea, whereas typhoid often causes headache, fever, and constipation. Diagnosis can be made through blood or feces culture but cultures can also be made of urine, bone marrow, vomitus, and pus. A positive culture 1 year or more after recovery indicates that the patient has become a carrier of *S. typhi.* Other laboratory indications of infection include passing leukocytosis in the first week of typhoid infection and leukopenia in the third week. As Fig. 3–1 shows, the case rate of salmonellosis excluding typhoid

Fig. 3–1. Salmonellosis (excluding typhoid fever); reported cases per 100,000 population, by year, United States, 1955–1983

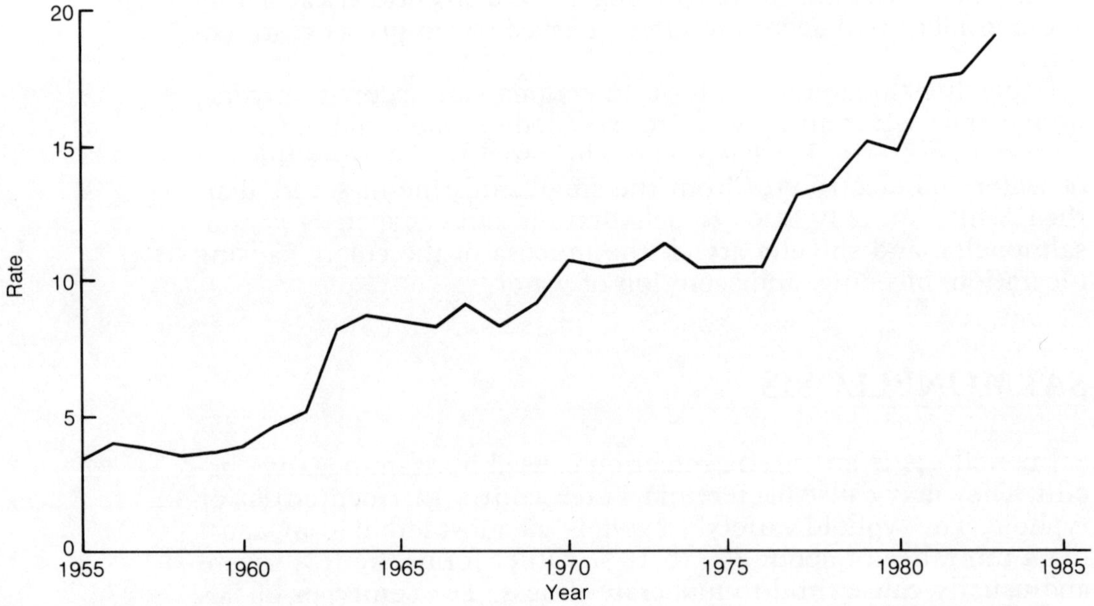

Source: Morbidity and Mortality Weekly Report, Annual Summary 1983

fever has been steadily increasing in the United States since the early 1960s. Although 40% of all cases occur in children younger than age 5 years, the increase in cases has occurred primarily in older age groups. Whether the rising tide of cases is due to more conscientious reporting or to more infections is unknown.

The number of cases reported for each state in 1981 is shown in Table 3–1. A total of 39,990 cases were reported for the United States and its territories.

TABLE 3–1. Salmonellosis (excluding typhoid fever): Reported cases, by Area and Age, United States, 1981

AREA	TOTAL	UNDER	1–4	5–9	10–14	15–19	20–24	25–29	30–39	40–49	50–59	60+	UNK.
United States	39,990	7,391	6,414	2,433	1,703	1,998	2,444	1,990	2,465	1,483*	1,454*	3,245*	6,607
New England	3,328	331	461	226	180	284	295	236	278	138	140	286	473
Maine	244	(					NA					)	244
N.H.	207	14	24	7	17	39	29	17	13	11	16	19	1
Vt.	166	3	17	7	8	16	14	11	17	13	14	42	4
Mass	1,736	181	243	136	105	159	169	130	171	68	73	149	152
R.I.	144	29	25	15	6	10	8	12	13	6	9	11	—
Conn.	831	104	152	61	44	60	75	66	64	40	28	65	72
Mid. Atlantic	6,795	1,204	1,203	500	353	462	425	338	418	263	297	718	614
N.Y. (excl. NYC)	1,525	160	279	120	92	147	135	104	121	69	73	167	58
N.Y.C.	1,458	375	276	94	38	48	41	36	51	30	32	94	343
N.J.	1,775	352	318	137	89	126	101	87	106	72	76	199	112
Pa.	2,037	317	330	149	134	141	148	111	140	92	116	258	101
E.N. Central	6,394	1,124	713	367	240	312	390	296	341	128*	109*	249*	1,762
Ohio	1,123	215	186	92	65	63	86	73	74	56	44	107	62
Ind.	623	95	92	45	24	30	39	24	42	22	24	56	130
Ill.	2,182	609	328	161	96	99	141	122	133	(	363	)	130
Mich.	1,364	(					NA					)	1,364
Wis.	1,102	205	107	69	55	120	124	77	92	50	41	86	76
W.N. Central	2,594	346	372	166	108	134	197	164	167	107	105	265	463
Minn.	712	57	91	49	33	48	74	70	50	46	38	86	70
Iowa	276	36	43	18	10	24	20	25	23	11	18	30	3
Mo.	700	123	100	34	25	20	33	20	32	26	21	72	194
N. Dak.	107	7	15	7	6	7	11	9	7	3	4	12	19
S. Dak.	165	30	21	10	5	10	6	6	10	6	7	9	45
Nebr.	203	16	30	21	13	12	13	11	13	6	3	24	41
Kans.	431	77	72	27	10	13	31	23	32	9	14	32	91
S. Atlantic	8,487	1,947	1,783	584	367	299	402	367	501	309	340	767	821
Del.	118	25	22	4	8	5	8	4	4	10	9	15	4
Md.	1,288	370	252	129	75	63	78	58	73	48	44	98	—
D.C.	191	49	44	10	6	1	4	4	6	6	3	10	48
Va.	1,572	335	289	132	72	78	78	76	110	62	56	120	164
W. Va.	176	31	15	21	7	8	8	2	10	6	7	9	52
N.C.	1,002	220	190	73	49	30	54	56	73	50	57	125	25
S.C.	545	106	54	27	21	12	21	17	36	17	29	51	154
Ga.	1,401	339	223	56	59	42	52	53	75	45	62	94	301
Fla.	2,194	472	694	132	70	60	99	97	114	65	73	245	73
E.S. Central	2,036	354	347	116	54	86	98	78	100	71	78	148	506
Ky.	347	55	37	15	16	17	15	14	23	13	11	19	112
Tenn.	598	124	125	47	18	42	56	43	45	20	27	51	—
'Ala.	603	42	116	32	10	15	14	15	14	21	28	32	264
Miss.	488	133	69	22	10	12	13	6	18	17	12	46	130
W.S. Central	3,759	968	719	172	131	111	148	128	169	149	132	304	628

TABLE 3–1. (Continued)

AREA	TOTAL	UNDER	1–4	5–9	10–14	15–19	20–24	25–29	30–39	40–49	50–59	60+	UNK.
Ark.	474	115	85	21	21	5	9	14	25	25	13	65	76
La.	237	85	43	8	12	10	8	11	7	10	8	14	21
Okla.	436	82	62	12	14	8	18	14	14	13	13	40	146
Tex.	2,612	686	529	131	84	88	113	89	123	101	98	185	385
Mountain	1,548	276	210	91	62	76	101	82	108	72	53	120	297
Mont.	124	21	17	9	1	10	12	9	14	5	1	11	14
Idaho	97	8	11	5	3	15	7	2	5	4	7	8	22
Wyo.	31	5	5	3	2	—	2	4	3	4	1	—	2
Colo.	407	45	58	29	11	22	31	29	33	16	21	39	73
N. Mex.	327	50	34	16	15	10	16	13	22	12	5	23	111
Ariz.	369	127	57	20	17	12	22	16	23	23	9	26	17
Utah	78	12	15	5	4	3	4	3	4	5	4	4	15
Nev.	115	8	13	4	9	4	7	6	4	3	5	9	43
Pacific	5,049	841	606	211	208	234	388	301	383	246	200	388	1,043
Wash.	574	77	94	41	30	27	64	39	57	35	32	57	21
Oreg.	302	44	37	9	17	15	27	29	41	19	9	31	24
Calif.	3,562	709	456	153	158	188	290	227	272	190	156	297	466
Alaska	102	11	19	8	3	4	7	6	13	2	3	3	23
Hawaii	509	(					NA					)	509
Guam	202	92	23	3	4	6	11	13	10	7	7	1	25
P.R.	436	(					NA					)	436
V.I.	9	3	2	1	1	—	—	—	1	—	—	—	1
Pac. Trust Terr.	174	(					NA					)	174
C.N.M.I.	—	—	—	—	—	—	—	—	—	—	—	—	—

*Does not include cases reported by state of Illinois

Source: Morbidity and Mortality Weekly Reports, Annual Summary 1981

As can be seen in Fig. 3–2, the incidence of typhoid fever has been declining in the United States since 1950 although there were large outbreaks in Florida in 1973 and in Texas in 1981. In 1983, there were 507 reported cases of typhoid fever but about one-half were acquired during foreign travel. Those acquired in the United States have often been transmitted through a chronic carrier and through laboratories.

Treatment for various salmonellosis infections include ampicillin, amoxicillin, chloramphenicol, and trimethoprimsulfamethoxazole in the severely toxemic patient. Antibiotics are given for enterocolitis if it causes septicemia or prolonged fever. Bed rest and maintenance of fluids are also standard therapy. With treatment, death rarely occurs; without it, fatality for typhoid is as high as 30%.

The major precautions to be taken to prevent salmonella infections is to promptly refrigerate meat and cooked foods and to avoid leaving foods for long periods of time at room temperature. Those handling raw meat should wash their hands before touching serving dishes or utensils. Any containers, dishes, or utensils used for raw meat should also be washed thoroughly before being used for

Fig. 3–2. Typhoid fever: reported cases per 100,000 population, by year, United States, 1955–1983

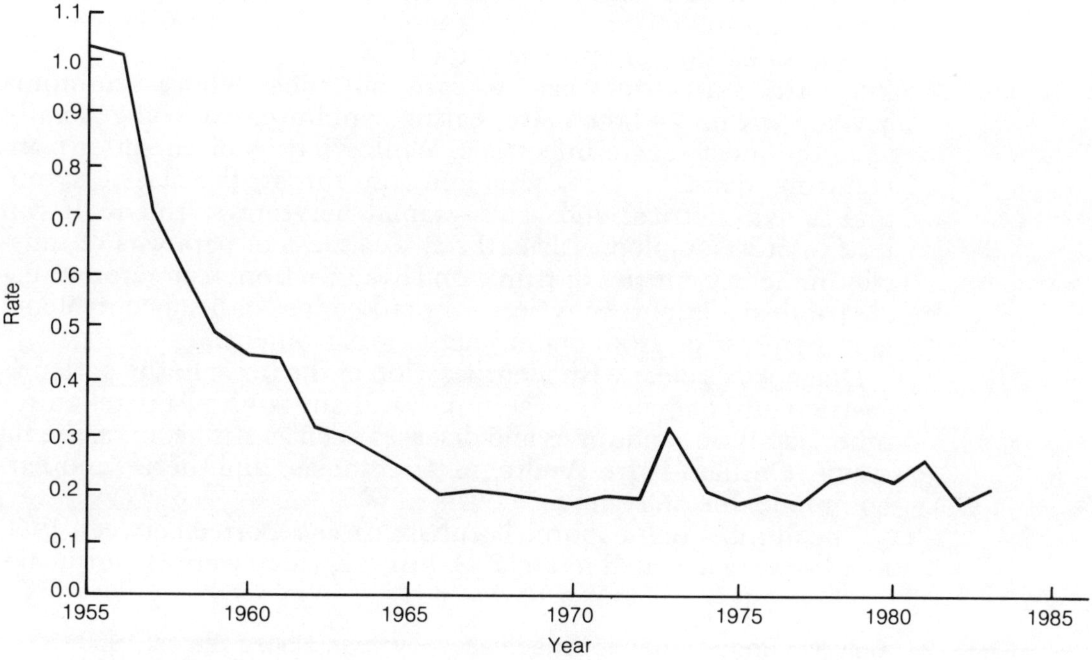

Source: Morbidity and Mortality Weekly Report, Annual Summary 1983

any other purpose. Proper cooking of meat, poultry, and eggs is also essential. Pasteurization of milk and purification of drinking water serve to reduce cases of typhoid.

BOTULISM

Botulism is caused by the anaerobic bacillus *Clostridium botulinum*. It is a gram-positive bacterium producing seven types of exotoxin in food that will cause severe food poisoning when consumed. The toxins that chiefly affect humans are types A, B, C, E, and F. Types A and B are highly poisonous. Most cases of botulism in the United States are type A followed by B and E. Type C toxin is often involved in wound and infant botulism. Western states generally report more type A, while eastern states report type B. Type E is more common in Alaska and the Great Lakes area. About 25% of those infected die.

Botulism is found in inadequately cooked, low acid-content foods, such as fruits and vegetables, especially those that are canned at home. Ingesting even a small amount as when tasting suspect food can be fatal. Botulism can also enter the body through a wound when handling foods. The symptoms develop from 6 hours to 8 days after eating contaminated food.

Severity varies from case to case, but those whose symptoms develop within 24 hours after eating contaminated food generally have the most severe infections. While victims often suffer from vomiting, diarrhea, weakness, and sore throat, the classic symptom is symmetrical and acute cranial nerve impairment. It can lead to ptosis, diplopia, dysarthria, weakness or paralysis of muscles in the extremities or trunk, and dyspnea from respiratory muscle paralysis. Infants may suffer a marked loss of head control and facial expression from cranial nerve involvement.

Diagnosis is clear with identification of the toxin in the patient's gastric contents, stool, or serum. Botulism is often mistaken for other paralytic syndromes and diseases such as stroke, myasthenia gravis, Guillain-Barré syndrome, trichinosis, diphtheria, and carbon monoxide poisoning.

The number of foodborne botulism cases reported between 1960 and 1982 are depicted in Fig. 3–3. In 1982, there were 18 outbreaks

Fig. 3–3. Botulism (food-borne): reported cases, by year, United States, 1960–82 Cases

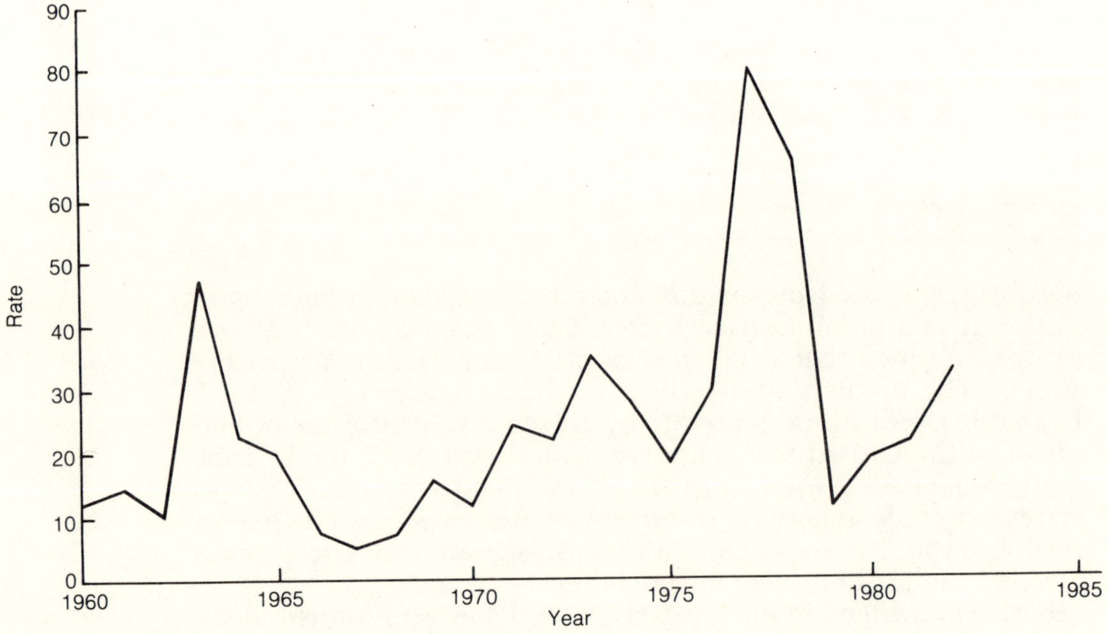

Source: Morbidity and Mortality Weekly Report, Annual Summary 1982

of botulism arising from home canned goods and three from commercially prepared foods. Type A toxin was involved in most cases.

Cases of infant botulism from 1975 through 1983 are shown in Fig. 3–4. There were 79 reported cases in infants ages 3 to 32 weeks. The cases occurred equally in males and females and were of both toxin A and B varieties.

The treatment for botulism involves either intravenous (I.V.) or intramuscular (I.M.) administration of antitoxin. The antitoxin is administered only to adults after allergic sensitivity (especially to horses) is ascertained. If contaminated food was eaten recently, vomiting is also induced and the bowels may be purged by enema. Hospitalization so that the patient can be watched for respiratory impairment is important. Respiratory distress is the symptom most often leading to death.

OTHER TOXINS

Botulism is not the only infection caused by a bacterial toxin. Two other toxins that cause gastroenteritis are those produced by *C. perfringens* and staphylococcus bacilli. The former is found in meat,

Fig. 3–4. Botulism (infant): reported cases, by year, United States, 1975–83

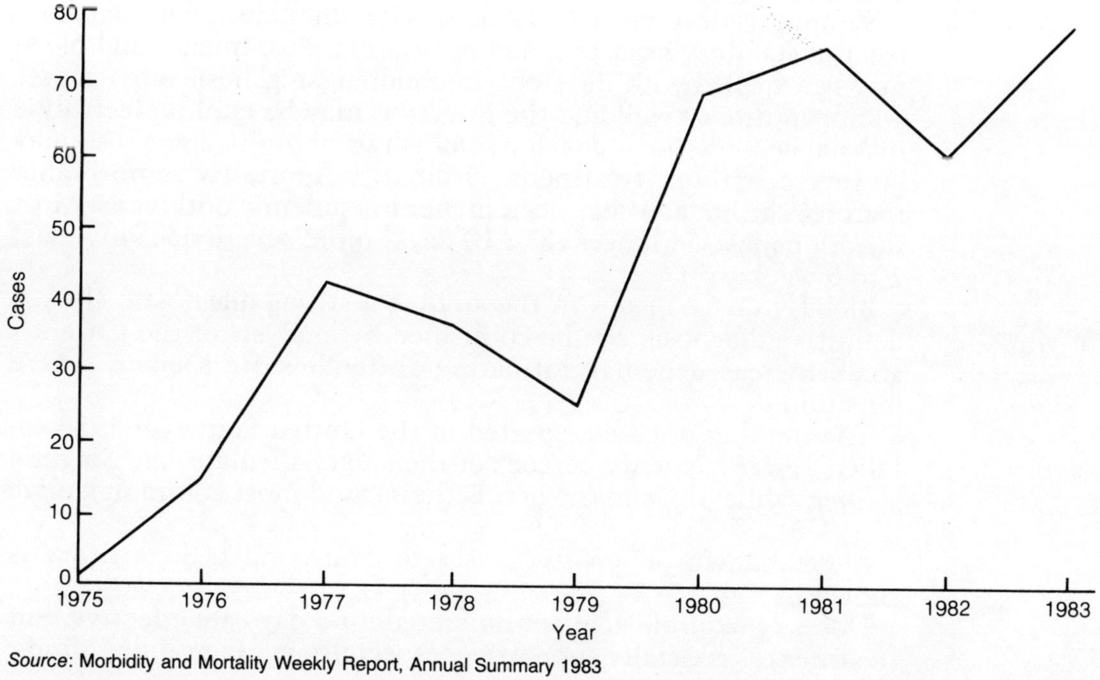

Source: Morbidity and Mortality Weekly Report, Annual Summary 1983

water, soil, air, and feces. Type A causes a mild self-limiting gastroenteritis, whereas type C strains cause a fatal gastroenteritis. Penicillin and supportive remedies comprise the usual treatment.

Staphylococcus enterotoxin is a common cause of food poisoning. When foods are left either at room temperature or in contact with infected food handlers, the staphylococci multiply and produce enterotoxins. Within 2 to 8 hours after ingesting contaminated food, victims develop abdominal cramps, vomiting, diarrhea, fever, and headache. Most episodes subside within 6 hours, but severe cases may deteriorate to prostration and shock and be fatal. For typical cases, fluid and electrolyte replacement usually brings relief.

SHIGELLOSIS

Also known as bacillary dysentery, shigellosis is caused by the gram-negative rod bacteria, shigella, and is endemic in the Tropics, Europe, and North America. Although it can be transmitted by the house fly, it is most commonly contracted through ingestion of impure water or food or by contact with fecally infected objects. It often occurs among institutionalized persons including the temporarily hospitalized.

Symptoms develop in 1 to 4 days. They include abdominal pain, rectal irritability, headache, and prostration. Pus, mucus, and blood may be expelled with the stool. In children, shigellosis often causes a temperature as well and the infection may be fatal if electrolyte imbalance and shock develop. Dehydration and weight loss may be severe without treatment. Ordinarily, mortality is no higher than 1%, although it has been higher in epidemic outbreaks. Most infections last no longer than 10 days; more severe ones may last 2 to 6 weeks.

Blood, mucus, or pus in the stool is a strong diagnostic clue. A definitive diagnosis can be confirmed by analysis of the patient's stool. Increased hemagglutinating antibodies are seen in severe infection.

The number of cases reported in the United States for 1983 totalled 19,719. Seventy percent of the shigella isolates are *Shigella sonnei,* while *Shigella flexneri* is the second most common isolate (Fig. 3–5).

A breakdown of reported cases by state and U.S. territory is shown in Table 3–2.

Doses of oxolinic acid administered for 5 days are effective. But treatment is generally supportive, especially in maintaining fluids.

Fig. 3–5. Shigellosis: reported cases per 100,000 population, by year, United States, 1955–83

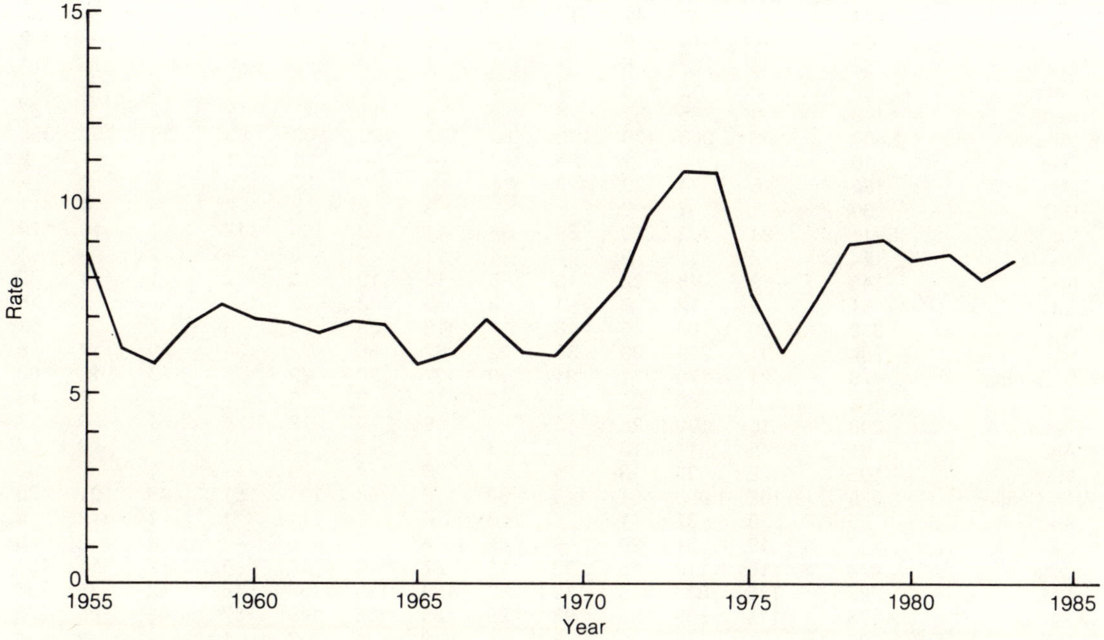

Source: Morbidity and Mortality Weekly Report, Annual Summary 1983

TABLE 3–2. Shigellosis: Reported Cases, by Area and Age, United States, 1981

AREA	TOTAL	UNDER 1	1–4	5–9	10–14	15–19	20–24	25–29	30–39	40–49	50–59	60+	UNK.
United States	19,859	892	6,045	2,755	941	671	1,284	1,327	1,479	540*	359*	482*	3,021
New England	921	28	239	174	52	35	00	05	90	37	10	10	69
Maine	21	—	1	—	—	—	1	4	3	1	1	2	8
N.H.	13	—	4	2	—	—	—	3	1	2	1	—	—
Vt.	6	2	1	1	—	—	1	—	1	—	—	—	—
Mass	351	5	67	72	18	11	43	41	43	18	7	7	19
R.I.	94	5	37	16	10	3	4	6	9	2	1	1	—
Conn.	436	14	129	83	24	21	37	31	33	14	9	9	32
Mid. Atlantic	1,516	51	377	177	70	58	97	130	158	68	30	43	257
N.Y. (excl. NYC)	405	13	117	61	27	21	37	35	39	16	9	15	15
N.Y.C.	573	14	98	47	21	10	20	55	61	19	10	13	205
N.J.	367	17	132	47	16	15	17	28	32	22	7	9	25
Pa.	171	7	30	22	6	12	23	12	26	11	4	6	12
E.N. Central	1,951	130	533	262	88	63	102	119	129	12*	15*	12*	423
Ohio	202	12	68	38	12	4	12	19	16	3	3	3	12
Ind.	225	6	71	36	14	12	12	15	14	4	1	3	37
Ill.	1,071	92	352	160	54	35	65	65	78	(.......	63	.......)	107
Mich.	256	(............					NA					............)	256
Wis.	197	20	42	28	8	12	13	20	21	5	11	6	11
W.N. Central	769	31	251	107	37	19	55	48	44	24	23	23	107
Minn.	130	1	21	12	13	5	19	7	10	8	11	6	17
Iowa	40	1	9	4	3	—	6	5	5	2	—	3	2

TABLE 3–2. (Continued)

AREA	TOTAL	UNDER 1	1–4	5–9	10–14	15–19	20–24	25–29	30–39	40–49	50–59	60+	UNK.
Mo.	271	11	107	42	10	7	9	20	12	8	7	4	34
N. Dak.	29	—	10	6	2	—	4	1	1	2	1	—	2
S. Dak.	68	5	27	6	1	1	4	2	2	—	—	6	14
Nebr.	52	5	12	6	4	1	4	2	3	2	2	—	11
Kans.	179	8	65	31	4	5	9	11	11	2	2	4	27
S. Atlantic	2,809	107	966	470	179	83	147	190	203	63	39	57	305
Del.	10	—	4	1	—	—	—	—	1	1	—	1	2
Md.	182	18	74	29	9	4	9	5	20	5	2	7	—
D.C.	30	1	1	2	1	—	3	2	3	2	—	4	11
Va.	1,211	24	422	260	89	36	41	72	59	12	7	10	179
W. Va.	54	2	18	9	7	1	1	2	6	—	2	—	6
N.C.	148	9	48	22	16	6	10	10	15	2	1	7	2
S.C.	51	2	12	8	1	3	3	2	2	—	—	2	16
Ga.	339	20	88	46	18	11	18	29	24	8	7	9	61
Fla.	784	31	299	93	38	22	62	68	72	34	20	17	28
E.S. Central	476	21	179	71	21	20	27	20	29	5	3	12	68
Ky.	102	4	30	20	5	5	10	3	5	—	—	2	18
Tenn.	208	10	109	28	11	9	8	9	12	4	1	6	1
Ala.	61	5	11	10	1	3	3	4	3	1	1	2	17
Miss.	105	2	29	13	4	3	6	4	9	—	1	2	32
W.S. Central	3,025	166	1,050	451	146	82	176	164	166	51	49	91	433
Ark.	95	8	37	11	5	3	6	1	11	1	1	3	8
La.	157	12	81	20	9	5	4	7	5	—	4	2	8
Okla.	474	18	112	45	20	12	27	18	14	4	2	11	191
Tex.	2,299	128	820	375	112	62	139	138	136	46	42	75	226
Mountain	2,233	115	809	289	98	89	135	115	145	57	45	66	270
Mont.	35	—	12	2	1	4	2	1	7	1	—	1	4
Idaho	149	5	38	19	5	9	14	8	9	2	3	—	37
Wyo.	12	1	4	3	1	—	2	—	—	—	—	1	—
Colo.	425	9	117	55	15	17	34	39	41	19	11	11	57
N. Mex.	419	24	121	71	14	13	14	16	20	7	7	10	102
Ariz.	962	68	442	101	52	39	49	45	54	23	19	36	34
Utah	192	8	64	36	10	6	13	4	12	4	3	4	28
Nev.	39	—	11	2	—	1	7	2	2	1	2	3	8
Pacific	6,159	245	1,641	754	250	222	459	456	515	223	136	159	1,099
Wash.	426	9	86	60	26	13	45	66	50	20	10	10	26
Oreg.	219	5	45	28	7	17	19	22	27	8	8	10	23
Calif.	5,259	229	1,498	659	215	185	392	365	434	195	117	138	832
Alaska	41	2	12	7	2	2	3	3	4	—	1	1	4
Hawaii	214	(					NA					)	214
P.R.	135	18	45	25	12	2	3	2	2	2	—	8	16
V.I.	4	—	3	—	—	—	—	—	—	—	—	1	—
Pac. Trust Terr.	—	—	—	—	—	—	—	—	—	—	—	—	—
C.N.M.I.	—	—	—	—	—	—	—	—	—	—	—	—	—

*Does not include cases reported by state of Illinois
Source: Morbidity and Mortality Weekly Report, Annual Summary 1981

Sometimes ampicillin, tetracycline, or sulfamethoxazole with trimethoprim is used in severe cases even though antibiotics are not generally regarded as useful because resistance to them has developed. *S. sonnei* is resistant to both ampicillin and tetracycline.

BRUCELLOSIS

Undulant fever, or brucellosis, is an infection caused by gram-negative coccobacilli that can contaminate unpasteurized dairy products and undercooked meat or be present in the secretions of infected animals. It is rare in the United States. Where prevalent, however, it mostly affects people who work with animals, such as farmers and veterinarians. *Brucella suis* is found in swine, *B. melitensis* in goats, *B. abortus* in cattle, and *B. canis* in dogs.

After the onset of illness occurs, infected persons in the initial acute phase develop fever, chills, sweating, headache, fatigue, and enlarged lymph nodes. Other symptoms include hepatosplenomegaly; weight loss; and granulomas in the liver, spleen, and lymph nodes. Many of these symptoms, including enlarged lymph nodes, persist in the chronic stage but abscesses form in the brain, testes, and other organs. Of those with brain involvement, 10% to 15% suffer hearing or vision losses.

Diagnosis is partially confirmed by multiple agglutination tests. Blood and bone marrow cultures or spleen biopsy make the diagnosis definitive. Laboratory tests usually reveal increased erythrocyte sedimentation rate and normal or decreased white blood count.

The number of reported cases between 1945 and 1983 in the United States is shown in Fig. 3–6.

Treatment involves a 3-week schedule of oral tetracycline and a 2-week regimen of streptomycin I.M. Corticosteroids are also given in severe cases.

TULAREMIA

Tularemia is a disease transmitted mostly by infected wild animals. It is contracted by eating undercooked, infected meat or contaminated water in 10% of all cases. Cases arising in hunters, furriers, farmers and butchers typically cause cutaneous whitish yellow lesions. Eyes can become infected in about 3% of all cases. Two percent are glandular with digestive symptoms, suggesting infection by ingestion and 8% are typhoidal with abdominal pain and fever.

Most victims become ill about 2 to 4 days after contact with an infected animal, contaminated meat or tainted water. They develop chills, vomiting, fever, headache, weakness, and profuse sweating. An atypical pneumonia may develop. Tularemic pneumonia may occur with delirium.

Fig. 3–6. Brucellosis: reported cases per 100,000 population, by year, United States, 1945–83

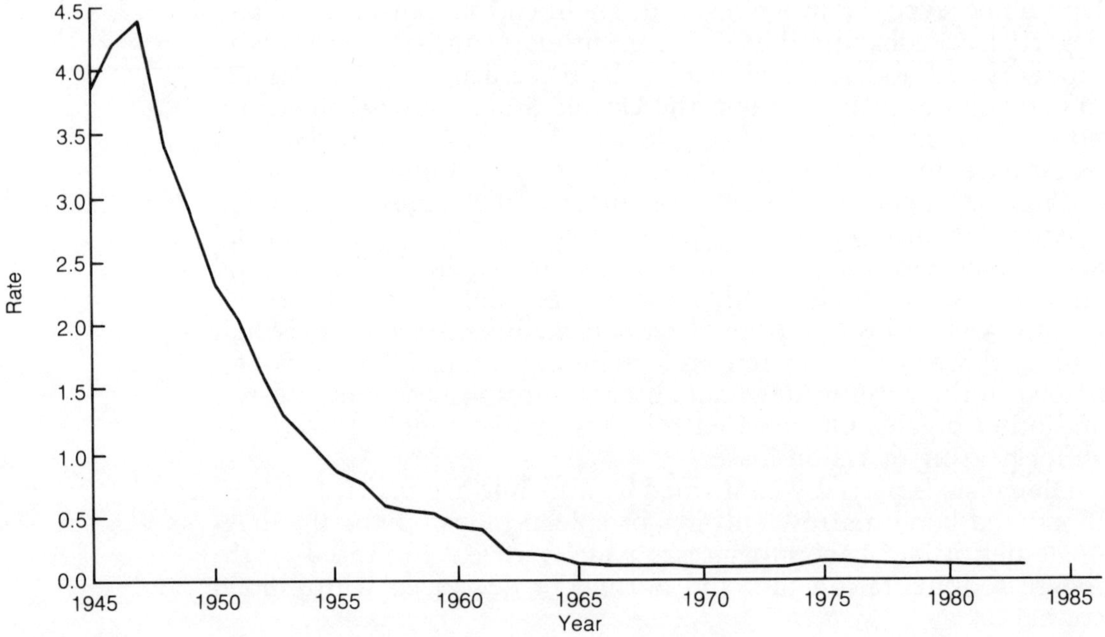

Source: Morbidity and Mortality Weekly Report, Annual Summary 1983

The number of cases has been increasing recently (Fig. 3–7). This is thought to be a real increase and not due to more conscientious reporting.

The locations of outbreaks in the United States during 1983 are shown in Fig. 3–8.

Treatment involves administration of streptomycin until fever subsides. Gentamicin, chloramphenicol, and tetracycline are also employed and wet saline dressings are used for skin lesions.

Prevention requires the utmost care when handling wild animals, especially rabbits and rodents. Protective clothing should be worn, and ticks removed promptly. Laboratory workers should not attempt to isolate the organism without protective hoods since it is so contagious.

TRICHINOSIS

Trichinosis is perhaps one of the best known foodborne diseases in the United States. Indeed, regulations affecting meat processing, the feeding of swine, and information about the importance of

Fig. 3–7. Tularemia: reported cases per 100,000 population, by year, United States, 1955–83

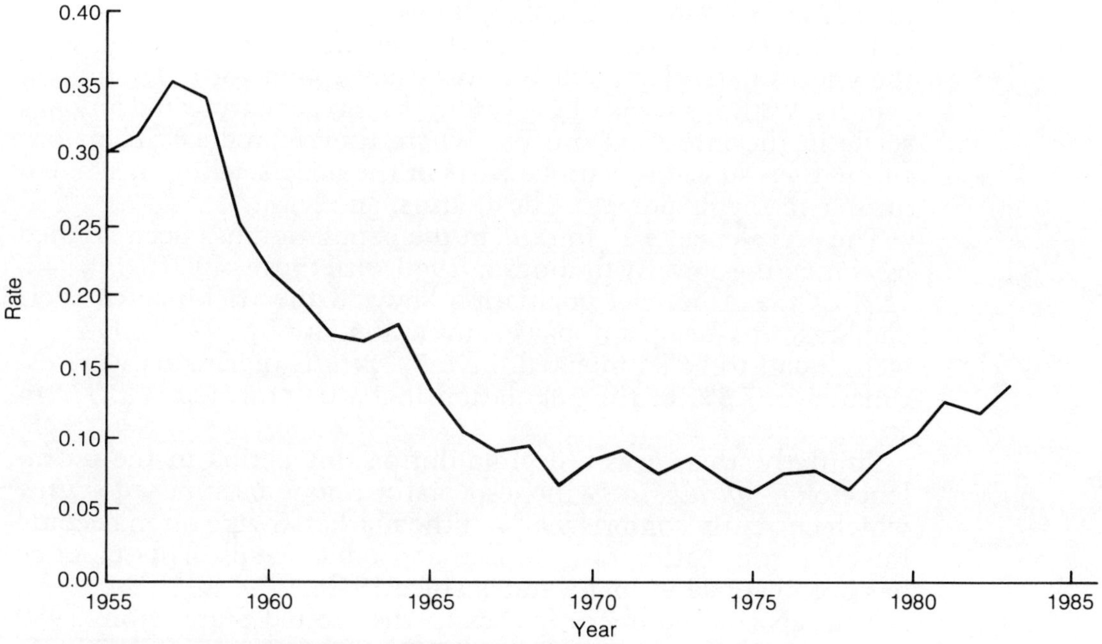

Source: Morbidity and Mortality Weekly Report, Annual Summary 1983

Fig. 3–8. Tularemia: reported cases, by county, United States, 1983

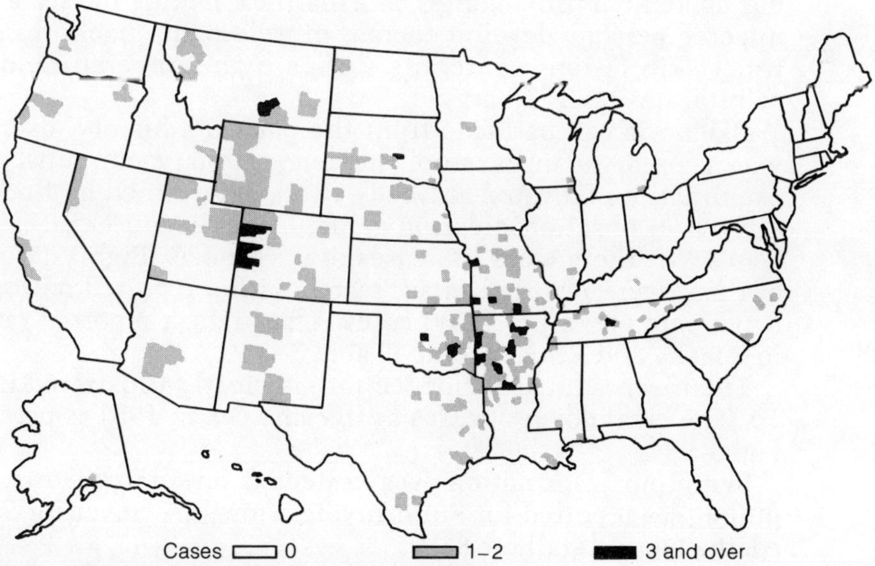

Source: Morbidity and Mortality Weekly Report, Annual Summary 1983

thoroughly cooking meat have led to a low incidence of this disease among Americans. Outbreaks in recent years have occurred mainly among new immigrant groups.

Trichinosis is caused by ingestion of meat contaminated with the encapsulated larvae of the intestinal roundworm *Trichinella spiralis*. Within a week of ingestion, the larvae mature and females settle in the intestinal mucosa where they reproduce. Their offspring then spread to various parts of the body settling in striated muscle in the diaphragm, chest, arms, and legs.

The prevalence of *T. spiralis* in the population has been studied by comparing autopsy findings in 1940 with those in 1970. In 1940, 12% of the American population showed the trichinae in their diaphragm tissue on autopsy examination. But by 1970, only 2.2% were found to be so infected. Live *T. spiralis* organisms were estimated in 7.3% of the population in 1940 compared to 0.7% in 1970.

Similarly, there was a decline during this period in the prevalence of *T. spiralis* in swine, especially among farm-raised swine, which currently comprise 95% of the market. Swine often become infected from eating raw garbage and table scraps. This practice has been banned in many states since 1940.

The reported number of cases in the United States from 1950 through 1983 is shown in Fig. 3–9. The spike of cases in 1975 was due to several large common source outbreaks. Since then, there have been less than 150 cases reported annually.

Symptoms include an initial phase of anorexia, nausea, vomiting, abdominal pain, cramps, and diarrhea. During the second phase, infected persons develop edema, muscle pain, diaphoresis, sometimes skin lesions or itching skin, a high temperature, delirium, palpitations, and lethargy.

Diagnosis can be made from the patient's history, discovery of worms or larvae in the stool, and encysted larvae in muscle biopsy examination. Elevated antibody titers determined by flocculation early after onset of infection confirm the diagnosis.

In 1981, there were 188 cases of trichinosis. Eighty-two percent of them were reported in six states with a reported national incidence rate of 5.8 per 1,000 cases. The highest reported rates were in Alaska and Rhode Island (Table 3–3).

The mean annual incidence rate is clearly illustrated in Fig. 3–10. The breakdown of cases by age and sex in 1981 is presented in Fig. 3–11.

Symptom information was collected on 145 patients. Eosinophilia was reported for 96%, myalgia for 94%, fever for 91%, and edema (periorbital) for 82%.

The source of infection was primarily from pork products, es-

Fig. 3–9. Trichinosis: reported cases, by year, United States, 1950–83

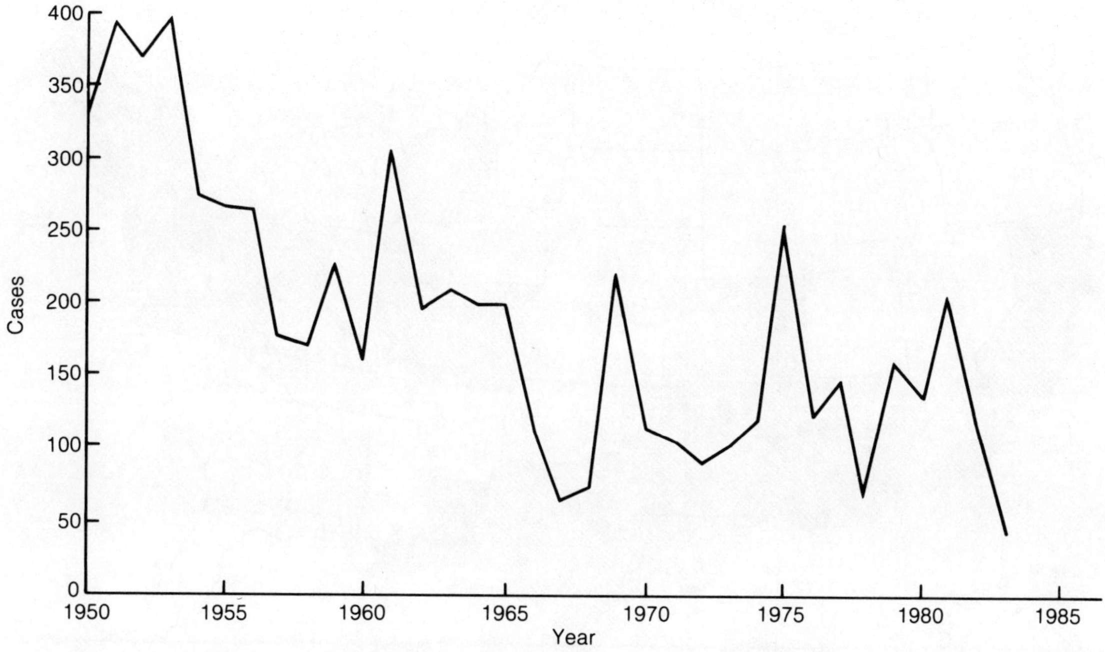

Source: Morbidity and Mortality Weekly Report, Annual Summary 1983.

TABLE 3–3. Trichinosis Cases, by State, United States, 1981

STATE	CASES	RATE PER MILLION POPULATION*
Connecticut	45	14.4
Rhode Island	35	36.7
New Jersey	25	3.4
New York	19	1.1
Pennsylvania	15	1.3
Alaska	14	33.9
Massachusetts	13	2.3
Illinois	7	0.6
California	5	0.2
Maryland	3	0.7
Virginia	3	0.6
Vermont	2	3.9
New Hampshire	1	1.1
Washington	1	0.2
Total	188	0.8

*Estimates of state populations on July 1, 1981.
Source: Morbidity and Mortality Weekly Report, Vol. 32, No.2SS

Fig. 3–10. Trichinosis mean annual incidence rate/1,000,000 population, by state, United States, 1977–81

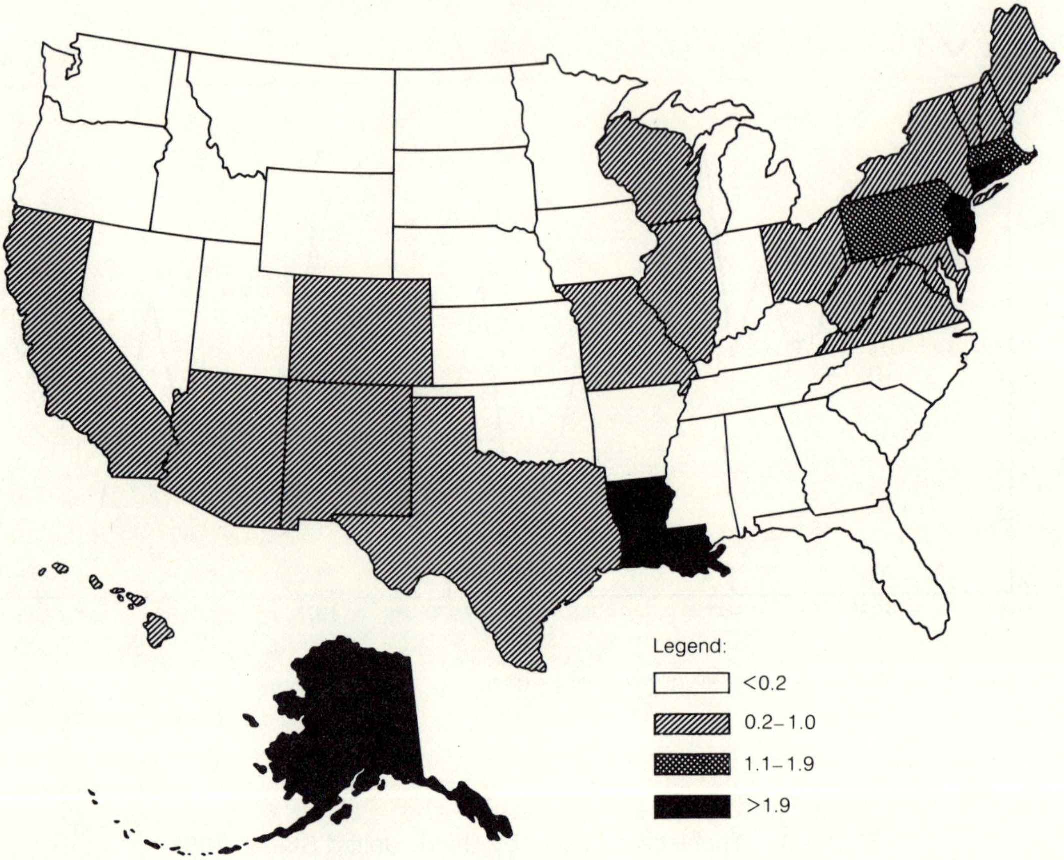

Source: Morbidity and Mortality Weekly Report, Vol.32, No. 2SS

pecially uncooked or undercooked pork sausage (Table 3–4). Other sources were hamburger meat, bear meat, and walrus meat. The meat was obtained from a supermarket or other commercial outlet in 58% of the cases, while 5% of patients had eaten at a restaurant. The walrus and bear meat obtained through hunting accounted for the cases in Alaska.

Alaskans sometimes eat frozen raw meat called "quaq," which has been implicated in trichinosis. Generally, freezing meat kills the trichinosis larvae in the United States, but recent cases in Alaska indicate that this does not occur in colder climates. Those infected are of ethnic backgrounds that typically eat raw meat, such as Germans and Italians. Sixty-three of the cases in 1981 were Kampuchean refugees who had eaten an undercooked pig pur-

Fig. 3–11. Trichinosis cases, by age and sex, United States, 1981

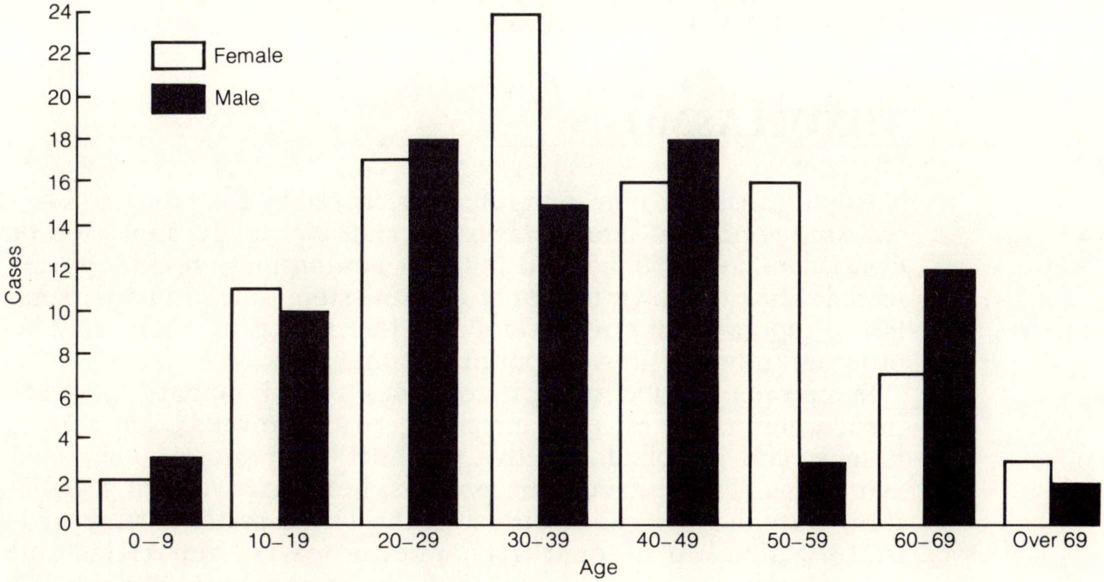

Does not include 11 cases of unknown age.

Source: Morbidity and Mortality Weekly Report, Vol. 32. No. 2SS

TABLE 3–4. Trichinosis Cases, by Source of Infection, United States, 1981

FOOD		CASES
Pork products		
Domestic swine:		
Sausage		93
Other products		44
Unspecified		9
	Subtotal	146
Meat products other than pork		
Hamburger		18
Bear meat		10
Other wild animals		7
	Subtotal	35
Unknown		7
	Subtotal	7
	Total	188

Source: Morbidity and Mortality Weekly Report, Vol. 32, No.2SS

chased a few days earlier from a local farm.

Treatment for the most part is supportive with bed rest and efforts to reduce fever and prevent bed sores. Thiabendazole is administered to eradicate the worms in the intestinal phase of the illness; occasionally glucocorticoids are prescribed to limit inflammation.

To prevent infection, the public is advised to thoroughly cook meats, including beef, to a temperature of at least 131° F and to avoid eating pork in poor areas where the swine may be fed garbage, contrary to local statutes.

TOXOPLASMOSIS

Toxoplasmosis is a common infection caused by the protozoa *Toxoplasma gondii.* In latent stages, it exists cystically; ingestion of cyst-laden raw or uncooked meat or contamination through infected cats are known modes of transmission. Since some persons fail to report these circumstances before infection, there may be other unknown routes of contamination.

Symptoms include (in localized cases) mild lymphatic involvement accompanied by fever, malaise, headache, myalgia, sore throat, fatigue, and lymphadenopathy. Patients with more generalized symptoms develop fever, encephalitis, headache, vomiting, delirium, convulsions, and a diffuse rash. These patients may ultimately develop myocarditis, pneumonitis, hepatitis, and polymyositis.

Diagnosis is confirmed by *T. gondii* antibodies in specimens of blood, body tissue, or fluids. *T. gondii* will also be isolated in mice after their inoculation with similar specimens.

Reported cases according to state in 1983 are shown in Table 3–5.

TABLE 3–5. Non-notifiable Conditions: Cases of Toxoplasmosis Optionally Reported by Certain Areas, 1983

	TOXO PLASMOSIS
No. Cases Reported	115
New England	—
Maine	NN
N H	NN
Vt	NN
Mass	NN
R I	—
Conn	—
Mid. Atlantic	15
N Y (excl NYC)	NN
N Y C	11
N J	NA
Pa	4
E.N. Central	3
Ohio	1
Ind	—

TABLE 3–5. (Continued)

	TOXO PLASMOSIS
Ill	2
Mich	—
Wis	—
W.N. Central	26
Minn	—
Iowa	NN
Mo	25
N Dak	—
S Dak	1
Nebr	NN
Kans	—
S. Atlantic	40
Del	NN
Md	—
D C	
Va	1
W Va	—
N C	NN
S C	2
Ga	26
Fla	11
E.S. Central	1
Ky	
Tenn	NN
Ala	
Miss	1
W.S. Central	8
Ark	6
La	1
Okla	1
Texas	NN
Mountain	7
Mont	1
Idaho	1
Wyo	
Colo	
N Mex	4
Ariz	1
Utah	
Nev	
Pacific	15
Wash	
Oreg	NN
Calif	8
Alaska	2
Hawaii	5

Source: Morbidity and Mortality Weekly Report, Annual Summary 1983

ANALYSIS OF ENTERIC DISEASE OUTBREAKS

In 1982, there were 656 outbreaks of foodborne disease resulting in 19,380 reported cases. These cases included diseases caused by bacteria, viruses, parasites, and chemicals.

Two hundred and twenty of the outbreaks were confirmed through identification of the etiologic agent, and information gathered on them was analyzed. Caveats were also published with the data, reminding readers that the cases, including fatal ones, were probably greatly underreported since many foodborne disorders, particularly those of viral origin, have lengthy incubations, which makes the clinical history difficult to establish. Most cases with identified etiology were due to bacteria and chemicals. The latter are perhaps the easiest to identify as causative agents because onset of illness is usually rapid, often less than 1 hour after ingestion of chemically contaminated food.

One hundred fifty-one outbreaks were caused by bacterial agents, with salmonella being the most frequent. It accounted for 55 outbreaks, while the second most common bacteria, *Staphylococcus aureaus* caused 28 outbreaks. Two outbreaks among patrons of a fast-food chain in two states had eaten hamburger meat contaminated with *E. coli* 157:H7, a pathogen not previously recognized as causing a problem. Analysis of the causative agent in the 220 confirmed cases is shown in Table 3–6.

Two large outbreaks of viral gastroenteritis from Norwalk virus occurred in Minnesota. In one case, 3,000 people became ill after eating frosted bakery goods; in the other, 2,000 had eaten cole slaw contaminated with the virus. Eleven deaths were related to *Vibrio cholerae* 01 (confined to Guam and the Trust territories). Eight others were salmonella related. Two were caused by *C. botulinum,* and two others were from an unknown source.

The vehicle of transmission for reported outbreaks is itemized in Tables 3–7. Identification of the vehicle or source of infection was made for 76% of the 220 confirmed outbreaks. Meat or a dairy product was the source in 52% of the outbreaks, while fish and shellfish were implicated in 57% of the cases caused by chemical contamination.

The reported outbreaks are indicated by state in Fig. 3–12. As shown, the greatest number of outbreaks occurred in New York City and in the states of New York and Washington, which accounted for about one-half of all the cases reported for the United States.

It should be remembered that the variability in reports from

TABLE 3–6. Confirmed Foodborne Disease Outbreaks, Cases, and Deaths, by Etiologic Agents, United States, 1982

	OUTBREAKS		CASES		DEATHS	
ETIOLOGIC AGENT	No.	(%)	No.	(%)	No.	(%)
Bacterial:						
Bacillus cereus	8	(3.6)	200	(1.8)	0	(0.0)
Brucella	1	(0.5)	3	(<0.1)	0	(0.0)
Campylobacter jejuni	2	(0.9)	31	(0.3)	0	(0.0)
Clostridium botulinum	21	(9.5)	30	(0.3)	5	(20.9)
Clostridium perfringens	22	(10.0)	1,189	(10.8)	0	(0.0)
Escherichia coli	2	(0.9)	47	(0.4)	0	(0.0)
Salmonella	55	(25.0)	2,056	(18.6)	8	(33.3)
Shigella	4	(1.8)	116	(1.1)	0	(0.0)
Staphylococcus aureus	28	(12.7)	669	(6.0)	0	(0.0)
Streptococcus Group A	1	(0.5)	34	(0.3)	0	(0.0)
Vibrio cholerae 01	1	(0.5)	892	(8.0)	11	(45.8)
Vibrio cholerae non-01	1	(0.5)	7	(0.1)	0	(0.0)
Vibrio parahaemolyticus	3	(1.4)	39	(0.4)	0	(0.0)
Yersinia enterocolitica	2	(0.9)	188	(1.7)	0	(0.0)
Total	151	(68.7)	5,501	(49.9)	24	(100.0)
Chemical:						
Ciguatoxin	8	(3.6)	37	(0.3)	0	(0.0)
Heavy metals	5	(2.3)	26	(0.2)	0	(0.0)
Monosodium glutamate	3	(1.4)	10	(0.1)	0	(0.0)
Mushrooms	4	(1.8)	9	(0.1)	0	(0.0)
Scombrotoxin	18	(8.2)	58	(0.5)	0	(0.0)
Shellfish	1	(0.5)	5	(<0.1)	0	(0.0)
Other	8	(3.6)	75	(0.7)	0	(0.0)
Total	47	(21.4)	220	(1.9)	0	(0.0)
Parasitic:						
Trichinella spiralis	1	(0.5)	4	(<0.1)	0	(0.0)
Total	1	(0.5)	4	(<0.1)	0	(0.0)
Viral						
Hepatitis A*	19	(8.5)	325	(2.9)	0	(0.0)
Norwalk virus	2	(0.9)	5,000	(45.2)	0	(0.0)
Total	21	(9.4)	5,325	(48.1)	0	(0.0)
Confirmed Total	220	(100.0)	11,050	(100.0)	24	(100.0)

* For full discussion of hepatitis A, see Diabetes, Liver, Renal and Digestive Disease
Source: Atlanta Centers for Disease Control

state to state depends not only on the actual number of outbreaks but also on the fastidiousness of state health personnel in investigating and reporting illness. The state of Washington has a reputation of strict reporting practices, which is one reason why it has the highest number of reported cases after New York.

Table 3–8 lists the place where the food outbreaks occurred. Restaurant food caused 44% of the outbreaks; 30% were caused by food prepared at home.

TABLE 3–7. Foodborne Disease Outbreaks, by Vehicle of Transmission, and Specific Etiology, 1982

ETIOLOGIC AGENT	BEEF	HAM	PORK	SAUSAGE	CHICKEN	TURKEY	OTHER MEAT	SHELL FISH	TUNA	MAHI-MAHI	OTHER FISH	MILK	EGGS	ICE CREAM
Bacterial:														
B. cereus	1	-	-	-	-	-	-	-	-	-	-	-	-	1
Brucella	-	-	-	-	-	-	-	-	-	-	-	-	-	-
C. jejuni	-	-	-	-	-	-	-	-	-	-	-	2	-	-
C. botulinum	1	-	-	-	-	-	-	-	-	-	1	-	-	-
C. perfringens	6	-	-	-	-	4	2	-	-	-	-	-	-	-
E. coli	2	-	-	-	-	-	-	-	-	-	-	-	-	-
Salmonella	1	-	2	1	2	4	1	-	-	-	1	1	2	4
Shigella	-	-	-	-	-	-	-	-	1	-	-	-	-	-
S. aureus	5	3	2	1	4	3	1	-	-	-	-	-	-	-
Streptococcus Group A	-	-	-	-	-	-	-	-	-	-	-	-	-	-
V. cholerae 01	-	-	-	-	-	-	-	-	-	-	-	-	-	-
V. cholerae non-01	-	-	-	-	-	-	-	1	-	-	-	-	-	-
V. parahaemolyticus	-	-	-	-	-	-	-	3	-	-	-	-	-	-
Y. enterocolitica	-	-	-	-	-	-	-	-	-	-	-	1	-	-
Other	-	-	-	-	-	-	-	-	-	-	-	-	-	-
Total	16	3	4	2	6	11	4	4	1	-	2	4	2	5
Chemical:														
Ciguatoxin	-	-	-	-	-	-	-	-	-	-	8	-	-	-
Heavy metals	-	-	-	-	-	-	-	-	-	-	-	-	-	-
Monosodium glutamate	-	-	-	-	-	-	-	-	-	-	-	-	-	-
Mushrooms	-	-	-	-	-	-	-	-	-	-	-	-	-	-
Shellfish	-	-	-	-	-	-	-	1	-	-	-	-	-	-
Scombrotoxin	-	-	-	-	-	-	-	-	3	5	10	-	-	-
Other	1	-	-	1	-	-	-	-	-	-	-	-	-	-
Total	1	-	-	1	-	-	-	1	3	5	18	-	-	-
Parasitic:														
Trichinella spiralis	-	-	1	-	-	-	-	-	-	-	-	-	-	-
Total	-	-	1	-	-	-	-	-	-	-	-	-	-	-
Viral:														
Hepatitis A	-	-	-	-	-	-	-	5	1	-	-	-	-	1
Norwalk virus	-	-	-	-	-	-	-	-	-	-	-	-	-	-
Total	-	-	-	-	-	-	-	5	1	-	-	-	-	1
Confirmed Total:	17	3	5	3	6	11	4	10	5	5	20	4	2	6
Unknown:	5	2	1	1	7	-	-	56	2	-	1	-	1	-
Total 1982	22	5	6	4	13	11	4	66	7	5	21	4	3	6

The most common reason for an outbreak in 1982 was improper holding temperature followed in order by origin of food from an unsafe source, inadequate cooking, and poor personal hygiene by a food handler (Table 3–9).

The profile of foodborne diseases presented in this chapter indicates that while such illnesses are not common they can occur easily without constant vigilance by those who prepare, handle, and consume food. Knowledge is a key factor. The decrease in trichinosis in the United States illustrates how important an informed population is in avoiding food-related illnesses.

The next chapter, which presents information on sexually transmitted disease, also points up the need for better dissemination of information about the serious effects of venereal disease and the growing problem of its spread.

Fig. 3–12. Outbreaks of foodborne disease reported to CDC, by state, 1982

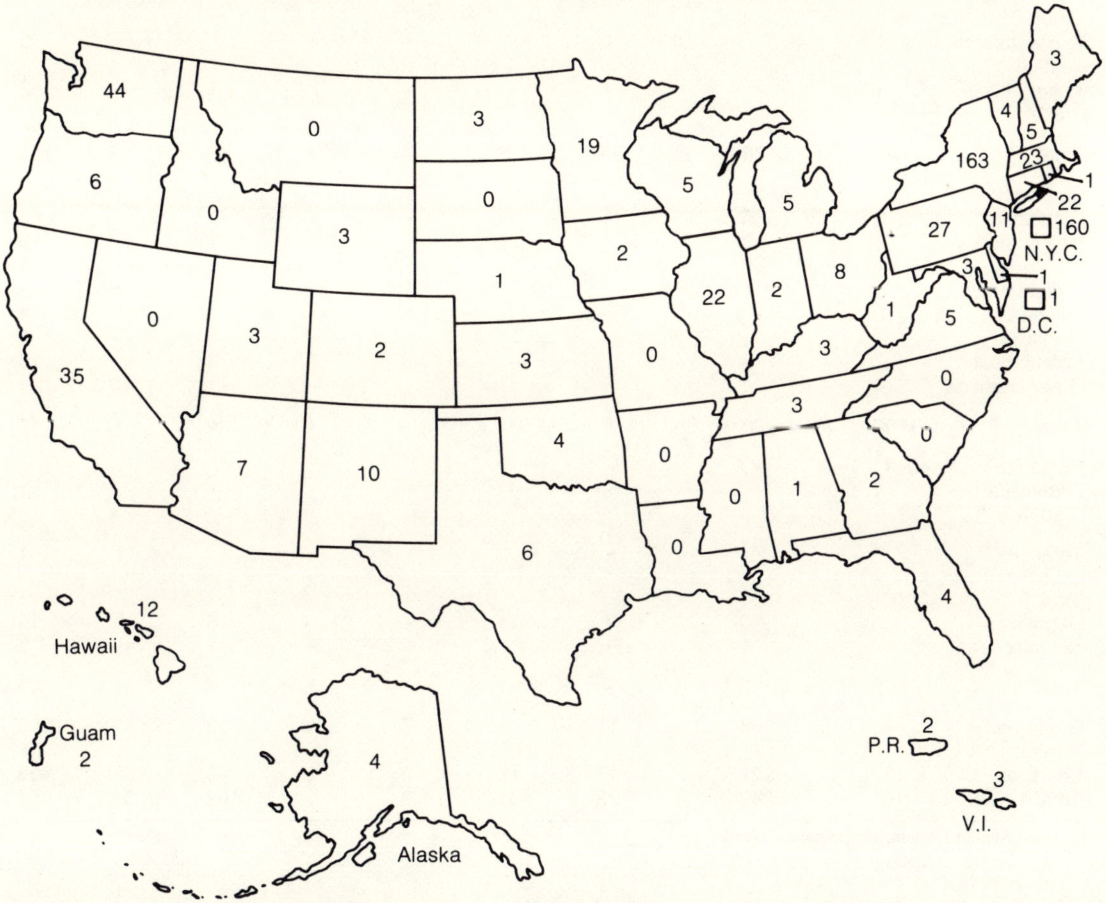

Source: The Atlanta Centers for Disease Control

TABLE 3–8. Foodborne Disease Outbreaks, by Specific Etiologic Agent and Place Where Food Was Eaten, United States, 1982

ETIOLOGIC AGENT	HOME	DELICATESSEN, CAFETERIA, OR RESTAURANT	SCHOOL	PICNIC	CHURCH	CAMP	OTHER	UN-KNOWN	TOTAL
Bacterial:									
B. cereus	-	3	2	-	-	1	2	-	8
Brucella	1	-	-	-	-	-	-	-	1
C. jejuni	1	-	-	-	-	-	1	-	2
C. botulinum	21	-	-	-	-	-	-	-	21
C. perfringens	-	9	1	-	-	-	12	-	22
E. coli	-	-	-	-	-	-	2	-	2
Salmonella	12	17	6	3	4	1	12	-	55
Shigella	1	2	-	-	1	-	-	-	4
S. aureus	4	7	2	2	2	1	10	-	28
Streptococcus Group A	-	-	-	-	-	-	1	-	1
V. cholerae 01	1	-	-	-	-	-	-	-	1
V. cholerae non-01	1	-	-	-	-	-	-	-	1
V. parahaemolyticus	1	-	-	1	-	-	1	-	3
Y. enterocolitica	1	-	-	-	-	-	1	-	2
Total	44	38	11	6	7	3	42	-	151
Chemical:									
Ciguatoxin	3	5	-	-	-	-	-	-	8
Heavy metals	1	3	-	-	-	-	1	-	5
Monosodium glutamate	1	2	-	-	-	-	-	-	3
Mushroom	3	-	-	-	-	-	1	-	4
Shellfish	1	-	-	-	-	-	-	-	1
Scombrotoxin	7	9	-	-	-	-	2	-	18
Other chemical	4	4	-	-	-	-	-	-	8
Total	20	23	-	-	-	-	4	-	47
Parasitic:									
Trichinella spiralis	1	-	-	-	-	-	-	-	1
Total	1	-	-	-	-	-	-	-	1
Viral:									
Hepatitis A	5	6	-	1	-	1	6	-	19
Norwalk virus	-	1	-	-	-	-	1	-	2
Total	5	7	-	1	-	1	7	-	21
Confirmed total	70	68	11	7	7	4	53	-	220
Unknown	127	221	17	16	2	1	49	3	436
Total 1982	197	289	28	23	9	5	102	3	656

Source: Atlanta Centers for Disease Control

TABLE 3–9. Foodborne Disease Outbreaks by Etiologic Agent and Contributing Factors, United States, 1982

ETIOLOGIC AGENT	NUMBER OF REPORTED OUTBREAKS	OUTBREAKS IN WHICH FACTORS REPORTED	IMPROPER HOLDING TEMPERATURES	INADEQUATE COOKING	CONTAMINATED EQUIPMENT	FOOD FROM UNSAFE SOURCE	POOR PERSONAL HYGIENE	OTHER
Bacterial:								
B. cereus	8	5	5	-	-	-	1	-
Brucella	1	-	-	-	-	-	-	-
C. jejuni	2	2	-	-	-	1	-	1
C. botulinum	21	4	1	-	-	-	-	3
C. perfringens	22	20	19	8	3	-	-	2
E. coli	2	1	1	-	-	-	-	-
Salmonella	55	34	16	18	6	6	7	4
Shigella	4	4	1	-	-	-	4	-
S. aureus	28	21	20	3	4	1	9	1
Streptococcus Group A	1	1	1	-	-	-	1	-
Streptococcus Group D	1	-	-	-	-	-	-	-
V. cholerae 01	1	-	-	-	-	-	-	-
V. cholerae non-01	1	1	-	1	-	-	-	-
V parahaemolyticus	3	2	-	-	-	2	-	-
Y. enterocolitica	2	-	-	-	-	-	-	-
Total	151	95	64	30	13	10	22	11
Chemical:								
Ciguatoxin	8	1	-	-	-	1	-	-
Heavy metals	5	4	-	-	2	-	1	2
Monosodium glutamate	3	2	-	-	-	-	-	2
Mushrooms	4	2	-	-	-	2	-	-
Shellfish	1	1	-	-	-	1	-	-
Scombrotoxin	18	9	5	-	-	5	-	-
Other	8	6	-	-	3	-	-	3
Total	47	25	5	-	5	9	1	7
Parasitic:								
Trichinella spiralis	1	1	-	1	-	1	-	-
Total	1	1	-	1	-	1	-	-

TABLE 3–9. (Continued)

ETIOLOGIC AGENT	NUMBER OF REPORTED OUTBREAKS	OUTBREAKS IN WHICH FACTORS REPORTED	IMPROPER HOLDING TEMPERA-TURES	INADEQUATE COOKING	CONTAMI-NATED EQUIPMENT	FOOD FROM UNSAFE SOURCE	POOR PERSONAL HYGIENE	OTHER
Viral:								
Hepatitis A	19	14	2	2	-	6	9	3
Norwalk virus	2	2	-	-	-	-	2	-
Total	21	16	2	2	-	6	11	3
Confirmed Total	220	137	71	33	18	26	34	21
Unknown	436	225	87	73	35	94	59	16
TOTAL 1982	656	362	158	106	53	120	93	37

Source: Atlanta Centers for Disease Control

Sexually Transmitted Diseases 4

Venereal, or sexually transmitted diseases (STD), are caused by infectious agents transmitted from one person to another by sexual contact. Although the prevention and control of STD have been a national priority of the Surgeon General of the United States for years, and widespread antibiotic use since the 1950s has made this a realizable goal, the overall incidence of STD cases continues to rise. The cases reported annually reached 10 million in the 1980s.

GROWING INCIDENCE OF STD

Efforts of the federal government to control and eliminate syphilis, which began in 1950, succeeded in reducing the 1950 rate of 146 cases per 100,000 to only 30 cases per 100,000 by 1978. The rate began to rise again, however, and was 32.9 by 1982. Alarmingly, the rate among women in their childbearing years is increasing in the 1980s, and syphilitic women who become pregnant have only a 20% chance of delivering a normal infant. Indeed, there is a 40% chance that the fetus will be delivered stillborn, die shortly after birth, or be born premature.

During the same period since 1950, gonorrhea incidence has increased from 192 to 468 cases per 100,000 by 1978, declining in the early 1980s to 418 cases per 100,000. By the same decade there were also 500,000 cases of genital herpes infection reported annually and 3 to 4 million cases of nongonoccocal urethritis, or chlamydial infection, which is the most common STD currently in the United States.

Eighty-six percent of reported STD cases are among people age 15 to 29 years old. This accounts in part for the increased incidences just mentioned. The number of people in this age bracket increased greatly between 1970 and 1980. Indeed, by the mid-1980s, 49 million Americans were between age 18 and 29 years.

But another reason for the increase in STD is the changed sexual mores of Americans. They are engaging in sex before marriage and with multiple partners to a much greater degree than they were before 1960. This trend increases as the number of singles increases. The number of single men and women has increased as the divorce rate has increased from 2.6 per 1,000 total population in 1967 to 5.3 per 1,000 in 1980. People are also engaging in sex at earlier ages and remaining single longer than in previous eras. All these developments have contributed to a higher incidence of STD and to the current national health problem.

The most common sexually transmitted infections and the organism causing them are listed in Table 4–1. As indicated, salpingitis, a form of pelvic inflammatory disease (PID) involving fallopian-tube inflammation is caused by the two most commonly transmitted organisms, *Neisseria gonorrhoeae,* the causative agent of gonorrhea and *Chlamydia trachomatis,* which causes chlamydia.

CHLAMYDIA

In 1985, public-health professionals estimated that annually 3 to 4 million Americans contract infections caused by *Chlamydia trachomatis.* Although these infections are not reportable by law, based on records from clinics in metropolitan areas, medical personnel note a sharp increase in chlamydial infections since 1975. Nongonoccocal urethritis, the most common chlamydia-caused infection, is reported in England and Wales, and the incidence there has doubled during the same period.

It has been difficult to isolate and identify infections caused by chlamydia because the organism, which is classified as a bacterium, also shares many properties in common with viruses. The organism must be cultured in the same expensive manner in which viruses are cultured and can grow only intracellularly.

The breadth of infections caused in adults and newborns by the chlamydia organism are listed in Table 4–2. Medical authorities now believe that many previously unidentified infections were caused by chlamydia and that one-half of the cases of nongonococcal urethritis among men and one-half of the 500,000 cases of epididymitis occurring in the United States annually are caused

TABLE 4–1. Major Syndromes of Sexually Transmitted Diseases

SYNDROME AND COMPLICATION	SEXUALLY TRANSMITTED ETIOLOGICAL AGENT
Salpingitis	Neisseria gonorrhoeae, Chlamydia trachomatis, Mycoplasma hominis
Infertility:	
Tubal damage following acute salpingitis	N. gonorrhoeae, C. trachomatis, M. hominis
Postepididymitis	N. gonorrhoeae, C. trachomatis
Ectopic pregnancy, postsalpingitis	N. gonorrhoeae, C. trachomatis, M. hominis
Pregnancy morbidity, including spontaneous abortion, stillbirth, premature labor/low birth weight, premature rupture of membranes, chorioamnionitis, and postpartum endometritis	Herpes simplex virus, Treponema pallidum, C. trachomatis, N. gonorrhoeae, Ureaplasma urealyticum
Congenital and perinatal infections:	
"TORCHES" syndrome*	Cytomegalovirus, herpes simplex virus, T. pallidum
Other infant and childhood morbidity, including—	
Sepsis	N. gonorrhoeae Group B Streptococcus?
Eye infection	C. trachomatis, N. gonorrhoeae
Pneumonia	C. trachomatis, T. pallidum
Otitis media	C. trachomatis
Cognitive impairment	Cytomegalovirus, herpes simplex virus, T. pallidum, Group B Streptococcus?
Male urethritis	N. gonorrhoeae, C. trachomatis, U. urealyticum
Epididymitis	N. gonorrhoeae, C. trachomatis
Lower genital tract infection in women:	
Vulvitis	Candida albicans, herpes simplex virus
Vaginitis	Trichomonas vaginalis, C. albicans, Gardnerella vaginalis
Cervicitis	N. gonorrhoeae, C. trachomatis, herpes simplex virus
Female urethritis	N. gonorrhoeae, C. trachomatis
Genital ulceration	Herpes simplex virus, T. pallidum, Haemophilus ducrey: Calymmatobacterium granulomatis, C. trachomatis (lymphogranuloma venereum)
Proctitis	N. gonorrhoeae, herpes simplex virus, C. trachomatis, Campylobacter fetus, Shigella spp., Entamoeba histolytica
Acute arthritis with genital infection	N. gonorrhoeae, C. trachomatis
Hepatitis	Hepatitis B virus, hepatitis A virus, cytomegalovirus, T. pallidum

* "TORCHES" syndrome refers to congenital infections caused by toxoplasmosis, rubella, cytomegalovirus, herpes simplex virus, and symphilis.
Source: Public Health Reports, Vol. 97 No. 5 p. 410, Sept./Oct. 1982

TABLE 4–2. Clinical Spectrum of *Chlamydia trachomatis* Infections[*]

MALES[†] ⇄	FEMALES[†] →	INFANTS
Infections[‡]	Infections[‡]	Infections[‡]
Urethritis	Cervicitis	Conjunctivitis
Postgonococcal urethritis	Urethritis	Pneumonia
Proctitis	Proctitis	Asymptomatic pharyngeal carriage
Conjunctivitis	Conjunctivitis	Asymptomatic gastrointestinal tract carriage
Pharyngitis?	Pharyngitis?	Otitis media?
Subclinical lymphogranuloma venereum	Subclinical lymphogranuloma venereum	
Complications[‡]	Complications[‡]	
Epididymitis	Salpingitis	
Prostatitis?	Endometritis	
Reiter syndrome?	Perihepatitis	
Sterility?	Ectopic pregnancy	
Rectal strictures[**]	Infertility	
	Dysplasia?	
	Postpartum endometritis?	
	Prematurity?	
	Stillbirth?	
	Neonatal death?	
	Vulvar/rectal carcinoma[**]	
	Rectal stricutes[¶]	

[*] Trachoma, the leading cause of preventable blindness in the world, is also caused by *Chlamydia* but has been excluded because it is not generally sexually transmitted.
[†] Arrow indicates direction of transmission of infection.
[‡] Question mark indicates that a relationship has not been firmly established.
[**] Associated with lymphogranuloma venereum.
Source: Morbidity and Mortality Weekly Report Supplement, Vol. 34, No 3S, Aug 1985

by chlamydia. One-half the cases of acute PID in women are also attributable to chlamydia. As Table 4–2 indicates, the effects on babies born to infected women range from death to multiple infections. Other infected women may be left infertile.

Each year more than 155,000 infants are born to women suffering from chlamydia-caused infections. Besides the physical and psychological pain and suffering that these infections cause, the economic burden they impose is over $1 billion a year.

The risk of becoming infected is directly related to the number of sexual contacts one has with different partners and inversely related to age. Sexually active teenage girls have an infection rate two to three times higher than that of older women. Similarly, teenage males have a higher rate of urethral infection than older men. There also appears to be a relationship between Chlamydia-caused infections and a lower socioeconomic status and membership in some ethnic groups. Homosexual men have a lower rate of urethral infection but a higher rate of rectal chlamydial infection than have heterosexual men.

The use of barrier-type contraceptives, such as a condom, diaphragm, and foam correlate with reduced risk of infection. Women taking oral contraceptives, however, have had a higher incidence of cervical chlamydial infection.

The tests currently available to detect chlamydial infections are intricate and not applicable to all infections. Cultures are time consuming and expensive, but new antigen detecting tests are cheaper. Antimicrobial treatment will vary, depending on the infection. Generally, uncomplicated urethral, endocervical, or rectal infection in adults can be treated by a regimen of tetracycline hydrochloride in a dose of 500 mg orally four times daily for 7 days. Doxycycline hyclate is also used alternatively as are the sulfonamides. Erythromycin base or erythromycin ethyl succinate is used to treat urogenital infections in pregnancy. Inpatient treatment for PID is often doxycycline at a 100-g I.V. dose twice daily.

GONORRHEA

Gonorrhea is at present the most common *reportable* infectious disease in the United States. Transmitted by vaginal, oral, or anal sexual contact, it is caused by the organism *Neisseria gonorrhoeae.* The infection is insidious in that 80% of infected females and 20 percent of infected males fail to experience any symptoms in the early stages. This leads to unsuspected spread of the infection and the development of serious complications as the untreated disease progresses.

When early symptoms do appear, the most common is a green yellow, vaginal discharge in females and urethral discharge in males. It develops within 1 or 2 weeks after sexual contact with an infected person. Infants passing through the birth canal of an infected mother may develop gonococcal ophthalmia neonatorum; adults who touch their eyes with contaminated hands may contract gonococcal conjunctivitis. Left untreated, the condition can cause blindness. Many of the women who fail to receive treatment within 8 to 10 weeks of the onset of their infection develop salpingitis (infection of the fallopian tubes) or PID.

Women whose infection deteriorates to salpingitis may develop fallopian-tube scarring, which can lead to an ectopic pregnancy or infertility. Symptoms of salpingitis or PID include dull-to-severe abdominal pain, fever, headache, nausea, or vomiting. Some women who are asymptomatic for months develop gonococcal septicemia. This disease can lead to a generalized septic arthritis causing joint destruction at various sites in the body.

Fig. 4–1. Gonorrhea: reported cases per 100,000 population, by year, United States and large cities, 1968–83

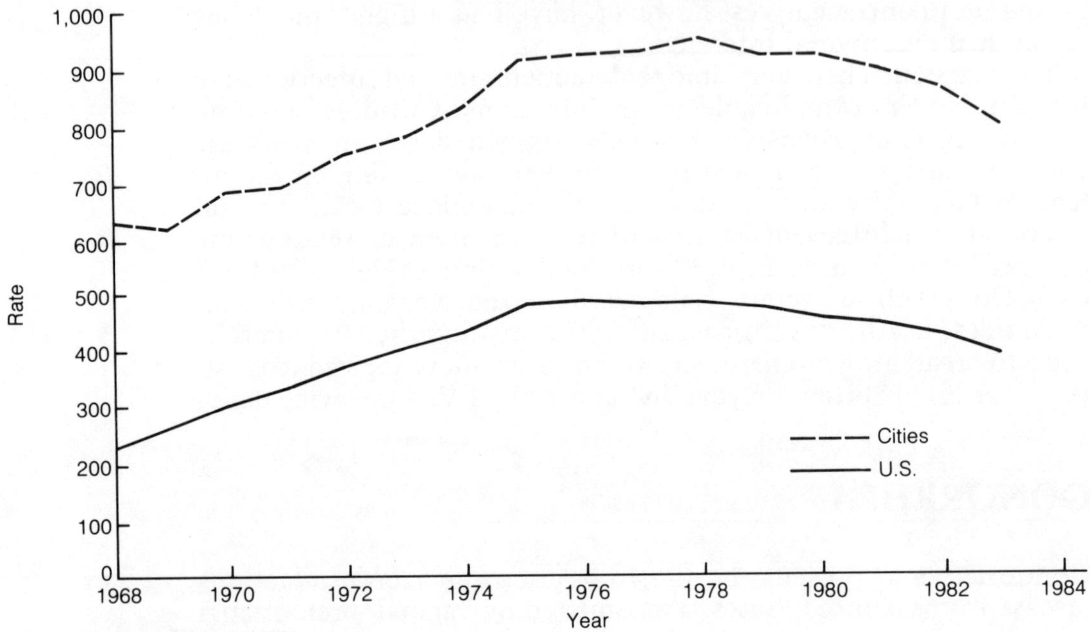

*Cities with population over 200,000.

Source: Morbidity and Mortality Weekly Report, Annual Summary 1983.

Because of the 12% average annual increase in gonorrheal incidence reported between 1965 and 1975, the federal government launched a gonorrhea control effort by the early 1970s, and gonorrhea morbidity began decreasing in 1975. The peak funds expenditure year was 1974. The number of office visits for PID also declined by 45% between 1973 and 1981.

The trend in gonorrheal incidence from 1968 through 1983 is shown in Fig. 4–1. The rate fell 17% in the United States as a whole and 12% in metropolitan areas.

The reported cases in each state per 100,000 population in 1983 is reflected in Fig. 4–2. The 1983 rates generally declined from those in 1982. But those reported by southeastern states remained high and fairly constant. Alaska also had high rates.

The reported incidence of gonorrhea and the 1990 public-health goal of 280 cases per 100,000 population are shown in Table 4–3.

The breakdown of cases and the rates for males and females by age during 1981 and 1982 are shown in Table 4–4.

Fig. 4–2. Gonorrhea: reported cases per 100,000 population, by state, United States, 1983

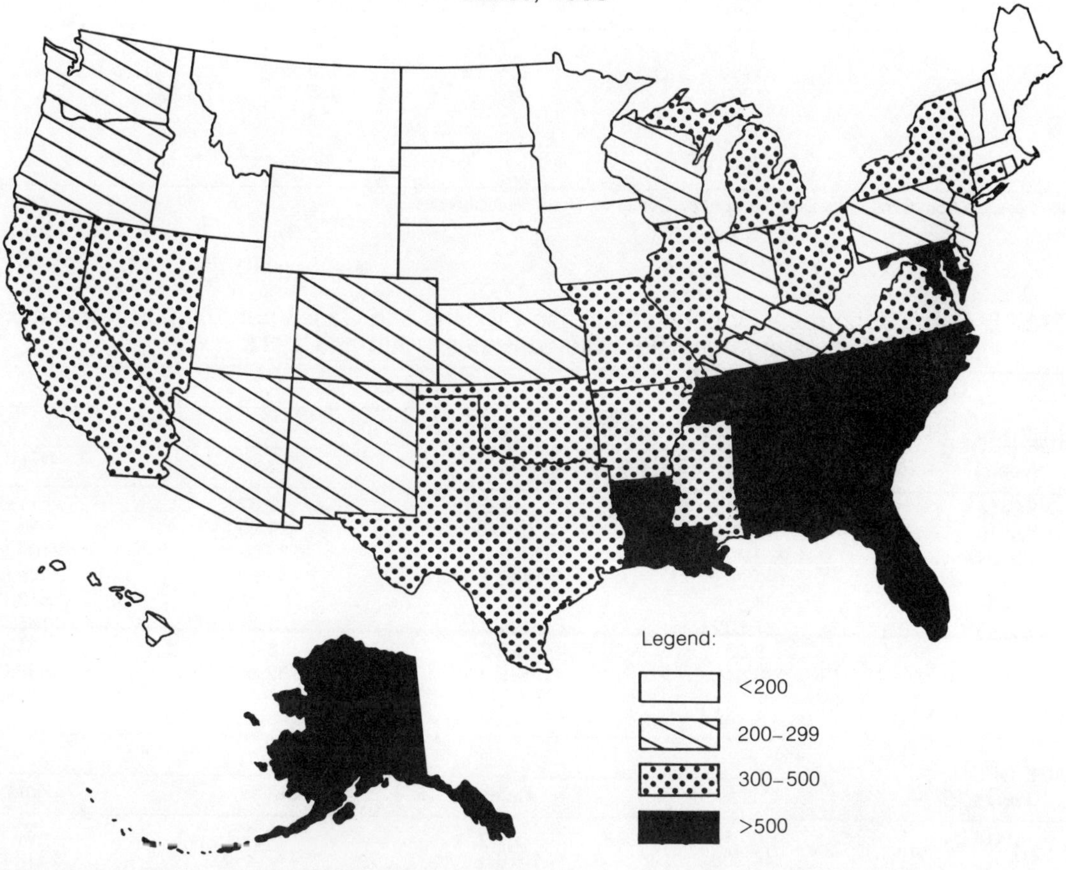

Source: Morbidity and Mortality Weekly Report, Annual Summary 1983

The case rate per 100,000 by age and sex shown for 1983 in Fig. 4–3 graphically reveals more clearly the prime ages at which gonorrhea is prevalent. Those subjects between ages 15 and 19 years accounted for 25% of all cases, whereas those age 20 to 24 years accounted for nearly 40% of all gonorrhea cases.

As indicated, the greatest proportion of gonorrhea cases occur in those subjects age 15 to 25 years but it should be noted that the case rate for those age 10 to 14 years jumped from 17.7 per 100,000 to 21.1 per 100,000 just between 1980 and 1981 alone. The spread of gonorrhea and PID—among American teenagers who are engaging in sexual activity at younger ages and in greater numbers than they have in the past—has alarmed the medical community. In 1981, more than 250,000 cases of gonorrhea were reported for American teenagers. It is widely believed that this number

TABLE 4–3. Reported Incidence of Gonorrhea, per 100,000

YEAR	REPORTED INCIDENCE
1979	459
1980	443
1981	435
1982	418
1990	280

Source: Data from Centers for Disease Control, Center for Prevention Services.

TABLE 4–4. Gonorrhea: Reported Cases in Civilians and Cases per 100,000 Population, by Age and Sex, United States, 1980 and 1981

AGE GROUP (years)	1981* Cases	1981* Rate	1980 Cases	1980 Rate
MALE				
0–14	2,846	12.0	2,877	11.0
15–19	99,224	924.0	99,994	930.0
20–24	222,399	2089.0	224,091	2102.2
25–29	139,603	1440.7	140,673	1449.8
30–39	94,613	609.7	95,345	613.7
40–49	21,532	194.3	21,717	195.7
50+	8,031	30.8	8,112	31.1
Total	588,248	535.2	592,809	538.8
FEMALE				
0–14	8,011	31.6	8,207	32.7
15–19	144,208	1370.5	147,245	1414.5
20–24	152,163	1413.2	155,365	1458.6
25–29	61,144	616.6	62,448	636.3
30–39	29,977	185.5	30,631	191.6
40–49	5,138	43.6	5,277	45.2
50+	1,975	5.9	2,047	6.2
Total	402,616	341.9	411,220	353.1
TOTAL				
0–14	10,857	21.1	11,084	17.7
15–19	243,432	1145.0	247,239	1168.3
20–24	374,562	1749.2	379,456	1780.5
25–29	200,747	1023.9	203,121	1040.7
30–39	124,590	393.3	125,976	399.7
40–49	26,670	116.6	26,994	115.6
50+	10,006	16.9	10,159	17.2
Total	990,864	435.2	1,004,029	443.3

* Age distributions are provisional.
Source: Morbidity and Mortality Weekly Report, Annual Summary 1983

Fig. 4–3. Gonorrhea: reported cases per 100,000 population, by age and sex, United States, 1983

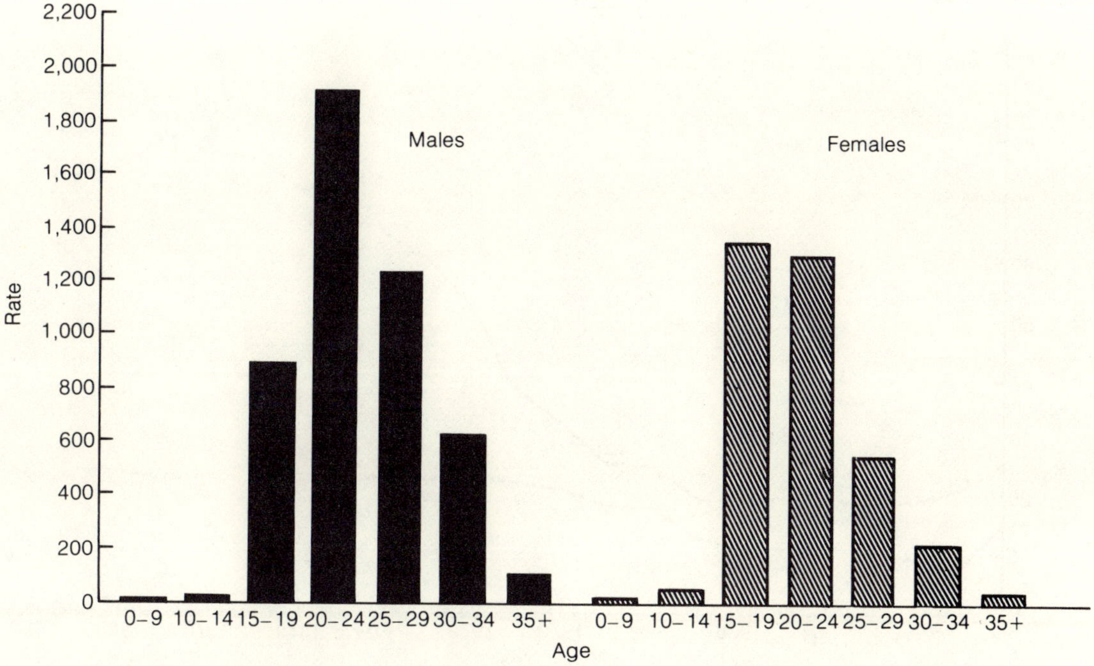

Source: Morbidity and Mortality Weekly Report, Annual Summary 1983

reflects only one-half of the actual number of cases. The peak number of cases for teenagers as well as for the population at other ages was reached in 1975. The dramatic increase in disease among teenagers since 1960 is shown in Table 4–5.

The pattern for teenagers age 10 to 14 years by sex reveals a higher incidence in females that increased sharply around 1970 (Fig. 4–4).

TABLE 4–5. Gonorrhea in the United States

YEAR (19')	10–14 Male	10–14 Female	15–19 Male	15–19 Female	Total
60	1,190	2,068	30,649	23,000	56,907
65	1,038	1,763	42,834	24,113	69,748
70	2,061	3,228	90,494	57,458	153,241
75	2,199	7,443	115,504	151,109	276,255
80	2,199	6,674	99,994	147,245	256,112

AGE GROUP (YEARS)

Source: Monthly Morbidity and Mortality Report, Vol. 32, No. 3SS

Fig. 4–4. Gonorrhea rates/100,000 population among teenagers ages 10–14 years, United States, 1960–81

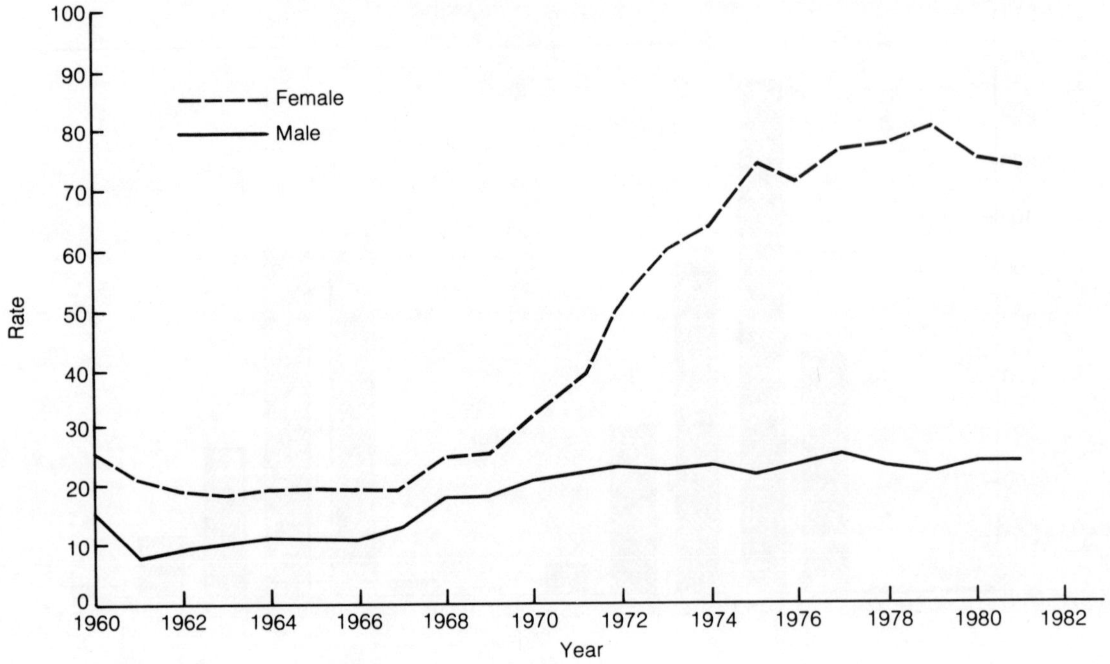

Source: Monthly Morbidity and Mortality Report, Vol. 32, No. 3SS

The pattern for males and females among older teenagers from 1960 through 1982 is shown in Fig. 4–5. Until 1972, the case rate was lower for females. But programs urging infected males to advocate treatment in their partners caused the reported case rate for females to increase and surpass that of males.

A common sequela of not only chlamydia but also gonorrhea in women is PID. It can cause sterility and sometimes lead to death in affected women. PID can also be fatal as well as cause mental retardation, loss of hearing or vision, and neurologic damage in the newborn. The estimated incidence of gonococcal PID for the years 1978 through 1982 and the projected case rate goal of no more than 60 cases per 100,000 is shown in Table 4–6.

Table 4–7 summarizes the cases of PID requiring hospitalization in females age 15 to 19 years by race between 1970 and 1980.

Changes in the rates of gonorrhea (GC) and PID for females ages 15 to 19 years between 1970 and 1980 are shown in Fig. 4–6.

Fig. 4–5. Gonorrhea rates/100,000 population among teenagers ages 15–19 years, United States, 1960–81.

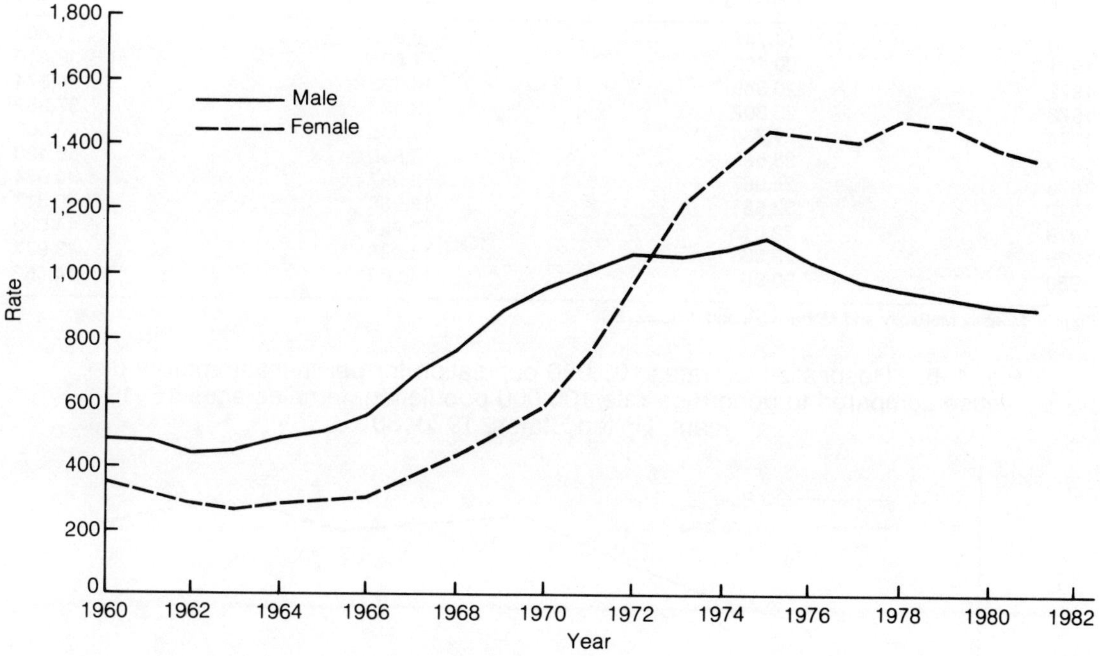

Source: Monthly Morbidity and Mortality Report, Vol. 32, No 333

THE GONORRHEA CHALLENGE

The standard treatment for gonorrhea is large doses of penicillin and probenecid; the latter drug inhibits the body's elimination of penicillin. Tetracycline is often used in patients allergic to penicillin except in pregnant women. Diagnostic cultures and follow-up cultures after treatment identify the gonococcal organism.

TABLE 4–6. Projected Case Rate Goal of Pelvic Inflammatory Disease for 1978–90, Per 100,000

YEAR	ESTIMATED INCIDENCE OF GONOCOCCAL PELVIC INFLAMMATORY DISEASE
78	133.8
79	131.7
80	127.1
81	123.1
82	116.6
90	60.0

Source: Data from Centers for Disease Control, Center for Prevention Services.

TABLE 4–7. Patients, Ages 15–19 Years, by Race, Hospitalized for Pelvic Inflammatory Disease, United States, 1970–80

YEAR	WHITES	OTHER RACES	TOTAL
1970	14,742	9,927	24,669
1971	20,909	11,501	32,410
1972	20,549	14,425	34,974
1973	23,802	13,587	37,389
1974	24,234	16,335	40,569
1975	23,585	12,838	36,423
1976	25,987	8,987	34,974
1977	32,651	13,966	46,617
1978	32,015	12,624	44,639
1979	29,501	14,436	43,937
1980	30,600	14,069	44,669

Source: Monthly Morbidity and Mortality Report, Vol. 32. 3SS

Fig. 4–6. Hospitalization rates/100,000 population for pelvic inflammatory disease compared to gonorrhea rate/100,000 population, females ages 15–19 years, United States, 1970–80

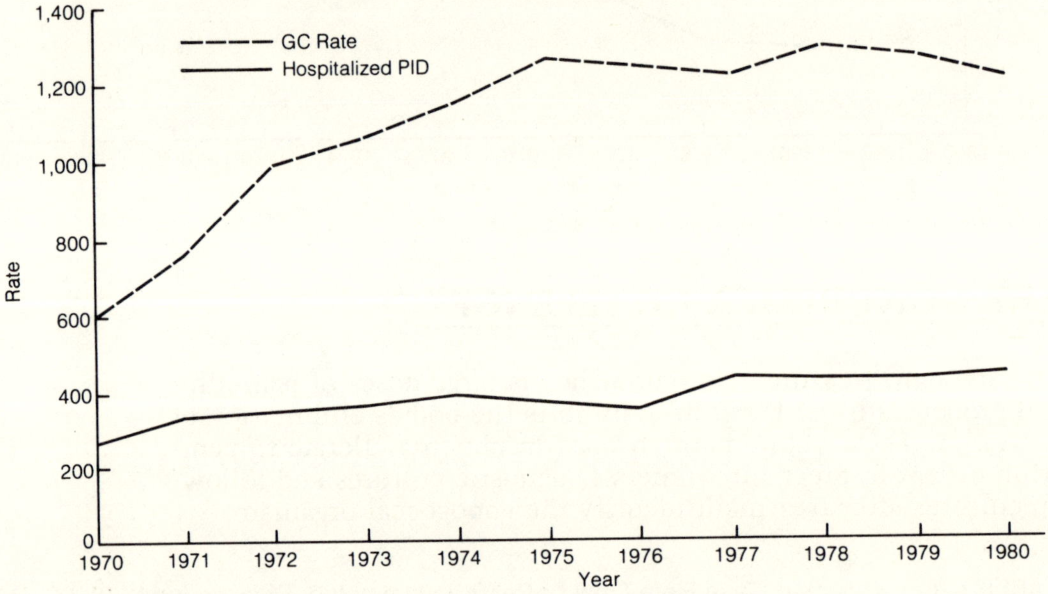

Source: Morbidity and Mortality Weekly Report, Annual Summary 1983

Epidemiologists are also concerned about the 241% increase in penicillinase-producing (penicillin-resistant) *Neisseria* (PPNG) *gonorrhoreae* infections. They were first isolated in the United States in 1976. The cases increased from 328 in 1979 to 1,118 in 1980 and then to 4,457 in 1982. The number in 1983 dropped to 3,737. These cases represent only a small proportion of all cases and seem to be confined to servicemen and immigrants entering the United States. But the increase in cases is making public-health officials apprehensive about their ability to keep local spread under control. Public-health resources are already spread thin by efforts to combat STD. The increase in cases through 1981 is graphically dramatic (Fig. 4–7).

In 1983, the first penicillin-resistant, nonpenicillinase producing strains of gonorrhea were reported in North Carolina. Currently, there are no standardized tests to identify this kind of strain even though it is fairly common in many parts of the world. Twenty percent of all gonococcal isolates in Southeast Asia are of this variety.

Physicians have been advised to suspect these strains whenever treatment failure not due to PPNG is noted. To control the spread of these infections, physicians can treat all patients whose urethral smears show gram-negative intracellular diplococci with spectinomycin, an effective replacement for penicillin.

Since February 1985, 12 isolates of *N. gonorrhoeae* have been identified as having high level resistance to tetracycline, but they are susceptible to penicillin.

Fig. 4–7. Gonorrhea: reported penicillinase-producing *Neisseria gonorrhoe.* United States, 1976–83

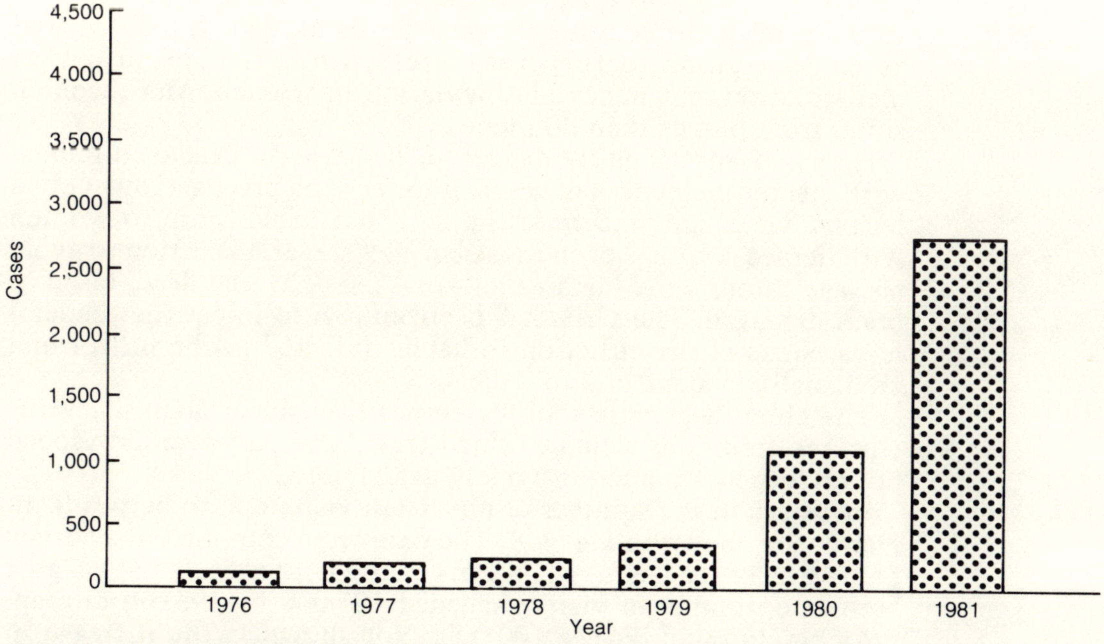

PPNG reporting began March 1976.

Source: Morbidity and Mortality Weekly Report, Annual Summary 1983

HERPES

Because of its rising incidence, genital herpes—also known as herpes simplex II—is now thought to be the second most common venereal disease in the United States although its existence was unknown until the middle of this century. Herpes type II produces symptoms similar to a closely related variant, herpes simplex I. The latter virus causes the common cold sore that occurs on or near the lips.

Herpes simplex II sores are similar in appearance but occur in the genital area (it is thought) when the virus has been transmitted from one person to another through sexual contact. The virus cannot survive outside the human body, and the exact mechanism of transmission is unclear since some persons seem to have contracted herpes II even though their sexual partner is uninfected. There have also been reported instances of the herpes I in genital sores and herpes II in oral sores.

The sores, which can last several weeks for a given outbreak, are usually painful or itchy. Those in the cervix are generally not painful, but cervical infections can cause a vaginal discharge. The lymph nodes in the groin may be swollen, and the herpes blisters may be accompanied by a low-grade fever and general malaise.

Typically, the sores heal within a few weeks, leaving the individual symptom-free until the next outbreak, which may be triggered by trauma to the area, stress, impaired immunity or menstruation, pregnancy and ovulation in women. More women suffer from herpes than do men.

Herpes II infections are dangerous because they have correlated with greater incidences of cervical cancer and precancerous vulval lesions. Of equal concern is the fact that babies born to women with herpes II virus—even those born by caesarian section to avoid passage through the birth canal—may be delivered dead, blind or brain damaged. The virus has been known to infect the prenatal fetus. Signs of the affliction in babies infected in the birth canal are usually evident in 4 to 7 days.

The chief diagnostic tool for herpes II is smear analysis. Virus cultures are not as reliable. Blood tests have also been developed but are expensive and not widely available.

Increases in the number of physician visits due to herpes II infection are shown in Fig. 4–8. The data were compiled in a survey of private, office-based, physicians in the United States. As can be seen, the number of visits exceeded 295,000 by 1981, a rate approaching around 35 per 100,000. Not shown is the increase in neonatal deaths from herpes II, which increased from 2.3 per mil-

Fig. 4–8. Genital Herpes: consultations, office visits and first office visits for genital herpes, United States, 1966–81

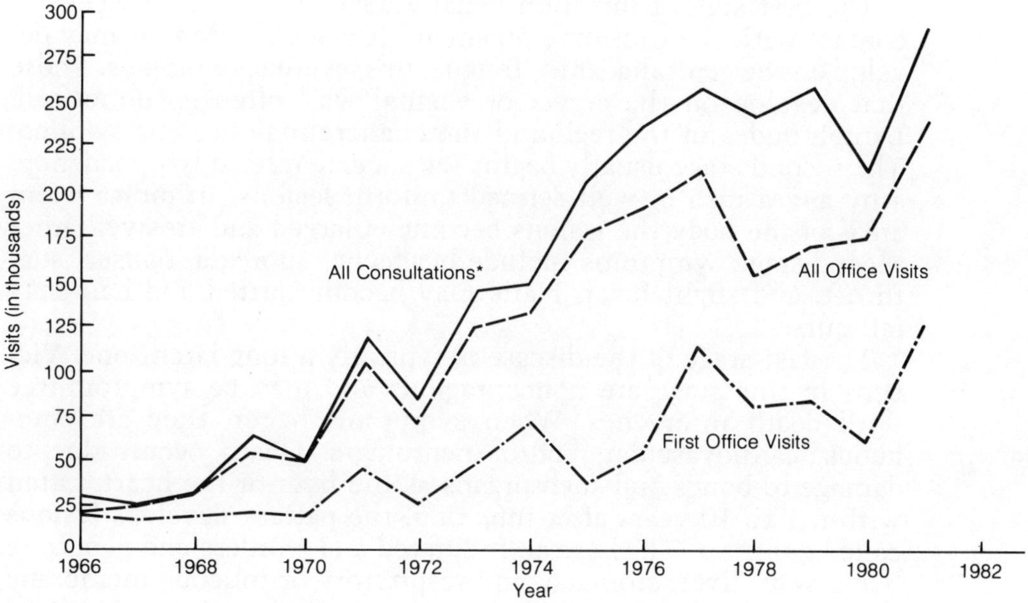

*Includes any type of patient/physician interaction, such as telephone calls, house calls, and office visits.

Source: Public Health Report, Vol. 97 No. 5: 413, Sept/Oct 1982

lion live births in 1968 to 9.0 per million by 1978 according to unpublished health data.

Treatment for herpes II is very limited and mostly topical until recent years. Now an antiviral medication called Zovirax, available as an ointment and a capsule, has proven effective in combatting the outbreak of sores. Makers of Zovirax capsules report that product-testing reflects prevention or reduction in recurrences in more than 95% of the patients who used the medication daily for 6 months.

SYPHILIS

Syphillis is a chronic venereal disease which begins in the mucous membranes. It quickly spreads through lymph nodes and the bloodstream. The causative organism is a spirochete, *Treponema pallidum.* The disease, if left untreated, progresses slowly through its primary and secondary stages. Eventually, crippling and death occur years after the infection is contracted.

The first sign of infection usually develops within 3 weeks of contact with the causative organism. It is a chancre that may develop on the genitalia, anus, tongue, lips, eyelids, or nipples. Those that develop on the cervix or vaginal wall often go unnoticed. Lymph nodes in the region of the chancre may become swollen. The second stage usually begins with a generalized lymphadenopathy and a rash of well-defined uniform lesions. In moist warm areas of the body the lesions become enlarged and erosive. Other second-stage symptoms include headache, anorexia, nausea, sore throat, and slight fever. Nails may become pitted and hair may fall out.

The last stage of the disease is typically a long latent one. Victims in this stage are noncontagious and may be symptom-free until death intervenes. When symptoms occur, they are cutaneous, cardiovascular, and/or neurologic. Death occurs due to damage to bones and such organs as the liver or the heart. Often within 1 to 10 years after infection, the patient develops lesions called *gummas*. They are an indurated and painless and penetrate bone, skin, liver, stomach, and respiratory or mucous membrane tissue to various extents. They can occur on almost any organ and lead to death with destruction of the organ or bones.

The aorta's elastic tissue may become fibrotic, ultimately leading to aortic regurgitation and sometimes aneurysm. About 10% of untreated syphilitics develop these cardiovascular symptoms in the last stage. Another 10% develop CNS impairment from 5 to 35 years after their initial infection. Trauma is manifested as personality changes, general paresis, and limb weakness. As with several other venereal diseases, infants born to infected women often have congenital syphilis.

The most sensitive test for diagnosing syphilis in all stages is the fluorescent treponemal antibody absorption test. This test can identify *T. pallidum* antigens in both tissue and various fluids. Efforts to diagnose and prevent the spread of syphilis were undertaken in the 1940s. These efforts led to an 87% reduction in incidence at all stages. The number of syphilis admissions to mental hospitals dropped 98%, whereas syphilis-related infant deaths declined 99%.

Primary and secondary syphilis cases increased again in the 1980s, rising 43% between 1980 and 1981. The trend in syphilis incidence in the United States between 1941 and 1983 is shown in Fig. 4–9. The reported cases by sex between 1956 and 1983 are indicated in Fig. 4–10.

Congenital syphilis reported for infants born in 1981 was 54%

Fig. 4–9. Syphilis (primary and secondary): reported civilian cases per 100,000 population, by year, United States, 1941–83*

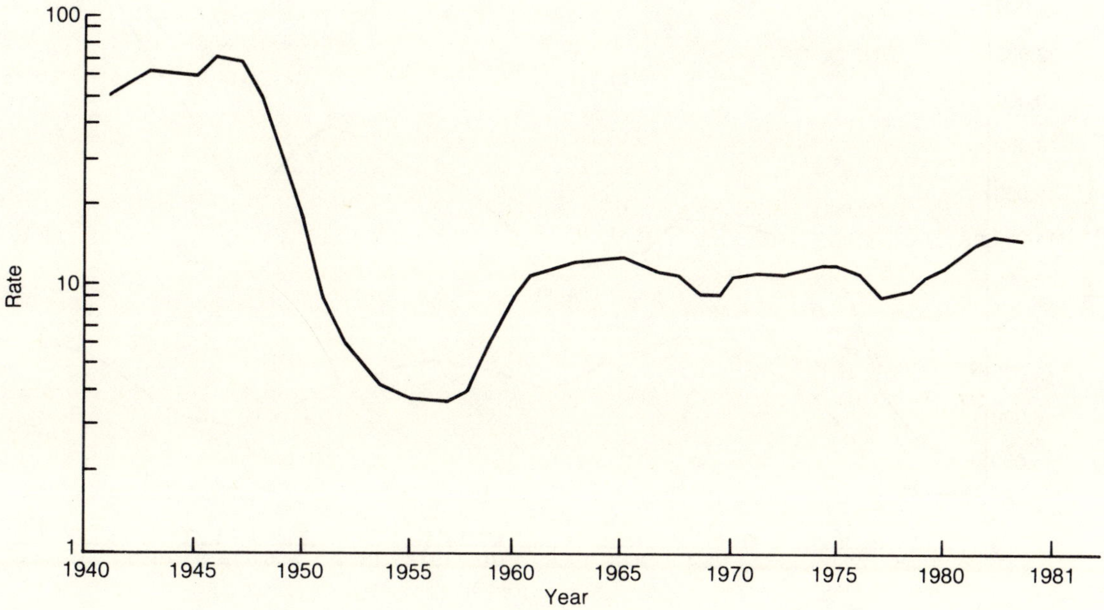

*1941–46 fiscal years (12 month period ending June 30). 1947–1983 calendar years.

Source: Morbidity and Mortality Weekly Report, Annual Summary 1983.

higher than the figures reported in 1978. These cases mostly reflected early congenital syphilis for children younger then age 1 year. The decline in total number of congenital cases reported reflects a drop in the late cases reported (Table 4–8).

The cases of primary and secondary syphilis and of congenital syphilis reported between 1979 and 1982 are summarized in Table 4–9 together with the 1990 incidence goals.

The relationship between funded control efforts and the incidence of reported cases is seen in Fig. 4–11. The inverse relationship between the two has long been noticed. Public-health analysts, however, believe that the new surge is not solely related to reduced funding of control efforts.

The usual treatment for syphilis is penicillin, often a single injection of penicillin G benzathine for early cases and 2.4 million units weekly for 3 weeks in cases of more than a year's duration. Tetracycline is used as a replacement for penicillin in those patients who are allergic to the latter.

Fig. 4–10. Syphilis (primary and secondary): reported cases, by sex, United States, 1956–83

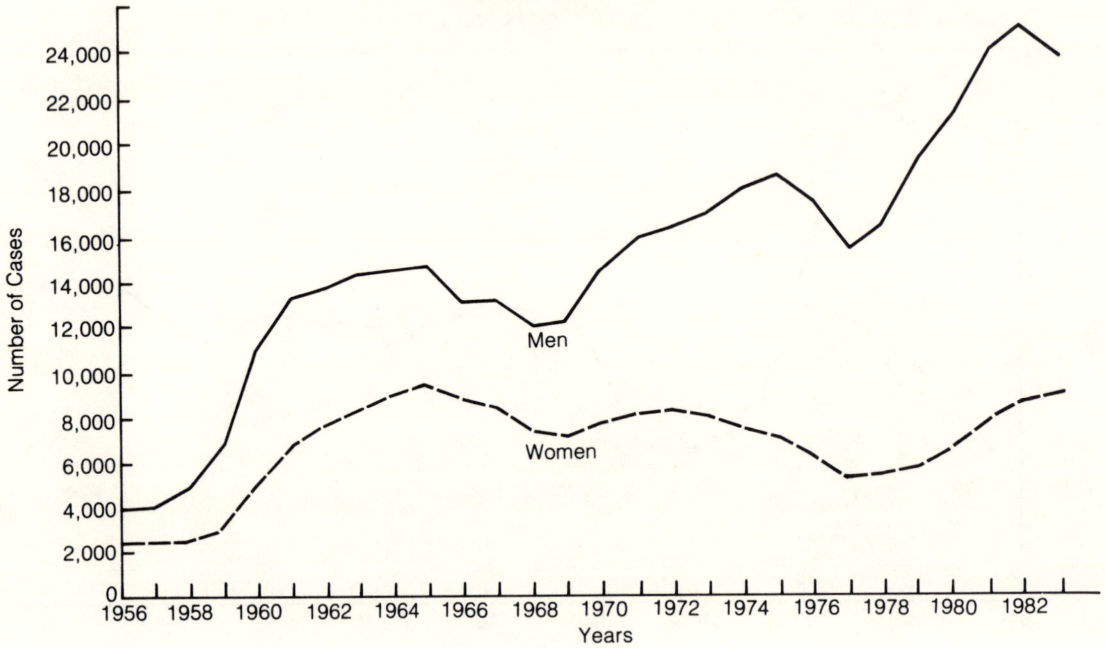

Source: Morbidity and Mortality Weekly Report, Annual Summary 1983

United States, 1982–83

AGE GROUP	CASES 1982	CASES 1983	TOTAL (%) 1982	TOTAL (%) 1983
<1	159	158	61.4	66.1
1–4	11	12	4.3	5.0
5–9	6	3	2.3	1.3
10+	71	62	27.4	25.9
Unknown	12	4	4.6	1.7
Total	259	239	100.0	100.0

Source: Morbidity and Mortality Weekly Report, Annual Summary 1983

AIDS

Acquired immunodeficiency syndrome (AIDS) results from impairment of the cellular immune system and leaves those affected open to opportunistic infections and rare cancers that are generally fatal. Only 20% of AIDS victims are alive 2 years after diagnosis.

TABLE 4–9. Primary and Secondary Syphilis and Congenital Syphilis in the United States, 1979–82

YEAR (19')	REPORTED INCIDENCE/ 100,000 OF PRIMARY AND SECONDARY SYPHILIS	REPORTED INCIDENCE/ 100,000 OF CONGENITAL SYPHILIS
79	11	3.5
80	12	3.0
81	14	4.4
82	15	4.3
90	7	1.5

Source: Data from Centers for Disease Control, Center for Prevention Services.

Fig. 4–11. Inflation and federal project grants to states for syphilis control, primary and secondary cases of syphilis versus federal project grants to states, in 1972 dollars* fiscal years 1964–81

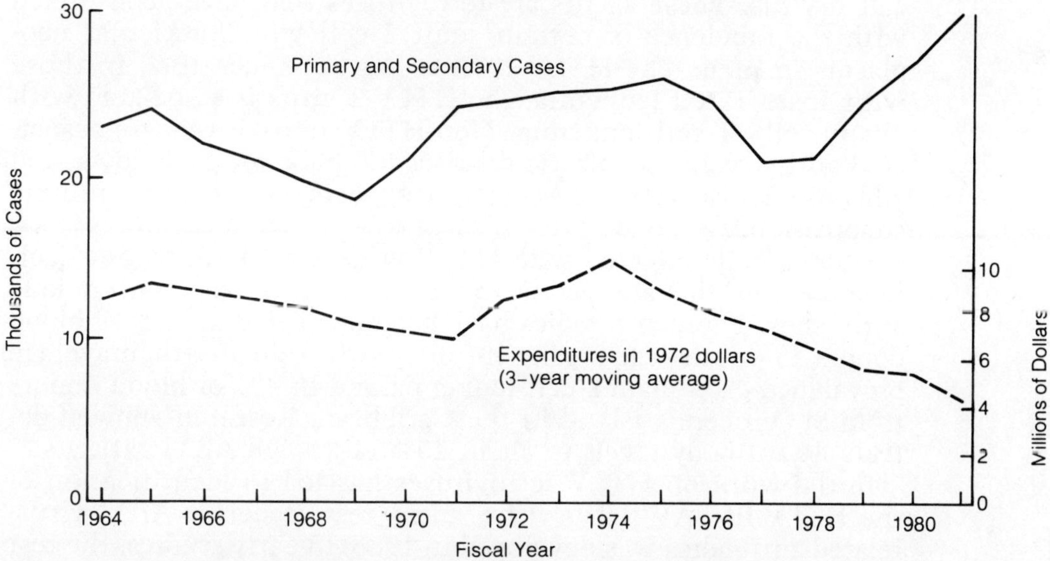

*Adjustments for 1972 dollars by price deflators to Federal Government purchases of goods and services.

Source: Public Health Report, Vol. 97, No. 5: 409 Sept./Oct. 1982

Diagnosis of a fully developed case of AIDS involves identification of an opportunistic infection, particularly Pneumocystis carinii pneumonia (PCP) and/or a malignancy, such as Kaposi's sarcoma, or B-cell lymphoma. Laboratory work-up often shows signs of impaired cellular immunity in ongoing reduction of T-helper cells, increased serum immunoglobulins, reduced cellular cytotoxicity, and reduced response to both mitogens and antigens. When no recognized cause of the immune suppression can be identified—such as a patient history of corticosteroid therapy, chemotherapy or radiotherapy, pre-existing malignancy, or a primary immunodeficiency syndrome—then a diagnosis of AIDS becomes more probable. Confirmation should be attempted by interviewing the patient to obtain information about risk factor exposure, such as a history of homosexuality in males, I.V. drug abuse, heterosexual relationship with an I.V. drug abuser or with persons at risk for or who currently have AIDS, and finally those who either are hemophiliacs or have been transfused within 5 years of manifesting AIDS symptoms.

The agent considered to be responsible for the development of impaired immunity is the HTLV-III/LAV virus, recently renamed the HIV virus. The letter designation of the former name stands for human T-lymphotropic virus, type III/lymphadenopathy-associated virus. These agents are retroviruses that have been linked with the incidence of certain adult T-cell lymphoreticular neoplasms in man. The HTLV-1 virus has been identified in those with acute T-cell leukemia; the HTLV-2 virus is associated with "hairy-cell" T-cell leukemia. Non-HTLV retroviruses are associated with several neoplastic diseases in chickens, cats, cows, and gibbons. Those retroviruses affecting cats also cause immune suppression.

Human cells infected with HTLV viruses exhibit antigens (cellular proteins) that are specific to the virus, which react with unique antibodies. These antibodies have been identified in 12% of blood donors in southwest Japan, an area with a greater-than-average prevalence of human T-cell leukemia and in 4% of blood donors from St. Vincent's island in the Caribbean. Research showed detectable antibody levels in about 25% of known AIDS patients.

Initial work on HTLV retroviruses has led to identification of the HTLV-III/LAV (HIV) virus, and a test to detect AIDS virus-related antibodies was developed in 1985. In early studies, the test identified antibodies in 86 of 88 AIDS patients. When used on the sera of 297 healthy adults, the test showed four false positive results. The test, however, does not predict whether someone with a positive antibody finding will in fact develop AIDS. Indeed, there are persons with the antibody who have developed lymphadenopathies but not the AIDS syndrome itself. The test, which has been approved for screening, is being used in particular to protect the blood supply of countries affected by AIDS. When testing persons, a repeat testing is recommended since commercially available tests, which are enzyme-linked immunosorbant assays (ELISAS) do yield a small proportion of false positive results. In addition to repeat testing, these tests can be used in combination with the Western blot test for greater accuracy.

Failure to detect the AIDS antibody in the blood of known AIDs patients may occur for several reasons. Victims may not mount an antibody defense to the AIDS virus. Difficulties with serologic testing or serum sampling at phases of the disease when these antibodies are not present may also account for failure to detect the antibody in known AIDS cases. Thus, protection of the blood supply or identification of AIDS-infected individuals is not 100%.

The first AIDS case was reported in the Atlanta Centers for Disease Control publications in the spring of 1981, although there were earlier reports among Haitians in the United States in 1980 (Fig. 4–12). Researchers now believe that some cases occurred in Haiti and the United States in the late 1970s.

The World Health Organization reported in its November 1983 Memorandum on the world AIDS situation published in Geneva that the earliest cases occurred in equatorial Africa and the Caribean. Cases reported later in the United States and western Europe seem confined to specific groups at high risk, namely homosexual and bisexual men, I.V. drug users, hemophiliacs, and recipients of blood transfusions, persons born in Haiti, the children of AIDS mothers, and sexual partners of AIDS victims.

Fig. 4–12. Reported cases of acquired immunodeficiency syndrome, by date of diagnosis, United States, 1979–82

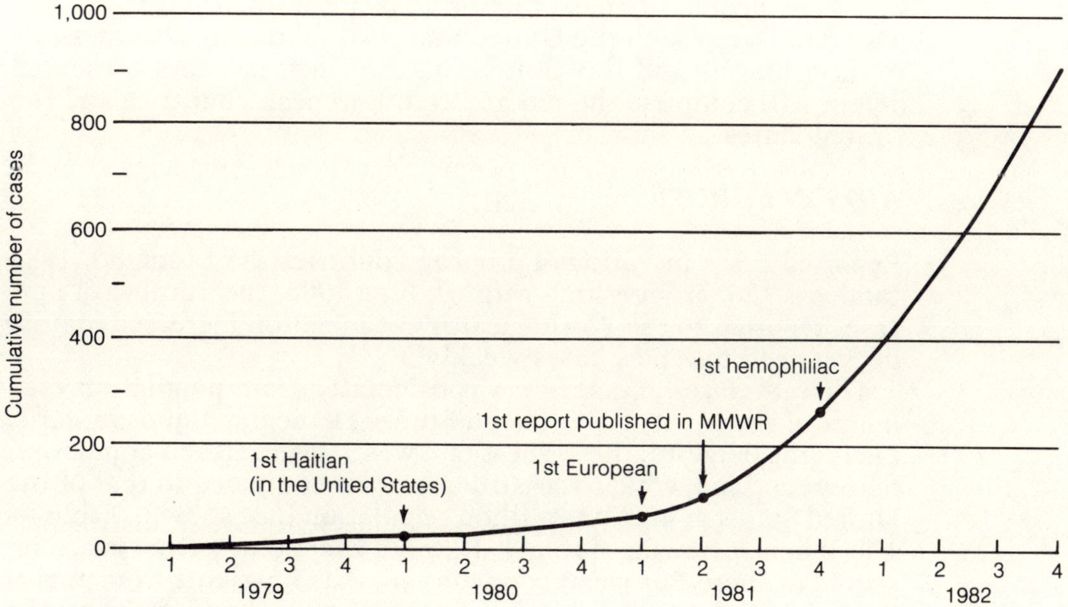

Note: 1st quarter of 1979 is cumulaive total from 1975.

Source: Public Health Report, Vol. 97, No. 5 Sept/Oct 1982

In the Caribbean, the pattern was similar except that 15% were women, some of whom had had blood transfusions. The use of unsterilized or contaminated needles for ordinary medical purposes (not I.V. drug abuse) is a suspected cause. The pattern in Africa, however, where 41% of the victims in one study of AIDS patients at two Kinshasa hospitals in Zaire were women is quite different. The patients were of both sexes and came from all strata of society. Here again, the role of heterosexual transmission is being studied. Researchers are also considering the level of bisexual activity among African men and the practice of anal intercourse among heterosexuals in Third World countries as a form of birth control. Anal intercourse has been long identified as a major mode of transmission for many diseases—viral, bacterial and parasitic. The immune impairment caused by sperm entering the body of the receiver through tears in rectal tissue has been under study for several years. This impairment takes place among Western homosexuals independently of AIDS infection. Western homosexuals also have a disease history that parallels that of many Third World peoples who have been exposed to hepatitis B, venereal pathogens, intestinal parasites, and other viruses. Both groups appear to be weakened hosts, perhaps more vulnerable to developing AIDS after exposure to HIV.

Records on patients in Haiti or Africa are difficult to obtain. Cases for people of these origins that are known have been reported in Europe and the United States while the afflicted persons were in Europe and the United States. Thus, the data presented herein will comprise the reports from European countries and the United States.

AIDS IN EUROPE

Reported cases in various European countries as of June 30, 1985 totaled 1,226. From March through June 1985, the number of new cases reported to the World Health Organization increased mainly in France (6 to 7 new cases weekly).

The rate for each country was calculated from population estimates of the Institut National d'Etudes Demographiques in Paris. Excluding Belgium, the highest rate was 9.7 per million population for Switzerland, which was still quite low compared to that of the United States at 48.2 per million population (not shown; Table 4–10). When reviewing Table 4–10, note that some of the cases reported in these European countries are AIDS patients from Africa or the Caribbean who had been visiting or had emigrated to the reporting countries. This is particularly true of Belgium where 74% of the reported cases originated in Africa.

TABLE 4–10. Reported Acquired Immunodeficiency Syndrome Cases and Estimated Rates per Million Population – 18 European Countries, July 1, 1984–June 30, 1985

COUNTRY	JULY 1984	DEC. 1984	MARCH 1985	JUNE 1985	RATES*
Austria	–	13	13	18	2.4
Belgium	–	65	81	99	10.0
Czechoslovakia	–	0	0	0	0.0
Denmark	28	34	41	48	9.4
Federal Republic of Germany	79	135	162	220	3.6
Finland	–	5	5	6	1.2
France	180	260	307	392	7.0
Greece	2	6	7	9	0.9
Iceland	–	0	0	0	0.0
Italy	8	14	22	52	0.9
Luxembourg	–	–	–	1	2.5
Netherlands	21	42	52	66	4.6
Norway	–	5	8	11	2.6
Poland	–	0	0	0	0.0
Spain	14	18	29	38	1.0
Sweden	7	16	22	27	3.3
Switzerland	28	41	51	63	9.7
United Kingdom	54	108	140	176	3.1
Total	421	762	940	1,226	

* Per million population based on 1985 populations

Source: Morbidity and Mortality Weekly Report, Vol. 34, No. 38 September 1985.

The breakdown of cases according to sex revealed an 11:1 ratio of men to women (Table 4–11). As also shown, 42% of the cases fell in the 30 to 39 age bracket. Thirty patients were children under age 15 years. Many had a parent either with AIDS or in a high risk group for AIDS. But 8 patients had contracted the disease from

TABLE 4–11. Acquired Immunodeficiency Syndrome Cases, by Age Group and Sex—18 European Countries, Through June 30, 1985

AGE GROUP	MALES	FEMALES	UNKNOWN	SEX RATIO	TOTAL No. (%)
0–11 mos	6	6		1:1	12 (1.0)
1–4 yrs	6	5		1:1	11 (1.0)
5–9 yrs	2	1	1	2:1	4 (0.3)
10–14 yrs	3				3 (0.2)
15–19 yrs	5				5 (0.4)
20–29 yrs	207	45		5:1	252 (20.6)
30–39 yrs	490	28		18:1	518 (42.3)
40–49 yrs	295	11		27:1	306 (25.0)
50–59 yrs	83	8		10:1	91 (7.4)
≥ 60 yrs	12	1		12:1	13 (1.1)
Unknown	11				11 (1.0)
Total	1,120	105	1	11:1	1,226 (100.0)

Source: Morbidity and Mortality Weekly Report, Vol 34, No. 38 Sept. 1985

blood transfusions and 4 had contracted the disease with no determined risk factor.

The origin of AIDS victims and their risk factor involvement is shown in Table 4–12. As can be seen, the greatest proportion of AIDS victims, 70%, were homosexual males. Twenty percent had no known or identifiable risk factor profile, i.e., they were not homosexual males, I.V. drug users, transfusion recipients, or children of an AIDS afflicted mother.

The proportion of deaths among AIDS victims compared to the number of cases is shown in Fig. 4–13.

The cause of death among AIDS patients is listed in Table 4–13. The disease generally takes one of four forms. The pulmonary pattern generally exhibits itself as pneumocystis carinii pneumonia, *Legionella pneumophilia*, and cytomegalovirus infection marked by chest pain and pulmonary infiltrates noticeable on chest films. Those with the gastrointestinal pattern have diarrhea and weight loss which either may be caused by an enteric infection with cryptosporidium or have an unknown cause.

Other victims develop a chronic fever and suffer from weakness, malaise, and weight loss. Evidence of *Mycobacterium avium intracellulare* infections have been detected in liver biopsy examinations and bone marrow specimens of some of these individuals. Still other patients exhibit CNS involvement with focal brain lesions, aseptic meningitis, cerebral hemorrhage, and subacute encephalitis.

The most common malignancy is Kaposi's sarcoma. It has been found in 30% of all AIDS patients worldwide. This cancer is clinically both more aggressive and more widespread than non-AIDS-

TABLE 4–12. Acquired Immunodeficiency Syndrome Cases, by Patient Risk Group Geographic Origin—18 European Countries, Through June 30, 1985

	ORIGIN				TOTAL
PATIENT RISK GROUP	Europe	Caribbean islands	Africa	Other	No. (%)
1. Male homosexual or bisexual	809	4	10	30	853 (70)
2. I.V. drug abuser	48	–	–	–	48 (4)
3. Hemophilia patient	38	–	–	1	39 (3)
4. Transfusion recipient (without other risk factors)	20	–	5	–	25 (2)
5. 1- and 2-associated	15	–	1	2	18 (1)
6. No known risk factor					
males	49	22	76	2	149 (12)
females	25	9	36	–	70 (6)
7. Unknown	7	1	13	3	24 (2)
Total	1,011(82%)	36 (3%)	141 (12%)	38 (3%)	1,226

Source: Morbidity and Mortality Weekly Report, Vol. 34, No. 38 Sept. 1985.

Fig. 4–13. Deaths from AIDS vs number of cases 1981–1985*

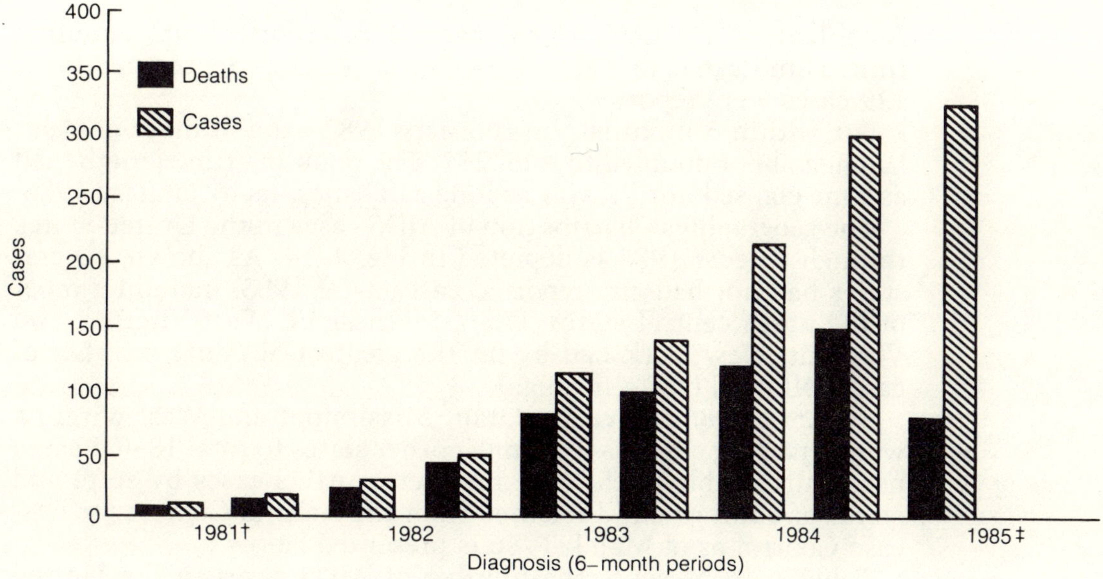

*Austria, Belgium, Czechoslovakia, Denmark, Federal Republic of Germany, Finland, France, Greece, Iceland, Italy, Luxembourg, Netherlands, Norway, Poland, Spain, Sweden, Switzerland, and the United Kingdom.

†Before 1981, 20 cases, including 12 deaths, were reported.

‡January–June 1985. An additional 12 cases (four deaths) with unknown dates of diagnosis were also reported.

Source: Monthly Morbidity and Mortality Report, Vol. 34, No. 38 Sept. 1985*

abetted Kaposi's sarcoma. Hodgkin's lymphoma and primary central nervous system lymphoma is also seen to a greater degree in AIDS patients than in nonaffected individuals.

Of the 626 European deaths analyzed in Table 4–13, 444 were from opportunistic infections, while 108 died of an opportunistic infection in combination with Kaposi's sarcoma, and 64 died of Kaposi's sarcoma alone.

TABLE 4–13. Acquired Immunodeficiency Syndrome Cases and Number of Deaths, by Disease Category — 18 European Countries,* Through June 30, 1985

DISEASE CATEGORY	CASES	(%)	DEATHS	(%)
Opportunistic infection	795	(65)	444	(56)
Kaposi's sarcoma	245	(20)	64	(26)
Opportunistic infection and Kaposi's sarcoma	171	(14)	108	(63)
Other	15	(1)	10	(67)
Total	1,226	(100)	626	(51)

*Austria, Belgium, Czechoslovakia, Denmark, Finalnd, France, Federal Republic of Germany, Greece, Iceland, Italy, Luxembourg, Netherlands, Norway, Poland, Spain, Sweden, Switzerland, and United Kingdom.
Source: Monthly Mortality and Weekly Report Vol. 34, No. 38 Sept. 1985

AIDS IN THE UNITED STATES

As of January 13, 1986, 16,458 cases were reported with doubling time as indicated in Table 4–14. Initially, as of September 1981, 129 cases were reported.

But within 5 months—by February 1982—the number of cases had just about doubled to total 257. The doubling time lengthened as time elapsed until it was as long as 11 months by January 1986.

The geographical distribution of AIDS cases in the United States through August 1983 is depicted in Fig. 4–14. As shown, several states had not had any reported cases as of 1983, including most of the north central states, Utah, Mississippi, West Virginia, and Vermont. New York had by far the greatest absolute number of cases followed by California.

By April 1986, however, Utah, Mississippi and West Virginia were reporting cases as were most other states to total 18,406 cases nationally (Table 4–15). The number of AIDS cases by state and status as adult or child released from the Atlanta Centers for Disease Control as of March 1986 is presented below.

Table 4–16 presents the number of AIDS cases in the United States according to the identified risk factor or mode of disease contraction. From the earliest period through the latest, the greatest proportion of AIDS patients were homosexual/bisexual men who had not been I.V. drug users. The next largest group consisted of I.V. drug users. As of September 1985, there were 485 adult cases that had no known or identified risk factor, no known mode of transmission. The reasons for this are several. Some cases lacked follow-up. Some patients died before interview. Others refused to be interviewed, while still others were from other countries where they may have contracted the disease through heterosexual contact. Ninety-nine on follow-up examination said that they were themselves prostitutes or had been to prostitutes before developing AIDS. Five percent of prostitutes tested for (HIV) in Seattle

TABLE 4–14. Doubling Times for Reported AIDS Victims

CASES REPORTED	DATE	(MONTHS)
129	September 1981	–
257	February 1982	5
514	July 1982	5
1,029	January 1983	6
2,057	August 1983	7
4,115	April 1984	8
8,229	February 1985	10
16,458	January 1986	11

Source: Morbidity and Mortality Weekly Report, Vol. 35, No. 2 January 1986

Fig. 4–14. Acquired immunodeficiency syndrome (AIDS) cases reported to CDC, by state—United States, as of August 1, 1983

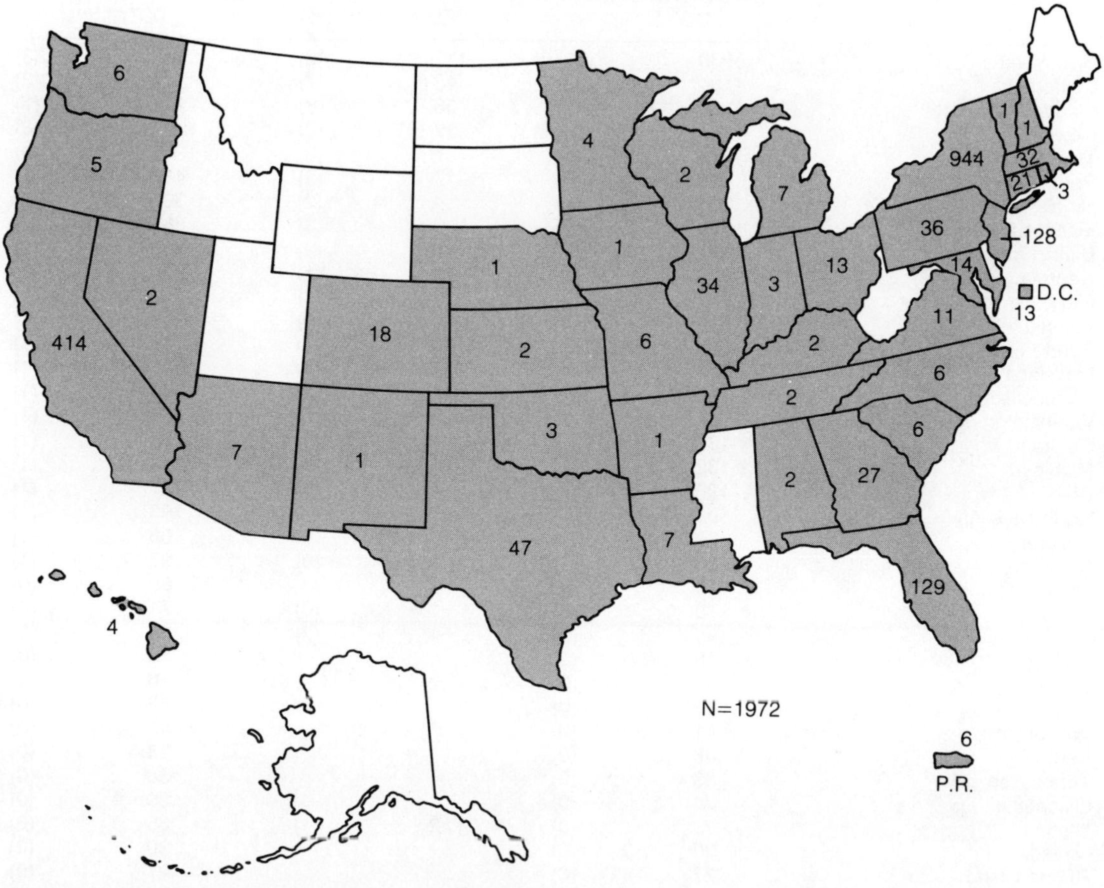

Source: Morbidity and Mortality Weekly Report, Vol. 32, No. 30 August 1983

had antibodies in their serum; 8 of 10 other prostitutes who tested positively said they were I.V. drug users.

Although HTLV-III/LAV (HIV) has been found in tears and saliva as well as in the blood and stool of infected persons, transmission of AIDS through tears or saliva is not documented. A case was reported in February 1986 of a mother who contracted AIDS while caring for her infant son who had contracted the disease through a blood transfusion. The child suffered from intestinal abnormalities, had undergone several surgical procedures, and his mother had frequent contact with the child's blood and other body fluids. She typically did not wear gloves or always wash her hands after contact but reported no needle sticks or exposure of open skin abrasions.

TABLE 4–15. AIDS Cases Reported to CDC

RESIDENCE	ADULT/ADOLESCENT (%)		PEDIATRIC†† (%)		TOTAL (%)	
New York	6030	(33)	111	(42)	6141	(33)
California	4194	(23)	18	(7)	4212	(23)
Florida	1189	(7)	35	(13)	1224	(7)
New Jersey	1077	(6)	32	(12)	1109	(6)
Texas	1005	(6)	7	(3)	1012	(5)
Pennsylvania	405	(2)	7	(3)	412	(2)
Illinois	391	(2)	4	(2)	395	(2)
Massachusetts	358	(2)	9	(3)	367	(2)
District of Columbia	337	(2)	4	(2)	341	(2)
Georgia	308	(2)	2	(1)	310	(2)
Maryland	261	(1)	2	(1)	263	(1)
Virginia	213	(1)	5	(2)	218	(1)
Puerto Rico	207	(1)	3	(1)	210	(1)
Louisiana	204	(1)	3	(1)	207	(1)
Connecticut	198	(1)	7	(3)	205	(1)
Washington	204	(1)			204	(1)
Colorado	163	(1)	1	(0)	164	(1)
Michigan	132	(1)	1	(0)	133	(1)
Ohio	126	(1)	1	(0)	127	(1)
North Carolina	109	(1)			109	(1)
Arizona	98	(1)			98	(1)
Missouri	96	(1)	1	(0)	97	(1)
Minnesota	85	(0)			85	(0)
Indiana	70	(0)	1	(0)	71	(0)
South Carolina	65	(0)	4	(2)	69	(0)
Oregon	66	(0)			66	(0)
Hawaii	56	(0)			56	(0)
Alabama	42	(0)			42	(0)
Wisconsin	41	(0)			41	(0)
Kentucky	38	(0)			38	(0)
Tennessee	38	(0)			38	(0)
Oklahoma	36	(0)			36	(0)
Utah	33	(0)	2	(1)	35	(0)
Nevada	30	(0)			30	(0)
Rhode Island	27	(0)			27	(0)
Delaware	24	(0)			24	(0)
New Mexico	22	(0)			22	(0)
Kansas	21	(0)			21	(0)
Iowa	19	(0)	1	(0)	20	(0)
Arkansas	18	(0)			18	(0)
Mississippi	16	(0)			16	(0)
Alaska	15	(0)			15	(0)
Maine	15	(0)			15	(0)
Nebraska	13	(0)			13	(0)
West Virginia	12	(0)	1	(0)	13	(0)
New Hampshire	11	(0)	1	(0)	12	(0)
Other States/Territories (9)	25	(0)			25	(0)
Total - USA	18143	(100)	263	(100)	18406	(100)

Source: Unpublished data Atlanta Centers For Disease Control

Health-care workers and those caring for AIDS patients have been advised to wear gloves routinely during contact with the mucous membranes or nonintact skin of AIDS patients and when

TABLE 4–16. Acquired Immunodeficiency Syndrome Cases Reported by Year and Yearly Percent Increases, by Patient Group — United States, Through January 13, 1986

	BEFORE 1/14/82	1/14/82–1/13/83		1/14/83–1/13/84		1/14/84–1/13/85		1/14/85–1/13/86		
PATIENT GROUP	No.	No.	(% Inc)*	No.	(% Inc)*	No.	(% Inc)*	No.	(% Inc)*	Total
Adult										
Homosexual/bisexual men and I.V. drug users	16	66	(312.5)	211	(219.7)	418	(98.1)	599	(43.3)	1,310
Homosexual/bisexual men not I.V. drug users	178	473	(165.7)	1,341	(183.5)	2,939	(119.2)	5,669	(92.9)	10,600
I.V. drug users	22	138	(527.3)	392	(184.1)	785	(100.3)	1,429	(82.0)	2,766
Hemophilia patients	0	7	(0.0)	10	(42.9)	38	(280.0)	69	(81.6)	124
Heterosexual contacts	1	10	(900.0)	18	(80.0)	53	(194.4)	100	(88.7)	182
Transfusion recipients	0	6	(0.0)	28	(366.7)	56	(100.0)	171	(205.4)	261
None of the above/other:										
No identified risks:	3	28	(833.3)	76	(171.4)	131	(72.4)	348	(165.6)	586
Born outside U.S.†	7	48	(585.7)	85	(77.1)	114	(34.1)	144	(26.3)	398
Subtotal	227	776	(241.9)	2,161	(178.5)	4,534	(109.8)	8,529	(88.1)	16,227
Pediatric	0	16	(0.0)	35	(118.8)	48	(37.1)	132	(175.0)	231
Total	227	792	(248.9)	2,196	(177.3)	4,582	(108.7)	8,661	(89.0)	16,458

* Percent increase
† Includes persons born in countries in which most AIDS cases have not been associated with known risk factors
Source: Morbidity and Mortality Weekly Report, Vol. 35, No. 2 Jan. 1986

handling anything soiled with blood or body secretions. They have been advised to follow the caution regimen for hepatitis B, since this virus and the AIDS virus appear to have a similar transmission pattern. Both of them are transmitted through sexual contact, especially anal intercourse among homosexual men, parenteral exposure to contaminated blood or blood products, including I.V. drug abuse, and perinatal transmission from mothers to offspring. Although many cases of hepatitis B are of unknown transmission—and transmission through insect bite is suspected—the latter has not at this time been listed for AIDS. The focal pattern of Kaposis sarcoma in tropical Africa and the positive reaction to the AIDS antibody test among malaria victims in Africa and Venezuela raise a question about possible insect transmission. Those who refuse to consider this possibility point to the lower density of the AIDS virus in blood compared to that of hepatitis B. The incidence of hepatitis-B infection following puncture wounds in health-care workers varies from 10% to 30 percent. But the risk for AIDS after such an exposure is estimated at only 1%.

The AIDS cases and the AIDS patients who have died in the United States between 1981 and 1986 are shown in Fig. 4–15. Those with AIDS in 1981 are almost all dead. Patients diagnosed between 1982 and 1983 reflect a greater proportion of survivors.

Fig. 4–15. Acquired immunodeficiency syndrome cases and known deaths, by 6-month period of report to CDC—United States, through January 13, 1986

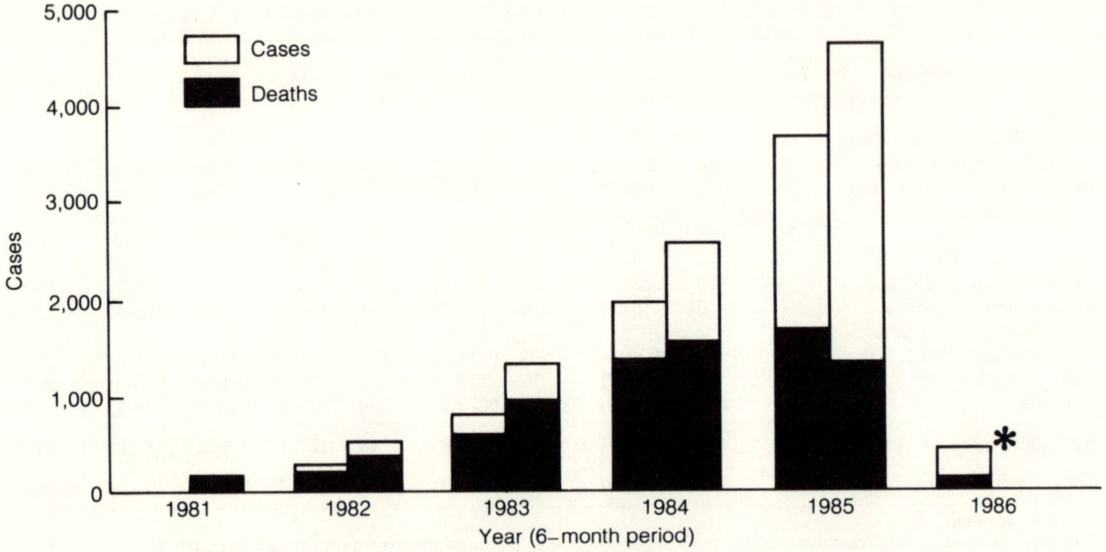

*Data incomplete.

Source: Morbidity and Mortality Weekly Report, Vol. 35, No. 2 Jan. 1986

The data show that AIDS victims survive as long as 5 years after diagnosis but not longer.

The treatment for AIDS is specific to the type of infection or malignancy that victims develop. Generally, pneumocystis carinii pneumonia is treated with TMP-SMZ or as second choice in the allergic, pentamidine-isetionate.

The World Health Organization noted in June 1986 that 10 million people throughout the world are now infected with the AIDS virus, which they can transmit to others. As AIDS cases approach epidemic proportions and include the heterosexual community in Africa, medical observers are growing uneasy about their knowledge of the disease. Its modes of transmissability and containability are of particular concern. The U.S. medical community has stressed the mutable nature of the virus and its non-casual transmissability. However, in a letter to *Lancet* in September 1985, 3 scientists at the Pasteur Institute reported that HIV can survive in a dry state at room temperature for as long as 10 days. These same 3 researchers, Sinouss, Nugeyre and Chermann, warned that added disinfectant precautions should be taken by hospitals, laboratories, and dentists to prevent the spread of AIDS.

Genetic engineering techniques are being employed by U.S. and French scientists to produce fragments of HIV so that a vaccine can be developed that will not employ the whole virus. Most researchers doubt that a vaccine will be developed before 1990, and efforts to control the spread of AIDS will likely be intensified.

As with many other infections discussed in this volume, venereal diseases are preventable. Most—with the exception of AIDS—are treatable. But the human suffering, pain, and debility and the billions spent to treat these diseases make prevention the best and first avenue of defense.

Nosocomial And Other Infections 5

Nosocomial infections are acquired by approximately 5% to 6% of all hospital patients in the United States. One percent of these infections cause death, while 3.6% contribute to death. The cost for treating patients who contract these infections is estimated at $1 billion annually.

NOSOCOMIAL INFECTIONS

Noscomial infections develop in patients for several reasons. Some wound infections develop after surgery; some opportunistic infections develop in patients receiving immune suppressing treatments; some are due to the superstrain microbial environment of hospitals where bacteria have developed resistance to frequently used antibiotics. Lack of proper sterilization procedures, isolative precautions, and meticulous housekeeping may also contribute.

In the mid-1980s, the National Nosocomial Infections Study (NNIS) group released its findings after analyzing hospital infection data reported by 54 hospitals across the country during 1983. Teaching hospitals were primarily included in the group of hospitals, but nonteaching institutions were also represented. They ranged in size from 80 to more than 1,200 beds and were state owned, for profit, and not for profit.

The data were stratified into three categories: data from nonteaching hospitals, small teaching hospitals, and large teaching

TABLE 5–1. Infection Rates (cases/1,000 discharges), by Hospital Category, 1983

HOSPITAL CATEGORY	INFECTIONS	DISCHARGES	RATE
Nonteaching	6,845	281,122	24.4
Small teaching	7,875	255,601	30.8
Large teaching	13,528	328,559	41.2
Total	28,248	865,282	32.7

Source: CDC Surveillance Summary Vol. 33, No. 2SS

TABLE 5–2. Infection Rates (cases/1,000 discharges), by Hospital Category and Service, 1983

HOSPITAL CATEGORY	SURG	MED	GYN	OB	NEW	PED
Nonteaching	32.1	27.8	13.5	10.3	8.9	2.2
Small teaching	42.6	35.0	35.6	15.6	11.0	11.0
Large teaching	57.5	47.5	31.4	16.9	18.4	16.8
Total	44.3	37.1	27.4	14.7	13.4	11.1

Key: SURG, Surgical; MED, Medicine; GYN, Gynecology; OB, Obstetrics; NEW, Newborn; and PED, Pediatrics
Source: CDC Summary Surveillance, Vol. 33, No. 2SS

TABLE 5–3. Infection Rates (cases/1,000 discharges), by Hospital Category and Site of Infection, 1983

HOSPITAL CATEGORY	UTI	SWI	LRI	CUT	BACT	OTHER
Nonteaching	11.1	4.0	4.1	1.3	1.3	2.5
Small teaching	13.0	6.3	4.6	1.5	1.7	3.9
Large teaching	15.0	7.0	7.5	2.7	3.8	5.2
Total	13.1	5.8	5.5	1.9	2.4	3.9

UTI, urinary tract infection; SWI, surgical wound infection; LRI, lower respiratory infection; CUT, cutaneous infection; and BACT, primary bacteremia
Source: CDC Surveillance Survey Vol. 33, No. 2SS

TABLE 5–4. Percentage Distribution of Infections at Each of Major Sites, by Hospital Category, 1983

	HOSPITAL CATEGORY			
Site	Nonteaching	Small teaching	Large teaching	Total
UTI	45.8	42.2	36.3	40.2
SWI	16.1	20.4	16.8	17.7
LRI	16.5	14.8	18.4	16.9
BACT	5.8	5.3	9.1	7.3
CUT	5.7	4.8	6.6	5.9
Other	10.1	12.5	12.7	12.0

UTI, urinary tract infection; SWI, surgical wound infection; LR, lower respiratory infection; CUT, cutaneous infection; and BACT, primary bacteremia
Source: CDC Surveillance Summary, Vol. 33, No. 2SS

TABLE 5–5. Site-specific Infection Rates (cases/1,000 discharges), by Service, 1983

NONTEACHING HOSPITALS

	SITE						
Service	UTI	SWI	LRI	BACT	CUT	Other	All sites
Surg	13.3	8.9	5.1	1.3	1.2	2.3	32.1
Med	15.3	0.4	5.6	2.2	1.3	3.1	27.8
Gyn	8.2	3.8	0.4	0.2	0.2	0.7	13.5
Ob	2.8	4.1	0.2	0.2	0.3	2.7	10.3
Ped	0.0	0.5	0.5	0.1	0.3	0.8	2.2
New	0.3	0.1	1.4	1.3	3.8	2.2	8.9
Total	11.1	4.0	4.1	1.3	1.4	2.5	24.4

SMALL TEACHING HOSPITALS

	SITE						
Service	UTI	SWI	LRI	BACT	CUT	Other	All sites
Surg	16.0	13.5	6.6	1.6	1.0	3.9	42.6
Med	19.1	0.7	6.7	2.6	1.5	4.5	35.0
Gyn	20.6	11.8	0.8	0.4	0.3	1.6	35.6
Ob	3.4	8.0	0.7	0.3	0.4	2.7	15.6
Ped	1.4	0.6	1.3	1.6	1.1	5.0	11.0
New	0.4	0.2	0.8	1.3	4.8	3.4	11.0
Total	13.0	6.3	4.6	1.7	1.5	3.9	30.8

LARGE TEACHING HOSPITALS

	SITE						
Service	UTI	SWI	LRI	BACT	CUT	Other	All sites
Surg	19.2	15.5	10.1	4.3	2.9	5.5	57.5
Med	21.1	1.3	10.2	5.5	2.9	6.4	47.5
Gyn	16.2	7.7	3.0	1.1	0.7	2.2	31.4
Ob	4.7	7.6	0.4	0.7	0.6	3.0	16.0
Ped	2.2	2.4	3.2	2.4	2.3	4.4	16.8
New	0.7	0.4	4.0	2.6	5.5	5.2	18.4
Total	15.0	7.0	7.5	3.8	2.7	5.2	41.2

*See key to abbreviations, Tables 5–2 and 5–4.

hospitals. Not surprisingly, the hospitals generally receiving the most difficult cases and doing the most invasive procedures—teaching hospitals—reported higher infection rates (Table 5–1).

The infection rates in each type of hospital were highest for the surgical service and lowest in the newborn and pediatric units (Table 5–2). Isolation precautions are often used in pediatric and newborn units, which may help to reduce the incidence of infection. Children also have shorter hospital stays. Their nosocomial infections are thought to be viral. Since only a small proportion of participating hospitals have diagnostic virology laboratories, many of these nosocomial infections may go undetected. In small teach-

Fig. 5–1. Distribution of infections, by etiology, 1983

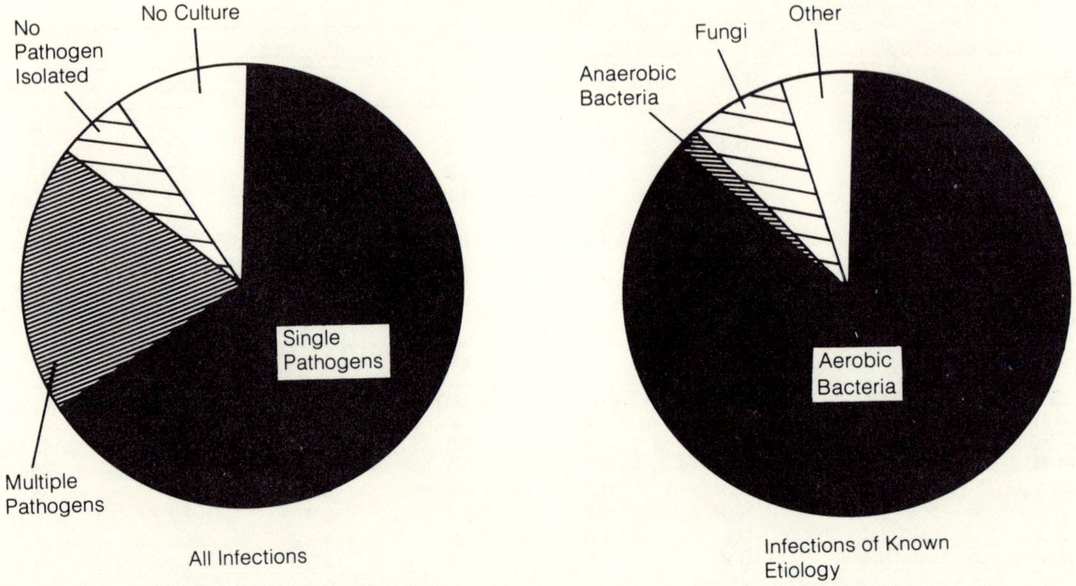

Source: CDC Surveillance Summary, Vol. 33, No. 2SS

TABLE 5–6. Most Frequently Isolated Pathogens and their Percentage Distribution on Each Service, 1983

PATHOGEN	MED†	SURG	OB	GYN	PED	NEW	TOTAL ISOLATES	%
E. coli	21.3	16.3	20.6	32.5	11.4	7.7	5,779	18.6
S. aureus	8.9	10.8	9.5	6.9	16.8	34.1	3,356	10.8
Enterococci	9.9	10.9	15.3	17.2	5.4	6.3	3,308	10.7
P. aeruginosa	10.8	12.4	1.2	3.2	7.4	4.4	3,286	10.6
Klebsiella spp.	8.7	7.0	2.8	5.5	7.7	5.4	2,288	7.4
Coagulase-negative staphylococci	5.1	6.1	6.7	4.9	12.4	14.6	1,892	6.1
Enterobacter spp.	5.2	7.3	2.0	3.7	1.5	2.1	1,811	5.8
Proteus spp.	5.9	5.6	3.2	4.7	2.4	1.0	1,667	5.4
Candida spp.	6.4	4.6	0.4	1.6	8.9	3.3	1,570	5.1
Serratia spp.	2.3	2.6	0.2	0.2	1.3	1.4	691	2.2
Other fungi	1.9	1.4	0.3	0.6	1.1	0.6	471	1.5
Bacteroides spp.	0.6	1.8	4.7	3.4	1.1	0.1	439	1.4
Group B *streptococcus*	0.7	0.7	9.6	4.2	1.1	5.6	418	1.3
Citrobacter spp.	1.5	1.4	0.8	0.4	0.4	0.5	403	1.3
Other anaerobes	0.9	0.9	4.1	2.2	0.9	0.6	337	1.1
All others*	9.9	10.2	18.6	8.8	20.2	12.3	3,296	10.6
Number of isolates	11,864	15,086	1,182	1,240	542	1,098	31,012	100.0

* No other pathogen accounted for more than 3% of the isolates on any service.
† See key to abbreviations, Table 5–2.
Source: CDC Surveillance Summary, Vol. 33, No. 2SS

TABLE 5–7. Fifteen Most Frequently Isolated Pathogens and their Percentage Distribution for Each Site of Infection, 1983

PATHOGEN	UTI[†]	SWI	LRI	BACT	CUT	Other	TOTAL ISOLATES	%
E. coli	31.7	11.4	7.1	9.5	7.7	7.3	5,779	18.6
S. aureus	1.6	19.0	12.8	12.8	33.3	16.4	3,356	10.8
Enterococci	14.9	11.4	1.6	7.3	9.5	7.3	3,308	10.7
P. aeruginosa	12.5	8.1	15.1	6.1	7.2	6.2	3,286	10.6
Klebsiella spp.	7.6	4.8	12.8	9.1	4.4	4.0	2,288	7.4
Coagulase-negative staphylococci	3.7	8.4	1.1	14.2	9.5	11.1	1,892	6.1
Enterobacter spp.	4.4	6.9	10.0	6.9	4.1	4.1	1,811	5.8
Proteus spp.	7.3	5.0	4.4	1.7	3.5	3.2	1,667	5.4
Candida spp.	5.1	1.4	4.2	5.6	4.5	13.4	1,570	5.1
Serratia spp.	1.2	2.0	5.6	2.8	1.8	1.8	691	2.2
Other fungi	2.0	0.4	1.8	1.0	0.4	2.3	471	1.5
Bacteroides spp.	0.0	4.4	0.2	3.4	1.0	1.9	439	1.3
Group B *streptococcus*	1.0	1.8	0.7	2.8	1.3	1.7	418	1.3
Citrobacter spp.	1.4	1.3	1.7	1.1	1.1	0.9	403	1.3
Other anaerobes	0.0	2.3	0.0	2.1	0.9	4.2	337	1.1
All others*	5.6	11.4	20.9	13.6	9.8	14.2	3,296	10.6
Number of isolates	13,165	6,163	4,490	2,292	1,798	3,104	31,012	100.0

* No other pathogen accounted for more than 3% of the isolates at any site.
† See key to abbreviations, Table 5–3.
Source: CDC Surveillance Summary, Vol. 33, No. 2SS

ing hospitals, the infection rate on the medical and gynecologic services was similar. After the surgical service, in the nonteaching and large teaching hospitals, the rates were highest for the medical service.

The most common infection site was urinary followed by surgical wound infections. The infection rates at the leading infection sites listed by type of hospital are shown in Table 5–3.

The percentage distribution of infections at each site according to hospital is presented in Table 5–4. As shown, the largest proportion of infections at each kind of hospital is that of urinary tract infections. At large teaching hospitals a greater proportion of infections were lower respiratory infections than surgical wound infections. This finding differed for non-teaching hospitals and small teaching hospitals.

Table 5–5 shows the distribution of infections by the service in which they occurred. At each type of hospital, urinary-tract infections developed most often on the medical service.

Information was available on the etiology of the infections and the agents were mostly aerobic bacteria (Fig. 5–1). Most infections were caused by a single pathogen.

TABLE 5–8. Five Most Common Pathogens Isolated and Percentage of Total within Each Site and Service, 1983

	SITE									
	UTI*		SWI		LRI		CUT		BACT	
SERVICE	Pathogen	%	Pathogen	%	Pathogen	%	Pathogen	%	Pathogen	%
Medicine	*E. coli*	32.7	*S. aureus*	15.7	*P. aeruginosa*	14.7	*S. aureus*	29.0	*S. aureus*	14.7
	Enterococci	14.2	Enterococci	13.4	*S. aureus*	14.1	Coag-neg *Staph.*	9.7	Coag-neg *Staph.*	13.9
	P. aeruginosa	11.1	*E. coli*	11.1	*Klebsiella* spp.	13.3	*P. aeruginosa*	8.9	*E. coli*	10.7
	Klebsiella spp.	8.2	*P. aeruginosa*	10.8	*Enterobacter* spp.	9.2	*Enterobacter* spp.	7.5	*Klebsiella* spp.	10.6
	Proteus spp.	8.0	*Enterobacter* spp.	8.0	*E. coli*	7.5	*E. coli*	7.1	*P. aeruginosa*	7.5
Surgery	*E. coli*	28.6	*S. aureus*	19.6	*P. aeruginosa*	15.6	*S. aureus*	19.2	Coag-neg *Staph.*	13.1
	P. aeruginosa	16.2	Enterococci	11.3	*Klebsiella* spp.	12.4	Enterococci	13.5	*S. aureus*	12.0
	Enterococci	14.4	*E. coli*	10.9	*Enterobacter* spp.	11.4	*P. aeruginosa*	10.0	*Enterobacter* spp.	10.3
	Klebsiella spp.	7.3	*P. aeruginosa*	9.0	*S. aureus*	11.1	Coag-neg *Staph.*	8.9	Enterococci	9.6
	Proteus spp.	7.1	Coag-neg *Staph.*	8.4	*E. coli*	6.9	*E. coli*	8.0	*E. coli*	8.8
Gynecology	*E. coli*	43.7	*E. coli*	17.2	*Klebsiella* spp.	17.2	Enterococci	25.0	*Bacteroides* spp.	14.7
	Enterococci	20.2	*S. aureus*	16.6	*S. aureus*	17.2	*E. coli*	20.8	*Klebsiella* spp.	11.8
	Klebsiella spp.	6.1	Enterococci	13.8	*P. aeruginosa*	10.3	*S. aureus*	20.8	*E. coli*	8.8
	Proteus spp.	5.2	*Bacteroides* spp.	9.5	*Enterobacter* spp.	10.3	*Proteus* spp.	8.3	Coag-neg *Staph.*	5.9
	Group B *Strep.*	4.5	Coag-neg *Staph.*	7.4	*E. coli*	3.4	*Enterobacter* spp.	4.2	*Proteus* spp.	5.9
					Coag-neg *Staph.*	3.4				
					Group B *Strep.*	3.4				
Obstetrics	*E. coli*	35.1	*S. aureus*	14.5	*S. aureus*	12.5	*S. aureus*	35.6	Group B *Strep.*	22.2
	Enterococci	27.0	*E. coli*	13.6	*E. coli*	8.3	*E. coli*	17.8	*S. aureus*	11.1
	Group B *Strep.*	7.1	Enterococci	10.0	*Klebsiella* spp.	8.3	Coag-neg *Staph.*	11.1	Coag-neg *Staph.*	11.1
	Klebsiella spp.	4.8	Group B *Strep.*	9.5	Enterococci	4.2	Enterococci	8.9	*Bacteroides* spp.	11.1
	Proteus spp.	4.5	Coag-neg *Staph.*	9.1			*Proteus* spp.	6.7	Other anaerobes	8.9
							Klebsiella spp.	6.7		
Pediatrics	*E. coli*	38.6	*S. aureus*	28.8	*Klebsiella* spp.	16.7	*S. aureus*	35.2	Coag-neg *Staph.*	18.0
	Candida spp.	16.9	Coag-neg *Staph.*	16.4	*P. aeruginosa*	13.0	Coag-neg *Staph.*	14.8	*S. aureus*	12.4
	P. aeruginosa	10.8	*E. coli*	8.2	*S. aureus*	13.0	Enterococci	8.0	*Klebsiella* spp.	10.1
	Enterococci	8.4	*P. aeruginosa*	6.8	*Candida* spp.	7.4	*E. coli*	6.8	*E. coli*	9.0
	Klebsiella spp.	8.4	Enterococci	6.8	*E. coli*	3.7	*Candida* spp.	6.8	*Candida* spp.	6.7
			Klebsiella spp.	6.8			*P. aeruginosa*	6.8		
Newborn	*E. coli*	25.5	*S. aureus*	30.4	*S. aureus*	21.1	*S. aureus*	60.2	Coag-neg *Staph.*	22.0
	Klebsiella spp.	15.7	Coag-neg *Staph.*	26.1	*P. aeruginosa*	16.7	Coag-neg *Staph.*	9.2	Group B *Strep.*	19.6
	Enterococci	9.8	Enterococci	13.0	Coag-neg *Staph.*	12.3	*E. coli*	6.3	Enterococci	8.9
	S. aureus	7.8	*Klebsiella* spp.	13.0	*Klebsiella* spp.	11.4	Enterococci	6.3	*S. aureus*	7.1
	Enterobacter spp.	5.9	*P. aeruginosa*	8.7	*E. coli*	7.0	*Klebsiella* spp.	2.9	*E .coli*	6.0

* See key to abbreviations, Table 5–3.
Source: CDC Surveillance Summary, Vol. 33, No. 2SS

TABLE 5–9. Percentage of Infections* with Secondary Bacteremia, by Service and Hospital Category, 1983

HOSPITAL	SURG†	MED	GYN	OB	NEW	PED	ALL SERVICES
Non teaching	3.8	5.1	1.2	3.7	1.1	0.0	4.2
Small teaching	4.4	6.3	0.6	2.6	3.0	6.7	4.7
Large teaching	6.5	7.5	2.6	3.6	9.9	12.1	6.8
All hospitals	5.2	6.5	1.6	3.2	6.0	9.6	5.5

* Excluding primary bacteremia
† See key to abbreviations, Table 5–2.
Source: CDC surveillance Summary, Vol. 33, No. 2SS

TABLE 5–10. Percentage of Infections with Secondary Bacteremia, by Site* and Hospital Category, 1983

HOSPITAL	SITE					
	UTI†	SWI	LRI	CUT	Other‡	All sites
Nonteaching	3.2	4.6	4.0	4.6	7.6	4.2
Small teaching	2.9	4.4	5.6	4.2	10.8	4.7
Large teaching	3.8	6.0	5.9	6.6	17.5	6.8
All hospitals	3.4	5.2	5.4	5.6	13.5	5.5

* Excluding primary bacteremia.
† See key to abbreviations, Table 5–4.
‡ Most frequently associated with cardiovascular (55.3%), arterial (8.7%), intra-abdominal (8.1%), central nervous system (6.1%), and burn infections (4.6%).
Source: CDC Surveillance Summary, Vol. 33, No. 2SS

A list of the most common pathogens is presented in Table 5–6. *E. Coli* accounted for the highest proportion of infections on each medical service. Enterococci were the causes of infection most often on the Ob and Gyn services. The distribution of pathogens according to the site of infection is presented in Table 5–7. *S. aureus* more than most other agents was responsible for surgical wound and cutaneous infections.

The breakdown for the pathogens responsible for specific infections occurring on each service is presented in Table 5–8.

The study defined secondary bacteremia as a bloodstream infection with an organism that was also isolated from an infection at another site. The pediatric, newborn, and medical services had the highest proportion of secondary bacteremia. Services with the fewest episodes of secondary bacteremia were obstetrics and gynecology (Table 5–9).

Urinary-tract infections resulted in the fewest secondary infections (Table 5–10).

Secondary infection developed most often with infections caused by Bacteroides spp., *S. aureus*, Acinetobacter spp. group B *Streptococcus,* and *Providencia* spp. (Table 5–11).

TABLE 5–11. Ten Pathogens with Highest Percentage of Associated Secondary Bacteremia, by Hospital Category, 1983

PATHOGEN	NONTEACHING		SMALL TEACHING		LARGE TEACHING		All hospitals	
	Number of infections	Percentage with secondary bact.	Number of infections	Percentage with secondary bact.	Number of infections	Percentage with secondary bact.	Number of infections	Percentage with secondary bact.
Bacteroides spp.	24	16.7	65	13.8	53	17.0	142	15.5
Serratia spp.	123	9.8	115	10.4	241	13.7	479	11.9
S. aureus	648	7.7	828	8.6	1,274	16.0	2,750	11.8
Acinetobacter	26	0.0	27	0.0	94	18.1	147	11.6
Group B *streptococcus*	57	7.0	87	8.0	100	16.0	244	11.1
Providencia spp.	14	7.1	13	7.7	19	15.8	46	10.9
Coagulase-negative staphylococcus	212	4.2	356	6.5	550	9.5	1,118	7.5
Enterobacter spp.	285	5.3	321	4.2	601	9.7	1,207	7.4
Klebsiella spp.	366	4.4	404	4.2	718	9.7	1,488	6.9
P. aeruginosa	773	5.0	644	7.6	1,209	5.7	2,626	6.0

Source: CDC Surveillance Summary, Vol. 33, No. 2SS

The number of resistant isolates divided by the number of sensitive or resistant organisms reflected the measure of resistance used in the study. Again, as in earlier studies methicillin-resistant

TABLE 5–12. Percentage of Infections Reported as Having Caused or Contributed to Patient Death, 1983

HOSPITAL CATEGORY	NUMBER OF INFECTIONS	PERCENTAGE THAT CAUSED DEATH	PERCENTAGE THAT CONTRIBUTED TO DEATH
Nonteaching	6,728	0.5	3.7
Small teaching	7,140	1.3	4.0
Large teaching	12,228	0.8	3.4
Total	26,096	0.9	3.6

Antimicrobial resistance of *S. aureus*, 1983:

HOSPITAL CATEGORY	NUMBER RESISTANT (%)									
	Methicillin		Gentamicin		Clindamycin		Chloramphenicol		Erythromycin	
Nonteaching	22	(4.1)	42	(8.1)	50	(7.8)	33	(6.0)	80	(12.3)
Small teaching	32	(3.6)	37	(4.9)	49	(6.0)	24	(2.8)	88	(9.5)
Large teaching	108	(7.8)	127	(12.3)	158	(10.6)	85	(6.4)	239	(15.9)

Antimicrobial resistance of *E. coli*, 1983:

HOSPITAL CATEGORY	NUMBER RESISTANT (%)									
	Gentamicin		Tobramycin		Amikacin		Cefotaxime		Moxalactam	
Nonteaching	23	(1.6)	18	(1.6)	26	(2.5)	3	(3.0)	1	(2.2)
Small teaching	42	(2.3)	25	(2.1)	18	(4.0)	5	(5.0)	4	(7.1)
Large teaching	48	(2.1)	47	(2.0)	28	(2.2)	8	(1.8)	6	(1.8)

Antimicrobial resistance of *K. pneumoniae*, 1983:

HOSPITAL CATEGORY	NUMBER RESISTANT (%)									
	Gentamicin		Tobramycin		Amikacin		Cefotaxime		Moxalactam	
Nonteaching	13	(3.3)	7	(2.2)	12	(4.2)	2	(4.2)	2	(7.4)
Small teaching	16	(3.3)	9	(2.7)	6	(4.9)	3	(11.5)	1	(4.3)
Large teaching	111	(13.2)	93	(11.0)	16	(2.8)	14	(4.6)	3	(1.6)

Antimicrobial resistance of *S. marcescens*, 1983:

HOSPITAL CATEGORY	NUMBER RESISTANT (%)									
	Gentamicin		Tobramycin		Amikacin		Cefotaxime		Moxalactam	
Nonteaching	7	(5.3)	12	(10.8)	3	(3.0)	0	(0)	3	(10.7)
Small teaching	5	(4.1)	8	(7.9)	5	(8.9)	4	(10.5)	2	(7.4)
Large teaching	38	(12.7)	38	(13.3)	16	(10.4)	10	(12.5)	11	(10.9)

Antimicrobial resistance of *P. aeruginosa*, 1983:

HOSPITAL CATEGORY	NUMBER RESISTANT (%)									
	Gentamicin		Tobramycin		Amikacin		Cefotaxime		Moxalactam	
Nonteaching	131	(17.5)	66	(9.3)	45	(7.7)	56	(72.7)	45	(38.8)
Small teaching	68	(9.3)	21	(3.5)	36	(10.8)	106	(51.2)	87	(46.5)
Large teaching	208	(16.2)	91	(6.7)	62	(6.3)	162	(44.5)	107	(26.5)

Source: CDC Surveillance Summary, Vol. 33, No. 2SS

S. aureus was most frequently reported by large teaching hospitals, and reported in increased proportion at nonteaching and small teaching hospitals. *S. aureus* resistance to gentamicin increased at small teaching hospitals. These findings, together with the resistances of other pathogens and the percentage of infections that directly or indirectly led to death in 1983, are shown in Table 5–12.

The report disclaims somewhat the resistance data for cefotaxime and moxalactam resistance since the numbers of tested *K. pneumoniae* and *S. marcescens* specimens were small. It also notes the increased number of primary infections due to coagulase-negative staphylococci, especially on pediatric and newborn wards and as the pathogen involved in more bacteremia on all services. Studies suggest that the increasing use of long-line catheters may be responsible for this trend.

OTHER COMMON INFECTIOUS DISEASES

Although many bacterial organisms commonly cause infection in hospital populations, evidence exists that undetected viral infections also affect pediatric and infant patients. Hence, the current picture of the incidence of nosocomial infections may be greatly underestimated. Since susceptibility of children to viral infections is of course well known, our discussion of infectious disease would be incomplete without considering the common viral childhood diseases.

Many of these diseases have a greatly reduced incidence today because of the development of vaccines during the last several decades. Figure 5–2 shows the decline in incidence of polio, pertussis, mumps, measles, and rubella in the United States since each vaccine became available. Especially marked is the decline in polio since the introduction of the vaccine in 1955 when about 29,000 cases were reported to the Atlanta Centers for Disease Control. By 1960, the reported cases had fallen to 3,000. By 1975, only 8 cases were reported. Between 1969 and 1982, only 40 cases were reported cumulatively; they occurred in three localized outbreaks, two of which were among nonimmunized religious groups.

MEASLES

The incidence of measles has fallen from 385,000 cases in 1963 to 22,000 by 1968. But there have been setbacks in 1971 and in 1976/

Fig. 5–2. Reported cases of selected diseases before and after availability of immunization, United States, 1940–80

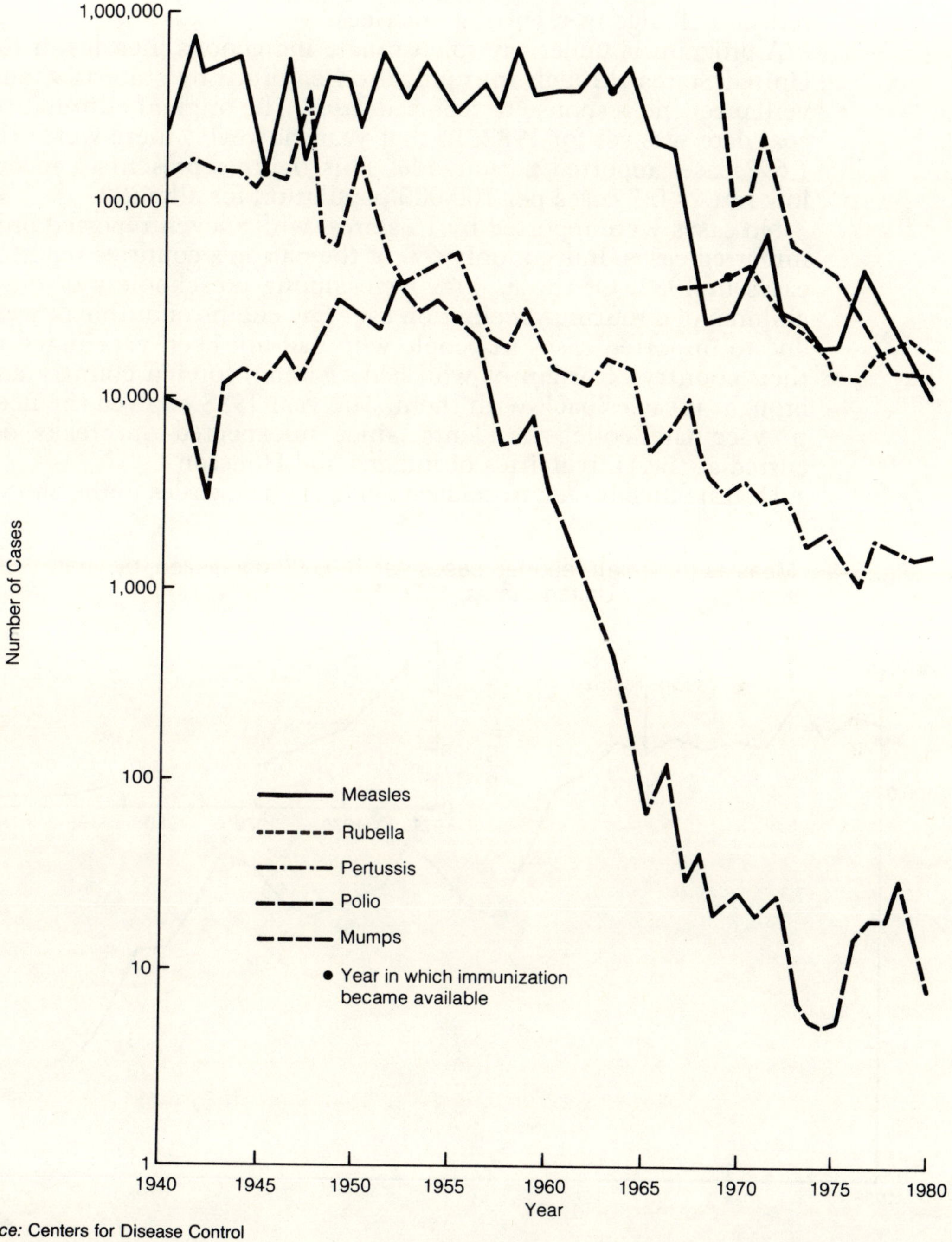

Source: Centers for Disease Control

77 (Fig. 5–2). It has not yet been determined if these outbreaks reflect failure to immunize high risk children or if they merely reflect a change in reporting practices.

A program is underway to eliminate indigenous measles in the United States through immunization enforced by state law, surveillance, and response to reported cases. The original elimination goal date was set for 1982. In that year, however, there were still 1,697 cases reported nationwide. This figure represents a record low rate of 0.7 cases per 100,000 population for all ages.

No cases were reported by 15 states, while seven reported only imported cases. Indeed, only 6% of the nation's counties reported cases in 1982. Of these, 60% were among preschoolers or older children of a routine vaccination age. The chains of outbreak were due to imported cases in people who had not been vaccinated in their country of origin or who had visited a foreign country and brought measles back with them. The year 1983 showed the need to vaccinate college students, since unexpected outbreaks occurred at the Universities of Indiana and Houston.

Health officials seek to eradicate indigenous measles in the United

Fig. 5–3. Measles (rubeola): reported cases per 100,000 population, by year, United States, 1955–82

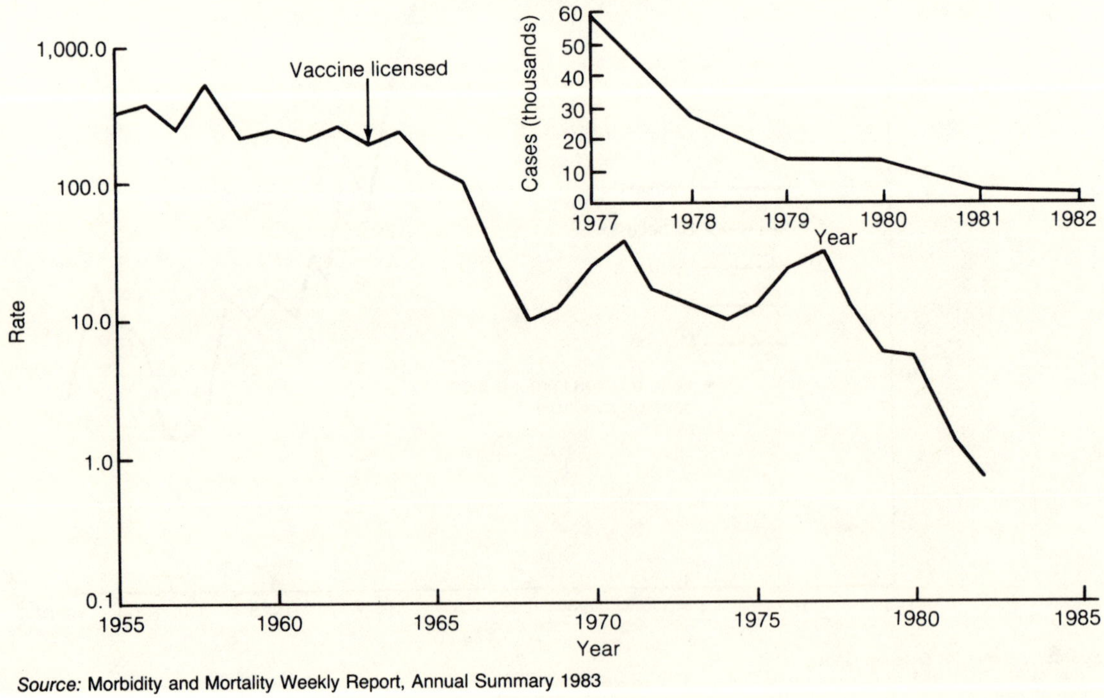

Source: Morbidity and Mortality Weekly Report, Annual Summary 1983

States because of the serious attendant complications. They can lead to developmental retardation and lifelong handicaps. In undeveloped countries, complications are often fatal, causing an estimated 900,000 deaths each year.

Reported cases between 1955 and 1982 are shown in Fig. 5–3.

The distribution of cases in 1983 by age is depicted in Figure 5–4.

About 10 days after exposure to the measles virus, patients develop prodromal fever, malaise, loss of appetite, conjunctivitis, photophobia, coryza, a hacking cough, and hoarseness just before the onset of Koplik's spots. The latter are red with a bluish center. Within 5 days, fever may rise sharply, and the spots are replaced by a pruritic rash that first appears behind the ears and on the face. Eventually it covers the body and then subsides. The sequelae in some cases include otitis media, pneumonia, and encephalitis.

Diagnosis is often possible from just the clinical evidence, i.e., the Koplik's spots and rash. But the virus can be identified as well in samples of blood or urine or from nasal secretions. Treatment

Fig. 5–4. Measles (rubeola): Reported cases per 100,000 population, by age group,* United States, 1980–82. [Estimated measles incidence has declined in all age groups. However, the greatest decreases have been among young school-age children. As a result, the highest estimated incidence in 1982 was for preschoolers, i.e., 2.8 cases/100,000 population.]

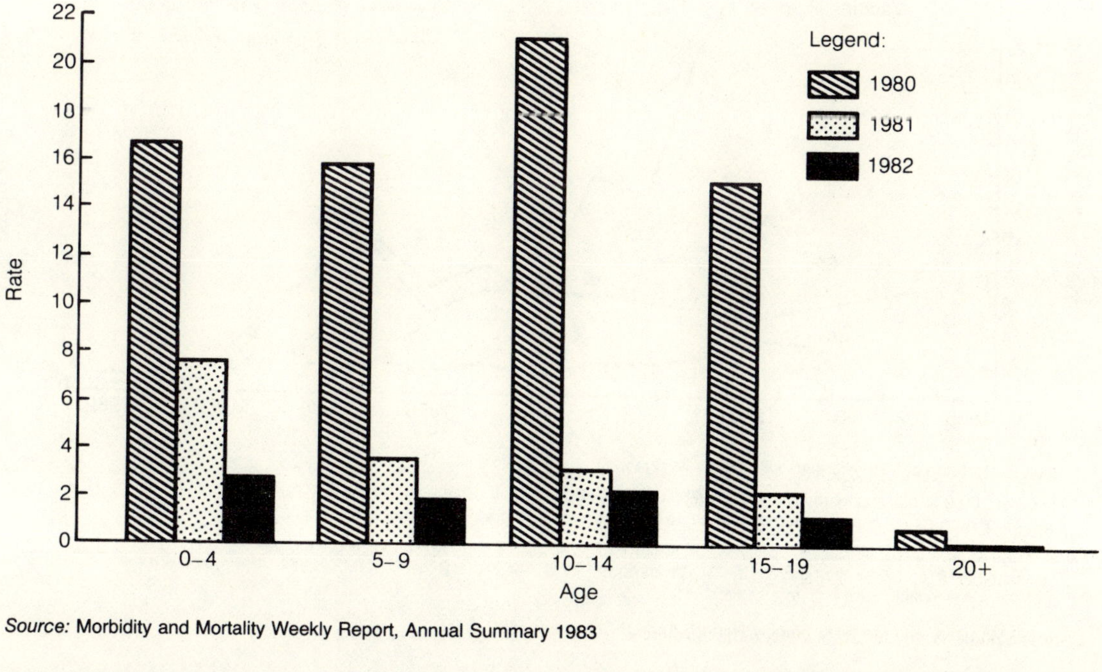

Source: Morbidity and Mortality Weekly Report, Annual Summary 1983

is supportive, requiring bed rest and symptomatic relief.

Scientists suspect a connection between multiple sclerosis (MS) and the measles virus. Epidemiologists will be watching the incidence of MS for the next several decades now that an entire generation has been immunized against the measles virus. If the measles virus is related to MS, the incidence of MS should decline in the United States. Meantime, the effort will be to keep Americans virtually free of measles and to try to eradicate it from the rest of the world. Once the latter end is achieved and foreign sources of infection are eliminated, Americans will no longer need to be immunized. This was the smallpox eradication strategy. And as of 1983 after the conquering of small pox worldwide, small pox vaccine is no longer available to the U.S. civilian population.

RUBELLA

Rubella, also known as German measles, is another virus-caused

Fig. 5–5. Incidence rate of reported rubella cases and congenital rubella cases, United States, 1966–82

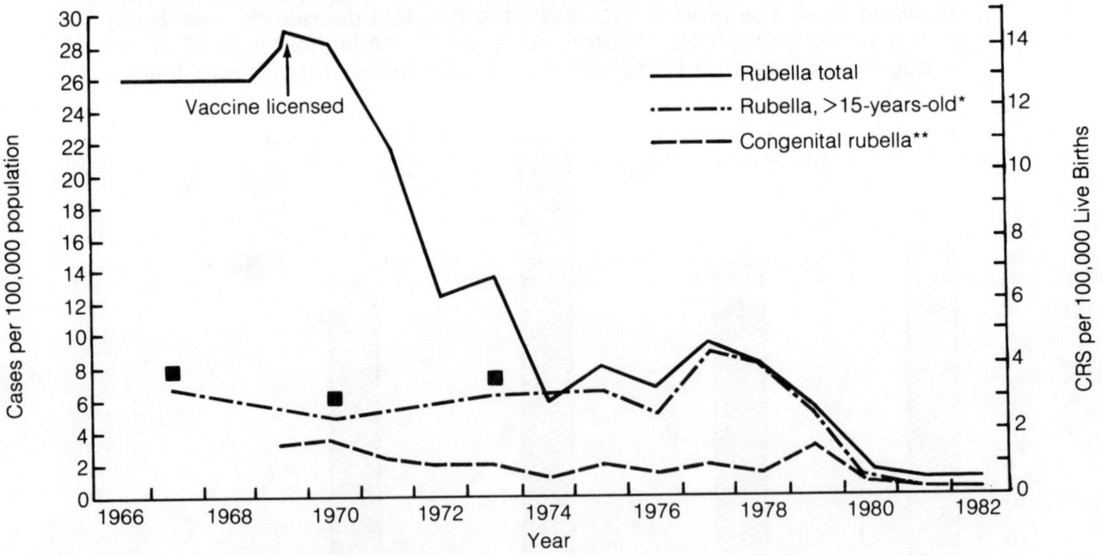

*Includes proration of >15-year-olds with unknown ages.

**Rate per 100,000 births confirmed and compatible cases of congenital rubella syndrome (CRS), by year of birth. Reporting for recent years is provisional, as cases may not be diagnosed until later in childhood.

■ Average annual U.S. estimate of rubella incidence in >15-year-olds, based on data from Illinois, Massachusetts, and New York City for the 3-year periods, 1966–1968, 1969–1971, 1972–1974. Age-specific data were not available for U.S. totals until 1975.

Source: Morbidity and Mortality Weekly Report, Annual Summary 1982

disease transmitted from person to person through nasal secretions, blood, urine, stool, and (possibly) the clothing of infected persons.

The onset of a maculopapular rash is usually preceded by malaise, headache, lymphadenopathy, coryza, low-grade fever, and loss of appetite. Enlargement of the suboccipital, postauricular, and postcervical lymph nodes is the most telling symptom.

The disease is seasonal, occuring most often in the spring. Figure 5–5 shows the steady and steep declinc of this disease since introduction of a vaccine in 1969. By 1981, the cases had been reduced 96% from the 1969 level.

Although not typically as serious as regular measles, rubella is feared because of the congenital injury it can cause to the fetus of a nonimmune pregnant woman. If mother and fetus are exposed, especially during the first trimester of pregnancy, the fetus may abort, be stillborn, or suffer heart damage, retardation, or blindness.

The factors for tragedy have been in place for generations since pregnant women who already have children are often exposed to the virus when their offspring contract the disease. Thus, the vac-

Fig. 5–6. Rubella (German measles): reported cases per 100,000 population, by age group*, United States, 1981 and 1980

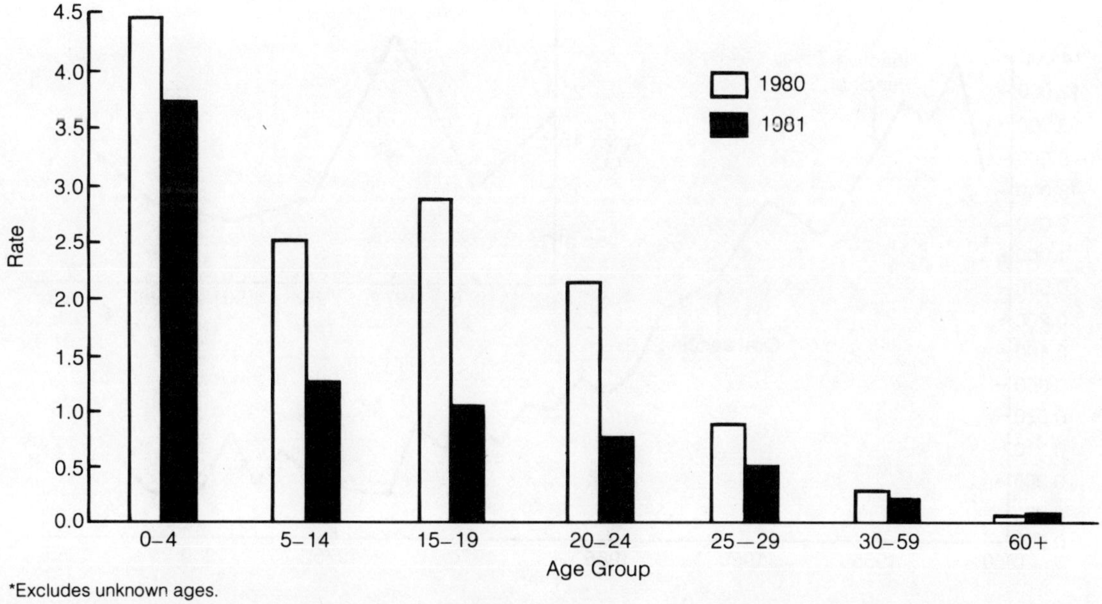

*Excludes unknown ages.

Source: Morbidity and Mortality Weekly Report, Annual Summary 1982

cine has helped children by preventing prenatal injury to them more than by preventing the disease postnatally. Between 1980 and 1981, rubella declined greatly for almost all ages but particularly for persons age 5 to 14 and 15 to 19 (Fig. 5–6).

Diagnosis can be confirmed by a rise in antibody titer but is usually determined clinically. Other than isolation, treatment consists of nothing more than administering a fever reliever.

POLIO

One of the most feared viral diseases often crippling children until the development of a vaccine was polio. The decline in polio is dramatic (Fig. 5–7). The peak shown in the box insert graph reflects an incidence of 90 cases reported for the years 1977–1983. Sixty-nine of the cases were related to the polio vaccine. Nine were subjects unexposed to the vaccine. Five were imported, while at least 6 were persons known to be immunodeficient.

Polio is endemic in the United States, and in other countries. When outbreaks occur, they are seasonal, occurring more in sum-

Fig. 5–7. Poliomyelitis (paralytic): reported cases per 100,000 population, by year, United States, 1951–83

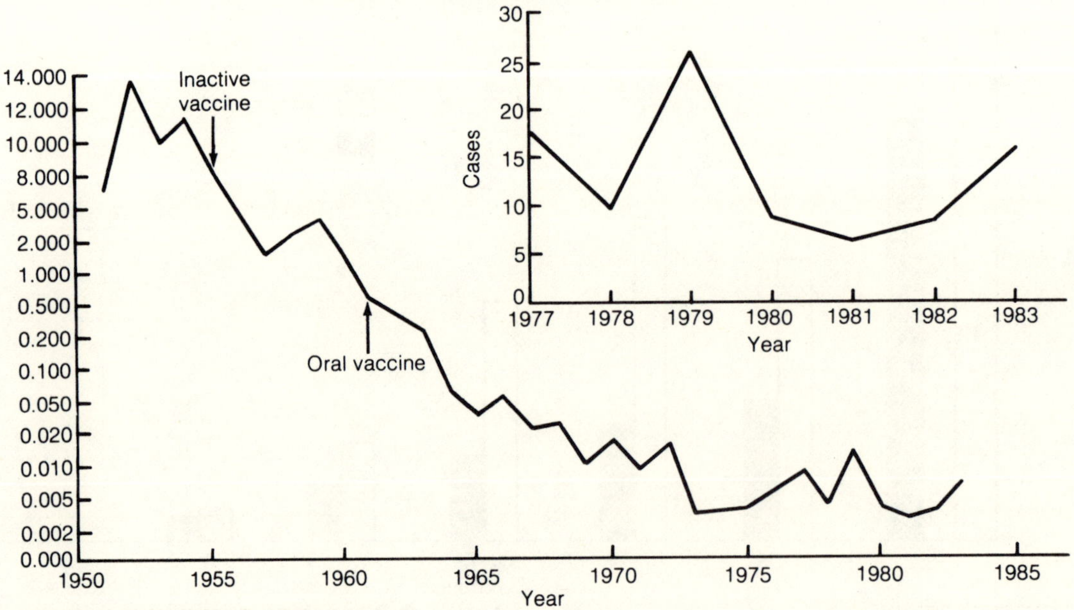

Source: Morbidity and Mortality Weekly Report, Annual Summary 1983

mer and fall. Children and pregnant women are most often stricken, and vaccination with the three strains of polio virus is recommended for all infants in three doses 1 to 2 months apart. In recent years there have been more cases among those older than age 15. The reported cases in 1983 are shown by state in Table 5–13.

When polio was common, major segments of the population were infected but were asymptomatic. A smaller percentage had the symptoms of a cold with possible digestive upset. The remaining cases with more severe infection had recognizable cases that either ended in complete recovery or in paralysis.

Diagnosis can be determined by isolating the virus from throat washings, CFS cultures, or stool specimens. Treatment can consist of administering analgesics and applying moist heat to muscles. When pain is intense the patient may be confined to bed rest. Rehabilitation requires extensive physical therapy.

The polio virus, which is absorbed orally, is stable and can survive for months outside the human body. Because of the disease's contagious nature, health-care personnel should be cautious in interacting with the patient, washing hands thoroughly after contact. Only hospital personnel who are vaccinated should be caring for such patients.

Until recently, the story of polio seemed over. In the past few years, however, former patients who had initially suffered paralysis that was overcome through physical therapy have begun to experience new disabling symptoms. These former patients, now in their 40s, have symptoms that mimic the earlier paralytic symp-

TABLE 5–13. Poliomyelitis (paralytic): Reported Cases, by Area and Age Group, United States, 1983

		AGE (YEARS)				
AREA	TOTAL	< 1	1–4	20–24	25–29	30–39
United States	15	10	1	1	1	2
California	1	–	–	–	–	1
Illinois	1	–	–	–	–	1
Indiana	3	1	1	1	–	–
Kentucky	1*	1	–	–	–	–
Louisiana	1	1	–	–	–	–
Missouri	2	2	–	–	–	–
N.Y.C.	1*	1	–	–	–	–
Ohio	1	1	–	–	–	–
Oregon	1	1	–	–	–	–
Pennsylvania	1	1	–	–	–	–
Texas	1*	1	–	–	–	–
Washington	1	–	–	–	1	–

* Onset of illness in 1982.

Source: Morbidity and Mortality Weekly Report, Annual Summary 1983

toms. This second manifestation of polio so many years after the original childhood bout has just been recognized as polio-related. Indeed, the medical community has little understanding or explanation for what seems to be renewed illness in former polio patients.

MUMPS

The incidence of another childhood disease, mumps, has been declining since the development of a vaccine in the 1970s (Fig. 5–8).

Its incidence is greatest in late winter and early spring. Most cases are children age 5 to 15 years (Fig. 5–9).

The number of cases, percentage and case rate for California, Massachusetts, and New York City from 1967 through 1983 are shown in Table 5–14. Consistently, the highest proportion of cases were among those age 5 to 14 years.

This highly contagious disease is transmitted through direct or indirect contact with the saliva or airborne droplets of a person infected with the paramyxovirus. An infected person is contagious

Fig. 5–8. Mumps: reported cases per 100,000 population, by year, United States, 1968–83

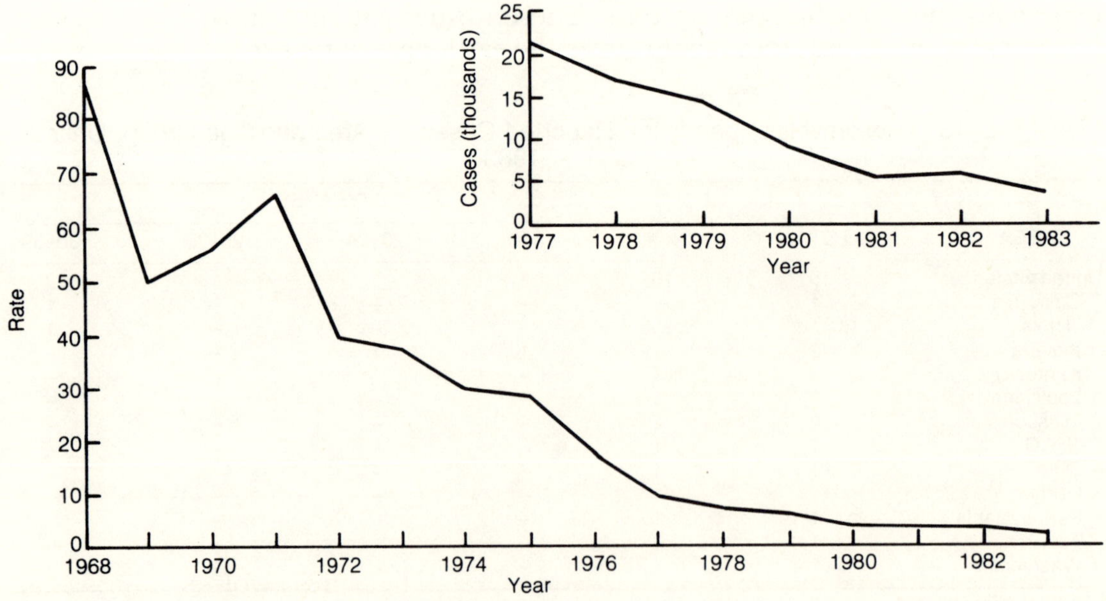

Source: Morbidity and Mortality Weekly Report, Annual Summary 1983

Fig. 5–9. Mumps: estimated* incidence of mumps, by age group, United States, 1981–83

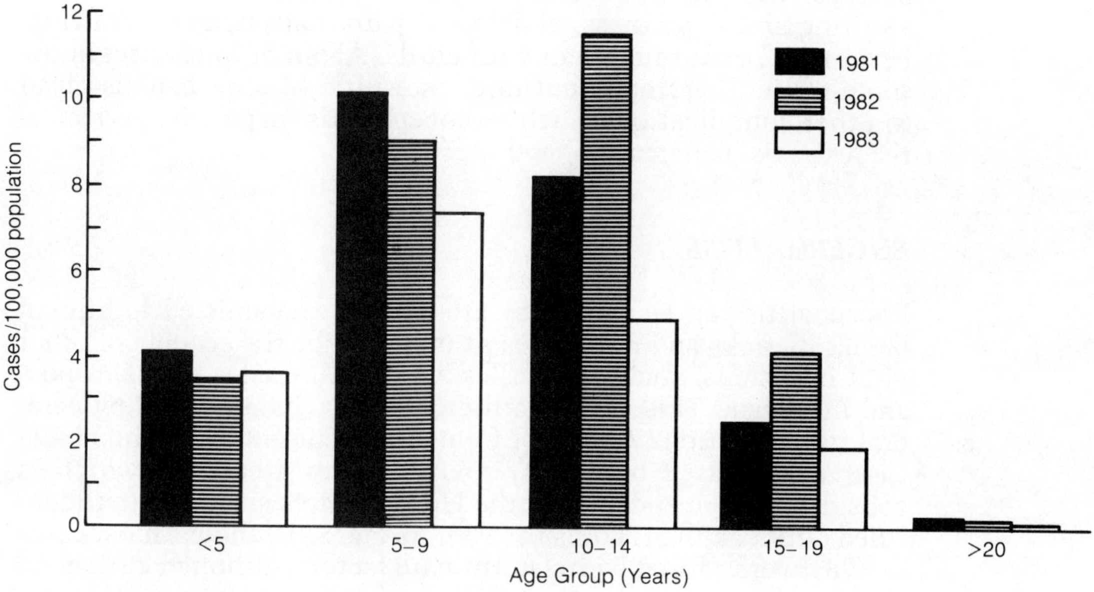

*Extrapolated from age distribution of cases with known age.

Source: Morbidity and Mortality Weekly Report, Annual Summary 1983

TABLE 5–14. Mumps: Age Distribution and Incidence* of Reported Mumps Cases,† California, Massachusetts, and New York City, 1967–1971,‡ 1972–76,** and 1979–1983

AGE GROUP (YEARS)	1967–1971			1972–1976			1979–1983**			PERCENTAGE RATE CHANGE 1967–1983
	No.	%	Rate	No.	%	Rate	No.	%	Rate	
0–4	2,932	17.1	102.5	1,125	18.7	41.2	96	17.1	3.8	−96.2
5–9	10,413	60.8	336.8	3,272	54.3	105.8	181	32.4	7.3	−97.8
10–14	2,372	13.8	75.5	992	16.5	31.6	132	23.6	4.8	−93.6
15**	1,418	8.3	5.8	633	10.5	2.6	150	26.8	0.5	−91.3
Total	17,135	100.0	51.1	6,022	100.0	18.0	559	99.9	1.5	−97.0

* Reported number of cases/100,000 population
† Cases of unknown age excluded
‡ Average annual figure over 5-year period
** These selected data accurately reflect changes using total U.S. data; 1980 population data used
(*Source:* Morbidity and Mortality Weekly Report, Annual Summary 1983

from 6 days before to 9 days after symptoms develop.

The initial symptoms may include myalgia, malaise, low-grade fever, headache, and loss of appetite. These are followed by an earache exacerbated by chewing. The parotid gland becomes swollen and tender, and temperature may rise to 104° F. Swelling may finally extend to the salivary glands. When adult males develop mumps, there may be testicular involvement characterized by swelling and tenderness, abdominal pain, nausea, and vomiting. Fever may occur in tandem with chills. About 50% of cases show some testicular atrophy but rarely sterility. Mumps can also lead to other complications, such as encephalitis, nephritis, pericarditis, arthritis, pancreatitis, and deafness.

ENCEPHALITIS

Encephalitis can be caused by arboviruses transmitted to human beings by ticks and mosquitos. It may also be the sequela of other viral infections, such as measles, German measles, chicken pox, and influenza. This "aftermath disease" is characterized by cerebral inflammation. When not following a common childhood disease, it is caused by an enterovirus or an arbovirus, which is considered to be endemic in the United States since its first identified outbreak in St. Louis in 1933. As Fig. 5–10 shows, most cases in 1981 were caused by indeterminate factors, although childhood

Fig. 5–10. Encephalitis: reported cases per 100,000 population, by etiology and age group, 1981

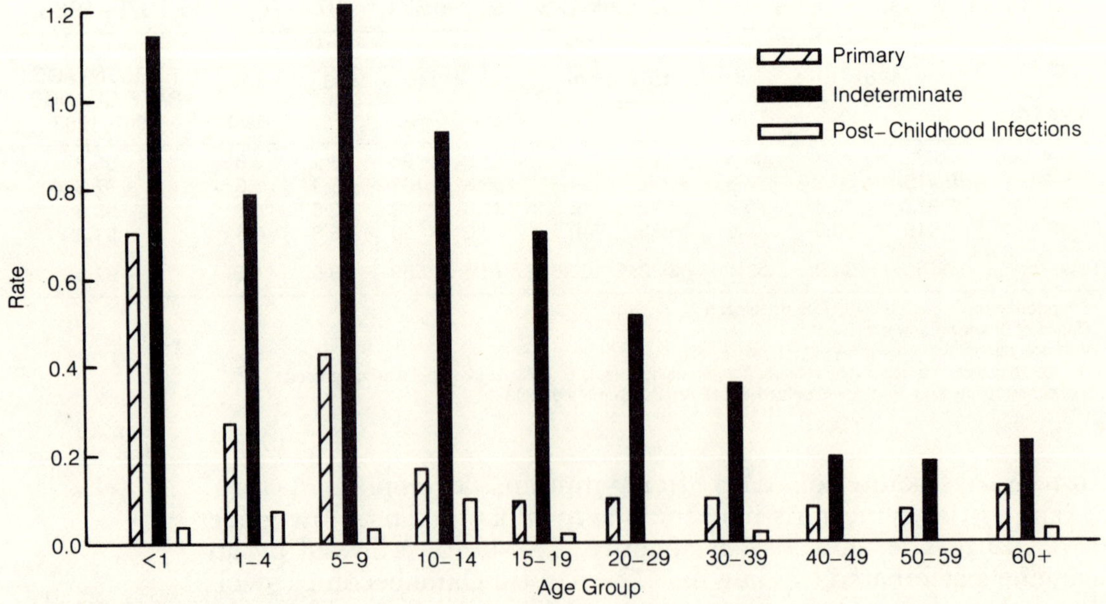

Source: Morbidity and Mortality Weekly Report, Annual Summary 1981

age categories show evidence of postinfection cases.

The symptoms of encephalitis often include fever; vomiting; aching head, neck, and back; drowsiness; coma; paralysis; and convulsions. The infection may be either subclinical or so severe that it can lead to death.

Diagnosis is confirmed through detecting the virus in CSF or blood. During outbreaks, cases may be identified through symptoms and history. Isolated cases may require laboratory work-up. The CSF pressure is elevated in all forms of encephalitis, and an EEG can reveal abnormalities. Treatment is supportive except in cases of herpes encephalitis. This latter is treatable by the antiviral agent vidarabine. Supportive treatment may include the anticonvulsant phenytoin and glucocorticoids for reduction of cerebral inflammation. Other agents to ease headache and fever are also prescribed.

Postinfection encephalitis is reduced by vaccination against several childhood diseases, a bonus gain in addition to protection from the diseases themselves. But in 1977, less than two-thirds of American children younger than age 15 years were immunized against

TABLE 5–15. Vaccination Status of Children Age 1–4 Years, According to Race and Standard Metropolitan Statistical Area (SMSA) Component: United States, 1976 and 1981 (data are based on household interviews of a sample of the civilian noninstitutionalized population)

YEAR, RACE, AND SMSA COMPONENT‡	VACCINATION				
	Measles	Rubella	DTP*,†	Polio†	Mumps
1976			Population (%)		
Total	65.9	61.7	71.4	61.6	48.3
Race					
White	68.3	63.8	75.3	66.2	50.3
All other	54.8	51.5	53.2	39.9	38.7
SMSA component					
Central city	62.5	59.5	64.1	53.8	45.6
Remaining areas in SMSA	67.2	63.5	75.7	65.3	50.7
Not SMSA	67.3	61.5	72.9	63.9	47.9
1981					
Total	63.8	64.5	67.5	60.0	58.4
Race					
White	65.7	66.6	71.0	63.8	60.5
All other	55.3	55.2	52.0	42.7	49.1
SMSA Component					
Central city	60.0	59.9	58.7	52.6	52.8
Remaining areas in SMSA	64.3	64.6	68.8	62.0	58.6
Not SMSA	65.9	67.5	72.2	63.0	61.9

* Diphtheria-tetanus-pertussis
† Three doses or more
‡ Standard Metropolitan Statistical Area
Source: Centers for Disease Control: United States Immunization Survey, 1981. Public Health Service, DHHS, Atlanta, Ga., to be published.

common and sometimes life-threatening diseases. President Carter, therefore, established a public health goal of 90% immunization to be reached by 1979. Through efforts by the states, the Atlanta Centers for Disease Control reported that data from the states for 1980–81 showed an immunization level of 90% for children entering kindergarten and first grade. The figures for children ages 1 to 4 years, however, show a significantly lower percentage vaccinated (Table 5–15).

REYE'S SYNDROME

Another sometimes fatal aftermath disease identified in the early 1970s is Reye's syndrome. Because of noticeable outbreaks at that time and the severity of the disease, national surveillance was established in 1976. Yet, reporting is still incomplete, particularly for milder cases in which symptoms may not be recognized as those of Reye's syndrome.

Most patients are younger than age 18 years, have had a respiratory viral illness or chicken pox, and have been treated during their illness with salicylates about 2 weeks before the onset of Reye's syndrome symptoms of vomiting, liver dysfunction, and coma. In 1982 and 1983, respectively, 80% and 79% were hospitalized in the precoma state. Data gathered since 1973 on this illness are shown in Table 5–16. As can be seen, the incidence of Reye's syndrome varies annually, possibly because of uneven reporting but also because of the annual variability of virus infec-

TABLE 5–16. Incidence of Reye's Syndrome, by Year — United States, 1973–74 and 1977–83

YEAR (DEC. 1–NOV. 30)	MAJOR INFLUENZA ACTIVITY	NUMBER OF CASES	INCIDENCE*	DEATH-CASE RATIO: Number of deaths/cases†	DEATH-CASE RATIO: Ratio (%)
1973–1974‡	B	379	0.58	157/379	41
1977	B	454	0.71	156/373	42
1978	A(H3N2/H1N1)	237	0.37	66/225	29
1979	A(H1N1)	389	0.62	113/349	32
1980	B	548	0.88	114/516	22
1981	A(H3N2/H1N1)	313	0.49	80/296	30
1982	B	222	0.35	72/208	35
1983**	A(H3N2/H1N1)	191	0.30	56/173	32

* Patients per 100,000 population < 18 years of age.
† With known outcome
‡ For the period December 15, 1973-June 30, 1974
** Preliminary count; reported cases as of January 15, 1984
Source: U.S. Department of Health and Human Services/Public Health Service

tions. Peak years have occurred when influenza-B virus was prominent, as in 1976–77 and 1979–80. The lowest occurrence was in 1977–78 and 1980–81 when influenza type A was most prevalent.

Detailed analysis of data for 1982 and 1983 reveals that Reye's syndrome occurs equally in boys and girls. But 93% of the cases were those of white children compared to 5% for blacks and 1% or 2% for oriental. Over one-half the cases occurred in children age 5 to 14 years, although as many as 3% occurred in persons older than age 18 years.

Since Reye's syndrome impedes liver function, interrupting in particular the urea cycle in which ammonia is changed to urea for excretion, diagnosis of the disorder can be determined by reading urea levels and liver function studies. Treatment has become more effective in recent years, reducing mortality from 90% to 20%. Improvement is due to monitoring of intracranial pressure as the CNS becomes depressed. Care is supportive.

Since Reye's syndrome sometimes follows chicken pox infection for which there is no administered vaccine, the incidence of chicken pox nationally is of interest as an important childhood disease that is still common.

CHICKEN POX

Chicken pox is the second most frequently reported infectious disease in the United States. Caused by the herpes virus, varicella-zoster, it maintains a constant seasonal pattern of high incidence from March to May (Fig. 5–11). In 1982, there were 167,423 reported cases nationally.

The predominant symptom is a pruritic rash preceded by a mild fever, malaise, and loss of appetite. The papules that develop on the trunk and face break and form scabs. The temptation to scratch them should be avoided to prevent infection and complications. The patient should be isolated until the scabs disappear. This usually occurs within 7 days of the onset of rash. Treatment involves symptomatic relief by administration of cool bicarbonate of soda baths, calamine lotion, and antipruritics.

Of the cases reported with known age in 1981, 53% were in children between ages 5 and 9 years. However, persons older than age 60 years can and do get chicken pox.

Fig. 5–11. Chicken Pox: reported cases per 100,000 population, by month, United States, 1978–82

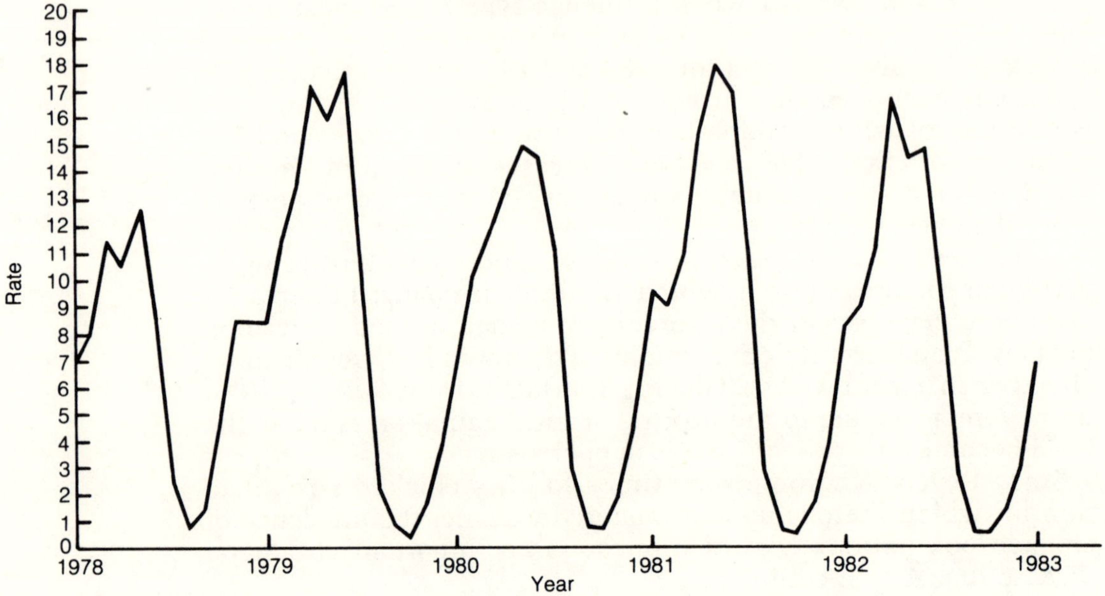

Source: Morbidity and Mortality Weekly Report, Annual Summary 1983

MENINGOCOCCAL INFECTIONS

Meningococcal infections most often affect children 6 months to 1 year old and are caused by a gram-negative bacteria, *Neisseria meningitidis.* Of the 7 serogroups, group A is responsible for most epidemics. As high as 40% of the population are carriers, transmitting the bacteria to uninfected persons through airborne saliva droplets.

Symptoms vary according to the infection. Persons infected with meningococcal bacteremia may suddenly develop a high temperature, sore throat, cough, headache, chills, myalgia, tachycardia, mild hypotension, and a maculopapular rash. The infection can deteriorate to a fulminant state if left untreated, leading to death in 6 to 24 hours.

Figure 5–12 shows the trend in meningococcal infections in the United States since 1930. In 1983, a full 52% of all cases were in children younger than 5 years.

Fig. 5–12. Meningococcal infections (total): reported cases per 100,000 population, by year, United States, 1930–83

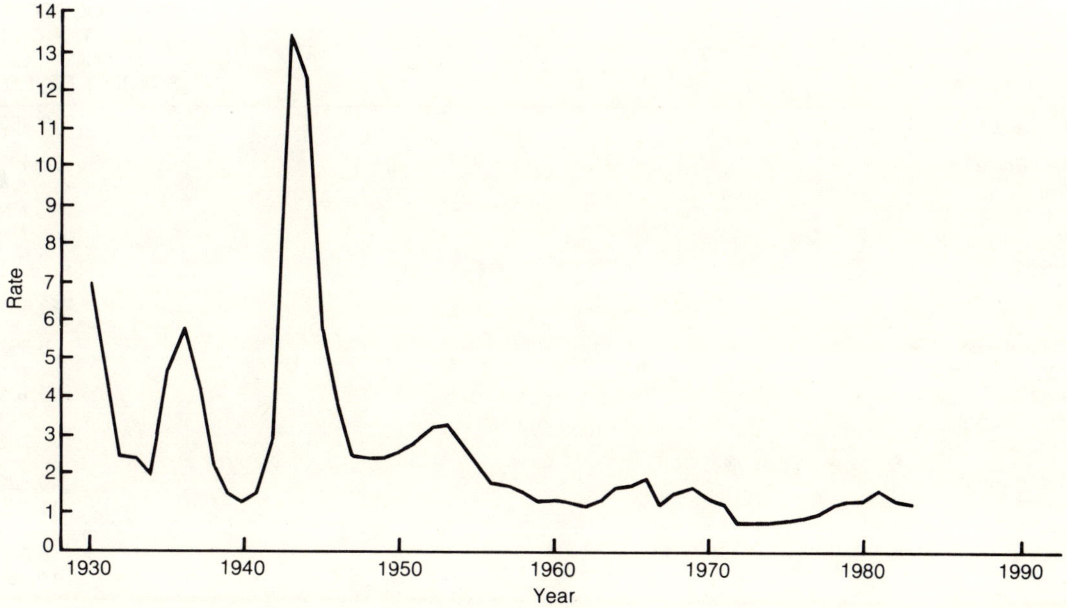

Source: Morbidity and Mortality Weekly Report, Annual Summary 1983

Diagnosis involves ruling out Rocky Mountain spotted fever and can be determined through isolation of *N. meningitidis* through a positive blood culture, CSF culture, noting of low WBC, adrenal hemorrhages, and decreased clotting levels.

As soon as possible after diagnosis, large doses of aqueous penicillin G or ampicillin should be administered. Allergic patients may be given chloramphenicol. Mannitol can be given for cerebral edema together with other agents for shock and congestive heart failure and to maintain fluid and electrolyte balance. Those caring for patients are sometimes given rifampin or minocycline prophylactically.

SCARLET FEVER

Another childhood disease occurring most often in subjects younger than 10 years is scarlet fever, or scarlatina, an acute infection caused by any of 40 strains of Group A *Streptococcus pyogenes.*

The usual symptoms are sore throat, strawberry tongue, and body rash. Patients may also experience nausea and vomiting.

TABLE 5–17. Non-notifiable Conditions: Cases of Streptococcal Scarlet Fever Optionally Reported by Certain Areas, 1983

AREA	STREPTOCOCCAL SORE THROAT AND SCARLET FEVER
No. Cases Reported	213,962
New England	36,499
Main	NA
NH	NN
Vt.	NN
Mass	–
RI	7,549
Conn	28,950
Mid. Atlantic	3,853
N.Y. (excl NYC)	NN
NYC	3,103
NJ	NA
Pa	750
E.N. Central	40,522
Ohio	11,120
Ind	–
Ill	18,245
Mich	11,157
Wis	–
W.N. Central	15,259
Minn	NN
Iowa	NN
Mo	NN
N. Dak	4,499
S. Dak	2,033
Nebr	3,049
Kans	5,678
S. Atlantic	28,720
Del	1,925
Md	11,819
DC	12
Va	75
W Va	11,704
NC	NN
SC	NN
Ga	3,185
Fla	NN
E.S. Central	3,458
Ky	2,522
Tenn	NN
Ala	
Miss	936
W.S. Central	38,982
Ark	
La	NN
Okla	

TABLE 5–17. (Continued)

AREA	STREPTOCOCCAL SORE THROAT AND SCARLET FEVER
Texas	38,982
Mountain	19,371
Mont	574
Idaho	NN
Wyo	14,590
Colo	NN
N Mex	
Ariz	83
Utah	4,064
Nev	60
Pacific	27,298
Wash	NN
Oreg*	NN
Calif	22,484
Alaska	NN
Hawaii	4,814
Guam	1,219
PR	7
VI	—
Pac Trust Terr	91
CNMI	53

* Cases reported by surveillance program for the period December 1, 1982-November ;30, 1983.
† Includes New York City
Source: Morbidity and Mortality Weekly Reports, Annual Summary 1983

Temperature is often elevated, and young children may be convulsive. As the rash subsides, typically within 3 days, temperature returns to normal. Incubation time is between 1 and 3 days, and the modes of transmission include direct contact and inhalation.

Scarlet fever is not a disease that must be reported by law to the Atlanta Centers for Disease Control. So, the numbers of cases presented by state in Table 5–17 provide an underestimate of the true number of cases because they represent only voluntary reports.

Diagnosis is often based on the clinically characteristic rash and strawberry tongue but can be confirmed by throat culture or gram strain identifying the causative organism. Treatment usually involves administering penicillin for at least 10 days to prevent rheumatic fever, which often follows strep throat infections (see Cardiovascular Disease). Bed rest and supportive measures, as needed, are also standard treatment.

INFECTIOUS MONONUCLEOSIS

Although children do contract infectious mononucleosis, it is often undetectable. It is notable in young adults, however, especially in American college students. Caused by the Epstein-Barr virus, it is thought to be transmitted by oral contact. Infected persons generally harbor the virus in their throat.

Incubation in young adults often takes as long as 50 days. Initial symptoms include headache, malaise, fatigue, and a mild fever. Many episodes also involve a rash and cervical lymphadenopathy. A small percentage of patients shows jaundice, splenomegaly, hepatomegaly, or pharyngitis.

The true incidence of this infection is unknown since physicians are not required to report it. Based on voluntary reports, however, the minimum number of cases in the United States in 1983 by state is presented in Table 5–18.

TABLE 5–18. Non-notifiable Conditions: Cases of Mononucleosis Optionally Reported by Certain Areas, 1983

AREA	INFECTIOUS MONONUCLEOSIS
No. Cases Reported	6,529
New England	2,405
Maine	NN
NH	NN
VI	158
Mass	NN
RI	37
Conn	2,210
Mid. Atlantic	2,472
NY (excl NYC)	2,472
NYC	–
NJ	NA
Pa	–
E.N. Central	4
Ohio	–
Ind	–
Ill	4
Mich	–
Wis	–
W.N. Central	229
Minn	NN
Iowa	213
Mo	3
N Dak	NN
S Dak	10
Nebr	NN
Kans	3

TABLE 5–18. (Continued)

AREA	INFECTIOUS MONONUCLEOSIS
S. Atlantic	903
Del	NN
Md	1
DC	—
Va	556
W. Va	346
N.C.	NN
S.C.	NN
Ga	—
Fla	NN
E.S. Central	377
Ky	293
Tenn	NN
Ala	
Miss	84
W.S. Central	3
Ark	3
La	—
Okla	
Texas	NN
Mountain	53
Mont	10
Idaho	NN
Wyo	—
Colo	NN
N Mex	—
Ariz	—
Utah	43
Nev	—
Pacific	83
Wash	NN
Oreg	NN
Calif	16
Alaska	2
Hawaii	65
Guam	12
PR	74
VI	—
Pac Trust Terr	NN
CNMI	NN

Source: Morbidity and Mortality Weekly Report Annual Summary 1983

Diagnosis is sometimes possible based on the symptoms of cervical lymphadenopathy, sore throat, and higher-than-normal temperature. But infectious mononucleosis resembles several other infections, including hepatitis. Hence, diagnosis is usually made by laboratory tests that, in the presence of disease, show elevated leukocyte count and heterophil antibody count. Liver function studies also are usually abnormal.

Treatment for this illness is nonspecific other than supportive measures to relieve symptoms and bed rest. If the spleen ruptures, surgical repair is required.

RABIES

Rabies is an acute central nervous system infection caused by an RNA virus, transmitted to human beings by animal bite. Animals infected include wild skunks, raccoons, foxes, bats, coyotes, and badgers. Because most dogs have been vaccinated, they no longer pose the threat they once did as transmitters of this dread disease.

Symptoms, which may take months to develop, include fever, malaise, nausea, loss of appetite, sore throat, headache, cough, nervousness, irritability, and increased sensitivity to light and noise. Respiration becomes shallow and the patient may salivate, perspire, and tear excessively. He may become phobic about water and tend to expel saliva from the mouth, resulting in dryness and

Fig. 5–13. Rabies: reported cases in wild and domestic animals, by year, United States, 1965–83

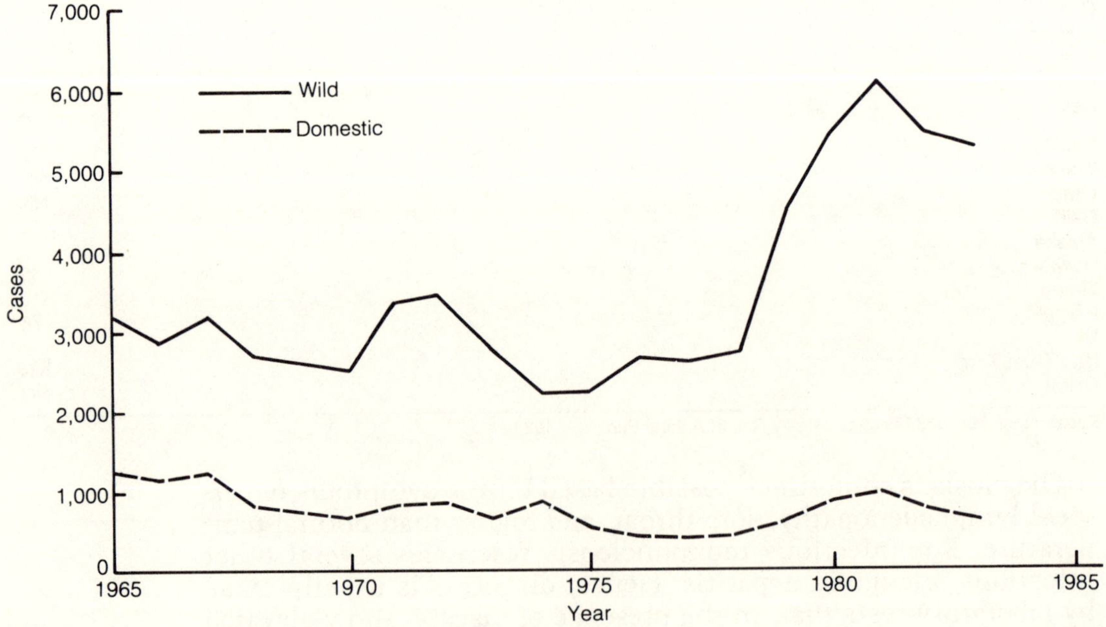

Source: Morbidity and Mortality Weekly Report, Annual Summary 1983

dehydration. He may froth at the mouth. Within days, paralysis ensues which causes circulatory collapse leading to death.

Reported animal cases in the United States between 1955 and 1983 show a great upsurge since 1978. The mid-Atlantic states reported an outbreak among raccoons that was especially marked (Fig. 5–13).

Table 5–19 shows the breakdown of reported animal cases by state in 1983. During 1983, there were only 2 human cases reported in the entire country, one of someone bitten by a rabid dog while traveling in Africa and one bitten by a rabid bat in Michigan.

A history of an animal bite that was unprovoked, together with laboratory tests that identify the virus in the patient's saliva or in the blood through fluorescent rabies antibody determination indicates rabies infection. Since rabies is fatal if not treated, any suspected case involves injection of rabies vaccine. Human rabies immune globulin is administered to those who have received multiple head wounds since spread of the virus to the CNS is often quicker when bites are above the neck. Some patients may be treated for tetanus as well.

TABLE 5–19. Rabies: Reported Cases in Animals, by Area and Species of Animal, United States, 1983

		DOMESTIC				WILD				
AREA	TOTAL	Cattle	Cats	Dogs	Other domestic	Skunks	Raccoons	Bats	Foxes	Other wild
United States	5,878*	204	168	132	80	2,285	1,906	910	111	82
New England	47	–	–	–	1	–	–	33	11	2
Maine	17	–	–	–	–	–	–	7	10	–
NH	5	–	–	–	1	–	–	3	1	–
Vt	2	–	–	–	–	–	–	2	–	–
Mass	15	–	–	–	–	–	–	15	–	–
RI	2	–	–	–	–	–	–	–	–	2
Conn	6	–	–	–	–	–	–	6	–	–
Mid. Atlantic	276	10	12	7	2	48	81	86	24	6
NY	84	7	2	2	1	19	–	29	24	–
NJ	24	–	–	–	–	–	–	24	–	–
Pa	168	3	10	5	1	29	81	33	–	6
E.N. Central	464	37	17	29	7	272	3	92	4	3
Ohio	60	3	1	2	1	26	1	25	1	–
Ind.	30	3	–	–	2	17	–	7	–	1
Ill	236	10	12	17	3	153	1	38	2	–
Mich	19	–	–	1	–	–	1	17	–	–
Wis	119	21	4	9	1	76	–	5	1	2
W.N. Central	856	94	62	32	24	604	5	33	1	1
Minn	171	23	11	3	1	120	3	9	–	1

TABLE 5–19. (Continued)

AREA	TOTAL	DOMESTIC				WILD				
		Cattle	Cats	Dogs	Other domestic	Skunks	Raccoons	Bats	Foxes	Other wild
Iowa	200	34	18	14	9	120	–	5	–	–
Mo	97	2	3	5	–	76	–	11	–	–
N Dak	92	12	5	5	3	67	–	–	–	–
S Dak	149	17	16	1	4	106	–	4	1	–
Nebr	64	5	4	3	2	48	1	1	–	–
Kans	83	1	5	1	5	67	1	3	–	–
S. Atlantic	2,146	12	32	3	1	90	1,768	190	30	20
Del	7	–	–	–	–	–	1	5	–	1
Md	828	3	9	–	–	28	732	43	5	8
DC	162	–	1	–	–	–	158	1	–	2
Va	625	3	6	–	–	33	545	17	15	6
W Va	120	3	6	1	–	14	88	7	1	–
NC	24	1	–	–	–	6	–	17	–	–
SC	35	–	2	–	–	1	20	9	1	2
Ga	214	1	6	1	1	7	168	22	8	–
Fla	131	1	2	1	–	1	56	69	–	1
E.S. Central	365	4	3	23	4	231	43	49	7	1
Ky	83	2	1	14	4	52	1	5	4	–
Tenn	190	1	2	8	–	171	–	5	2	1
Ala	83	1	–	1	–	8	42	30	1	–
Miss	9	–	–	–	–	–	–	9	–	–
W.S. Central	1,004	40	35	24	36	734	2	114	16	3
Ark	160	7	1	4	2	128	–	16	2	–
La	34	–	2	1	1	23	–	7	–	–
Okla	107	9	5	6	6	78	–	3	–	–
Tex	703	24	27	13	27	505	2	88	14	3
Mountain	279	1	5	3	2	112	–	152	2	2
Mont	119	1	4	3	2	94	–	15	–	–
Idaho	17	–	–	–	–	–	–	17	–	–
Wyo	10	–	–	–	–	–	–	10	–	–
Colo	36	–	–	–	–	–	–	36	–	–
N Mex	15	–	1	–	–	7	–	7	–	–
Ariz	33	–	–	–	–	10	–	19	2	2
Utah	11	–	–	–	–	1	–	10	–	–
Nev	38	–	–	–	–	–	–	38	–	–
Pacific	391	5	2	3	2	194	4	161	16	4
Wash	10	–	–	–	–	–	–	10	–	–
Oreg	3	–	–	–	–	–	–	3	–	–
Calif	358	5	2	1	2	194	4	148	1	1
Alaska	20	–	–	2	–	–	–	–	15	3
Hawaii	–	–	–	–	–	–	–	–	–	–
Guam	–	–	–	–	–	–	–	–	–	–
P.R.	50	1	–	8	1	–	–	–	–	40
VI	–	–	–	–	–	–	–	–	–	–

* Includes corrections reported through October 31, 1984

Source: Morbidity and Mortality Weekly Report Annual Summary 1983

TETANUS

Tetanus is caused by the anaerobic gram-positive bacillus *Clostridium tetani.* It is commonly found in soil and on old rusty objects. The infection is a response to the toxin produced by the bacilli. This infection has become less frequent in the United States since 1955 because of mass vaccination of the population (Fig. 5–14). In other countries where the population is unprotected by vaccination and many people work with the soil, tetanus fatalities even among infants are not uncommon.

In 1983, there were 91 cases reported throughout the country. Most of them occurred between April and September, the warm months when people work outdoors. The age breakdown for the 91 reported cases in 1983 is shown in Fig. 5–15. The skewing of the age distribution suggests to authorities that older people either need booster shots or have never been vaccinated. They recommend that persons in age ranges older than 60 years be vaccinated.

Symptoms may develop from 2 to 10 days after a puncture wound that allows *C. tetani* to enter the body. Usually, the sooner the symptoms develop, the more severe the infection. Symptoms in-

Fig. 5–14. Tetanus: reported cases per 100,000 population, by year, United States, 1955–1983

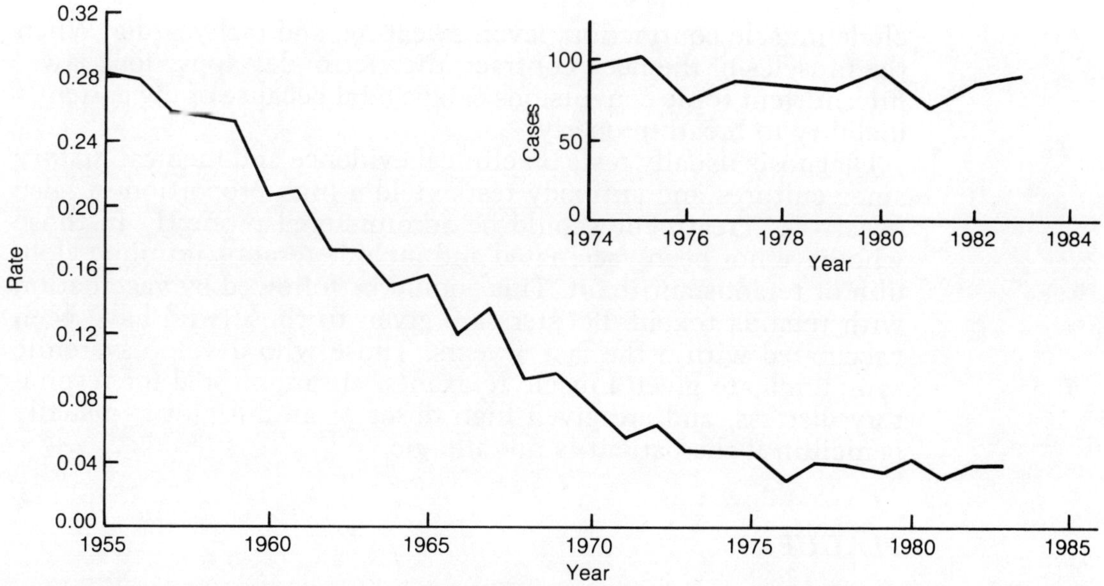

Source: Morbidity and Mortality Weekly Report, Annual Summary 1983

Fig. 5–15. Tetanus: reported cases, by age group*, United States, 1983

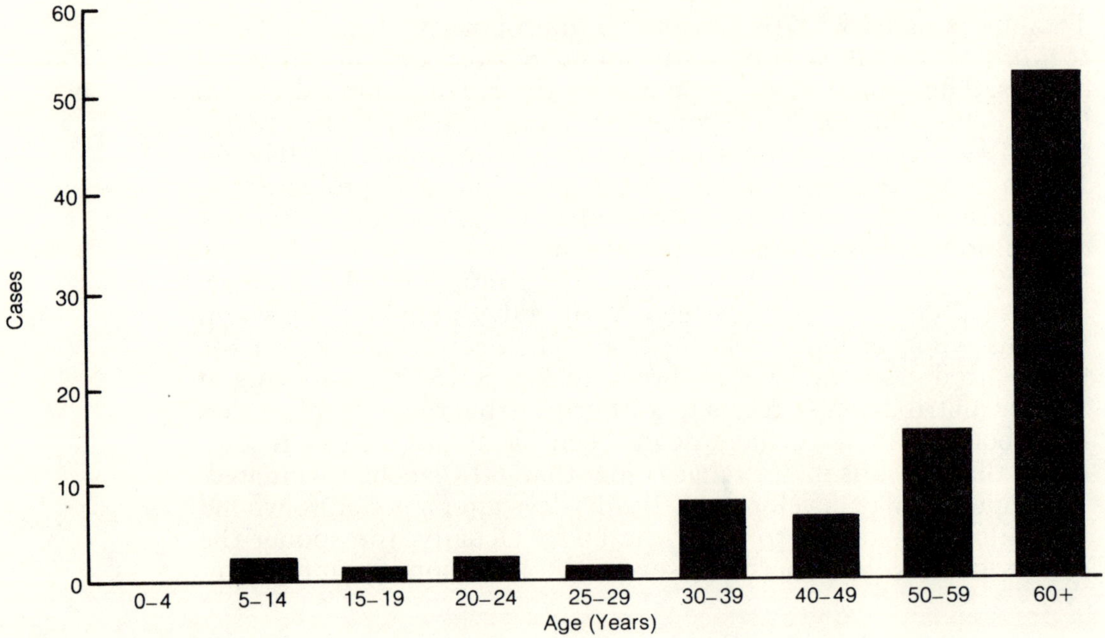

*Excludes unknown ages.

Source: Morbidity and Mortality Weekly Report, Annual Summary 1983.

clude muscle contraction, fever, sweating, and tachycardia. When the muscles of the neck contract, the victim develops "lock jaw." Intermittent tonic convulsions can be fatal because of the patient's inability to breath properly.

Diagnosis usually rests on clinical evidence and medical history since cultures and antibody tests yield a high proportion of false negatives. Treatment should be administered promptly in those who have not been vaccinated and include tetanus immune-globulin or tetanus antitoxin. This should be followed by vaccination with tetanus toxoid. Boosters are given to those who have been vaccinated within the last 5 years. Those who develop systemic symptoms are given muscle relaxants, are monitored for respiratory distress, and are given high doses of an antibiotic—usually penicillin if the patient is not allergic.

PLAGUE

Unlike many of the diseases reviewed in this chapter that have a much lower incidence today than 30 years ago, plague has been increasing in the United States, reaching a level in 1983 that was the highest since 1920 (40 cases confirmed and reported).

Plague is caused by the gram-negative bacillus *Yersinia pestis* and occurs in several forms. The most common form is bubonic plague. Others are septicemic plague and pneumonic plague, which either follows bubonic or septicemic plague or occurs as a severe primary infection that often leads to death within 2 or 3 days after symptoms first appear. Like pneumonic plague, septicemic plague has a mortality of 100%, whereas bubonic is 60% fatal.

Septicemic plague does not usually involve the lymph nodes but causes convulsions, shock, and disseminated intravascular coagulation with resultant widespread tissue damage. Bubonic plague causes pain and tenderness in the lymph nodes and fever. Painful buboes develop, and hemorrhagic areas turn black as they become necrotic. This has led to the popular name of "the black death" for bubonic plague. Other symptoms include chills, myalgia, headache, prostration, and delirium. Digestive symptoms may also develop. If pneumonic plague develops secondarily, a cough with bloody sputum develops with respiratory distress. This form is contagious since the infection can be passed through airborne saliva droplets.

Ordinarily, bubonic plague is transmitted to man through the bite of infected fleas that have lived on infected rodents, squirrels, or rabbits. Although still widespread in many parts of the world, such as South America, the Near East and Africa, plague is generally confined to the western part of the United States. It is especially common among the Navajo Indians. In 1983, 53% of the 40 reported cases were among Navajos. A few cases also occurred among Pueblo Indians. Sixty-five percent of all cases were males, and 46% developed in persons younger than age 19 years.

Figure 5–16 shows the rising incidence of plague in the United States in recent years.

Bubonic plague is usually diagnosed by the conspicuous buboes. They signify that the patient was in contact with rodents or other disease-bearing animals. Pneumonic plague can be diagnosed by chest X-ray films and examination of smear and culture of sputum. If pneumonic plague is suspected, treatment should be initiated without waiting for culture results.

Treatment includes administration of streptomycin as a first choice medication with tetracycline, chloramphenicol, or sulfamethoxazole as second choice backups. Other medications are often given for relief of fever, restlessness, toxemia, or shock.

Fig. 5–16. Plague: reported cases in humans, by year, United States, 1955–83

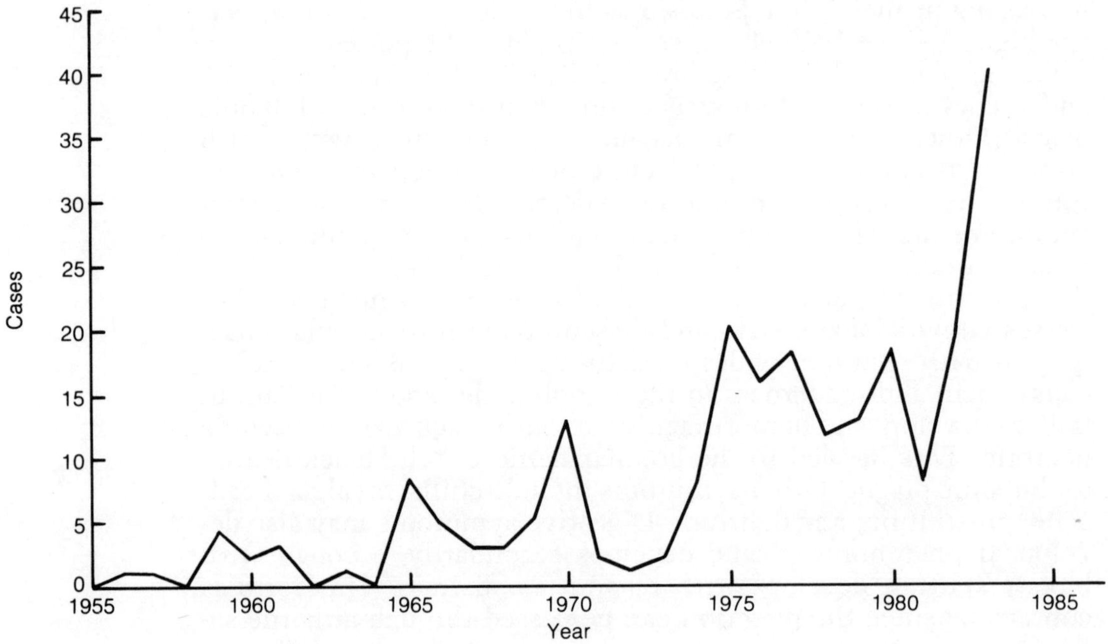

Source: Morbidity and Mortality Weekly Reports, Annual Summary 1983

LEPROSY

Also known as Hansen's disease, leprosy is a chronic infection caused by *Mycobacterium leprae*, an acid-fast bacillus. The organism attacks cutaneous tissue and peripheral nerves. Lesions develop and deteriorate to deformities. Today, it is not commonly fatal. Although transmission is thought to be via airborne respiratory droplets containing *M. leprae* or through open lesions, it is no longer thought to be highly contagious: close contact over an extended interval is considered to be necessary for its contraction.

Three varieties of leprosy are known. One is a *respiratory type*, which also affects the eyes, testes, skin, and nerves. This form is both the most common and the most severe. *Tuberculoid leprosy* affects the skin around peripheral nerves on the face, legs, buttocks, and arms. This form may be self limiting. The third variety is a mixture of the other two.

The incidence of leprosy, like that of plague, has been increasing in the United States continuously since the 1950s (Fig. 5–17). The number of indigenous cases has been level since the mid-70s. The

Fig. 5–17. Leprosy: reported cases, by year, United States, 1955–83

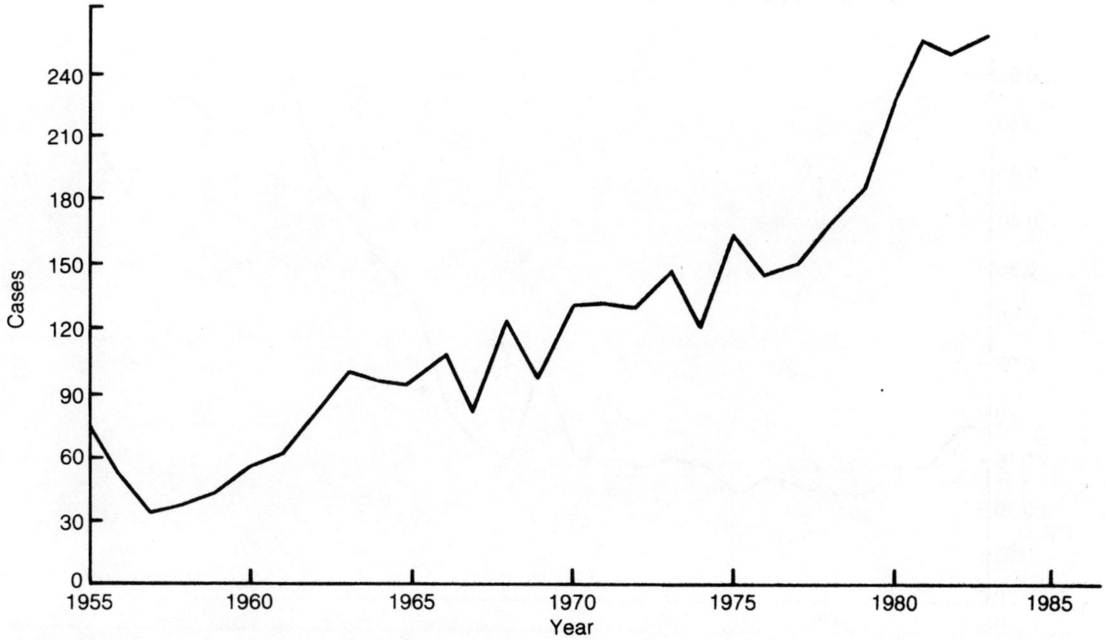

Source: Morbidity and Mortality Weekly Report, Annual Summary 1983

sharp total number of reported cases is due to an influx of Southeast Asians into the United States since 1976.

Clinical features usually allow diagnosis but biopsy examination can confirm it. Antimicrobials, such as dapsone and sulfoxone, are used to treat the disease. When these agents fail, or patients show intolerance, streptomycin and isoniazid are used. Drug administration may require a regimen as long as 5 years until all the skin lesions clear. The tuberculoid form may require treatment for several years after skin lesions subside. Deformities may also be corrected surgically.

TYPHUS FEVER

Typhus fever, also called Rocky Mountain spotted fever, is caused by the prolonged (up to 6 hours) bite of a tick carrying *Rickettsia rickettsii.* Occasionally, the infection can be contracted through inhalation of dried tick feces. As many as 5% of the ticks in heavily wooded areas are infected with *R. rickettsii*, and the incidence of typhus is rising. As Fig. 5–18 shows, a rise began in the late

Fig. 5–18. Typhus fever, tick-borne (Rocky Mountain spotted fever): reported cases per 100,000 population, by year, United States, 1955–83

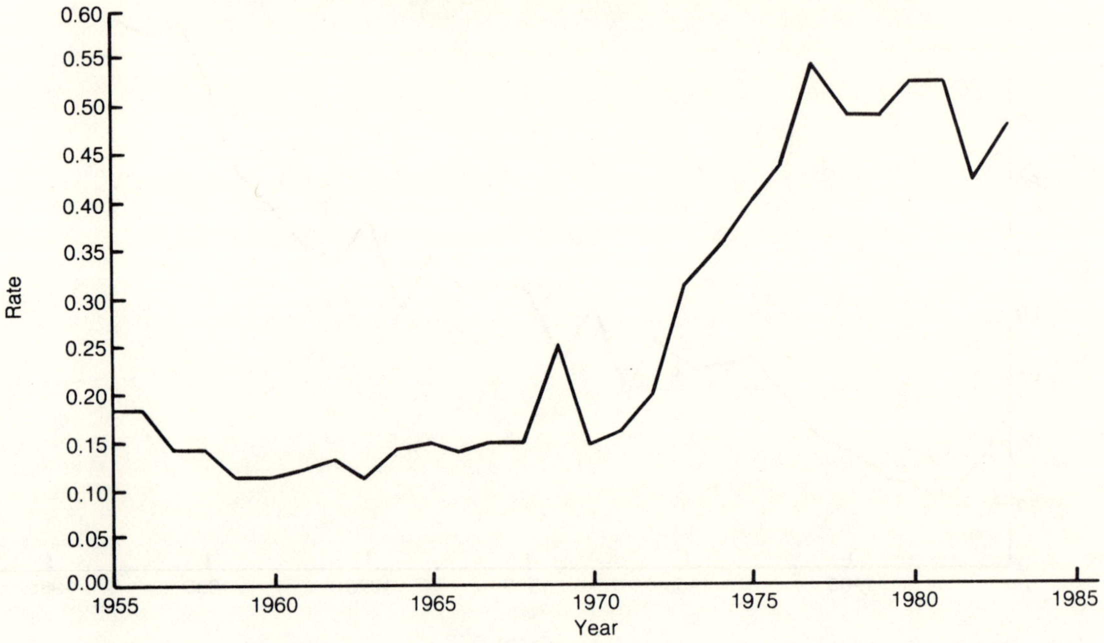

Source: Morbidity and Mortality Weekly Report, Annual Summary 1983

Fig. 5–19. Typhus fever, tick-borne (Rocky Mountain spotted fever): reported cases, by county, United States, 1983

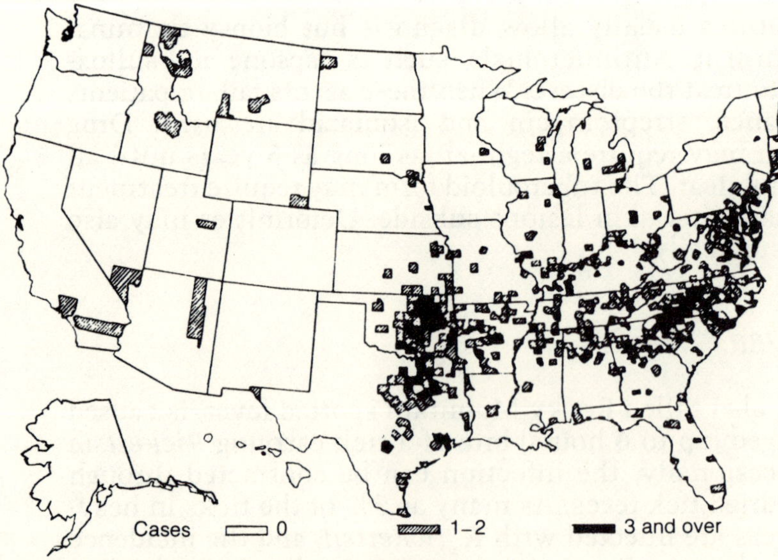

Source: Morbidity and Mortality Weekly Report, Annual Summary 1983

1960s, and epidemiologists believe it is due to the increased interest in camping and outdoor hiking in the United States. Cases in 1983 totaled 1,126.

As Fig. 5–19 shows, the greatest concentration of cases is in the South Atlantic states. In 1983, a large proportion (33%) was reported for the West and South central states: Oklahoma with 22 cases, Texas with 108, and Arkansas with 41.

The first symptom after an incubation that can range from 2 days to 2 weeks is a sudden high fever, severe headache, and generalized achiness. The tongue develops a white coat, which eventually turns brown, and a rash appears on the forehead, wrists, or ankles. The rash may become petechial and maculopapular if untreated and, by the third week, gangrenous. If the patient's blood pressure is low and pulse rapid, death may ensue from circulatory collapse. There may be digestive symptoms and a cough as well.

Diagnosis can be made from antibody titer tests but is often made from the clinical picture, especially if the patient has been in a wooded area just before falling ill. Treatment involves removal of the tick and antibiotic administration. The typical antibiotics are chloramphenicol or tetracycline. Other medications, including heparin, are supportive. Patients are watched closely for signs of circulatory or renal collapse. About 5% of all cases are fatal.

MALARIA

Malaria is caused by a protozoa of the Plasmodium genus, which is transmitted to human beings by female *Anopheles* mosquitos generally found in warm, swampy areas. After Plasmodium sporozoites enter the body, they migrate to the liver where they encyst. They emerge as merozoites and invade red blood cells where they feed on hemoglobin. Indigenous cases in the United States are rare; they have resulted from blood transfusions and the use of dirty needles among drug addicts. Nonindigenous infections have led to case totals as high as 4,230 in the early 1970s among returning soldiers from Vietnam.

Infected persons can survive with treatment, and their symptoms subside. But they are often chronic carriers, repeatedly exposed to bouts of the disease throughout life. Without treatment, about 10% of patients die. The most serious strain of malaria is *P. falciparum*. It causes high fever and massive erythrocytosis. Other symptoms include convulsions, delirium and coma, coughing and hemoptysis, vomiting, abdominal pain and diarrhea, and renal complications (oliguria, anuria, and uremia, among others).

Fig. 5–20. Malaria: reported cases per 100,000 population, by year, United States, 1930–83

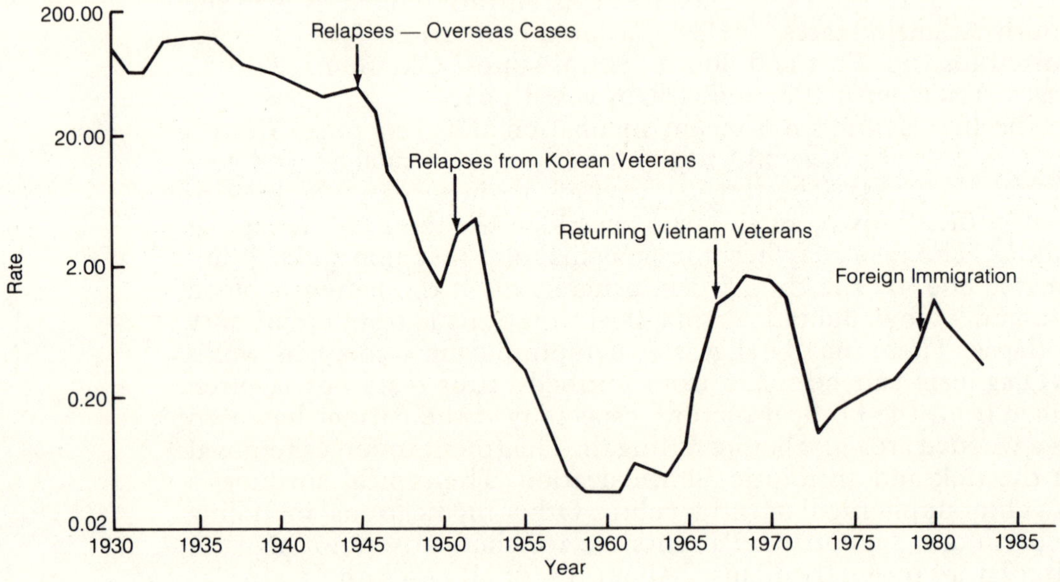

Source: Morbidity and Mortality Weekly Report, Annual Summary 1983

Figure 5–20 shows the reported cases in the United States since 1930 and their relation to episodes of involvement of the American population in foreign areas, such as Southeast Asia, where the disease is endemic.

Diagnosis is confirmed by identification of the parasites on multiple blood smears. Chloroquine is given orally for all forms of malaria with effective results except against the chloroquine-resistant *P. falciparum*. For the latter, patients receive oral doses of quinine concurrently with pyrimethamine and sulfadiazine. Quinine alone or with tetracycline is used to treat relapses. Patients are generally monitored for side effects.

The profiles of malaria and other diseases in this volume vividly portray the interaction between host, environment, and other common exogenous agents. People are more susceptible to some diseases, such as mononucleosis or chicken pox, at certain ages rather than at others. Those working in dust-creating occupations more often than others succumb to chronic lung disease. Developing respiratory ailments in turn can be exacerbated by another environmental agent—cigarette smoke. Diseases can be directly related to certain activities, such as sexual intercourse, or situations in which infectious vectors, such as fleas, transmit illness to healthy persons.

Yet, sometimes the reason for illness is endogenous and lies with the host, as in allergic persons who react to environmental agents abnormally and fall ill when others in the same circumstance do not.

The interplay of these many factors makes the profile of disease in man fascinating and the battle against disease difficult. Nevertheless, the profile of respiratory and infectious disease shows more successes than that of any other disease group.

A Note On Methodology

This volume and the others in this series are concerned with the demographics of disease, and the disease patterns of different groups of people considered on the basis of age, sex, or cultural grouping. The study of these patterns and the causes of disease in large and small populations is called *epidemiology*.

For thousands of years, people believed that sickness was a punishment for transgressions against the gods. The pattern of sinfulness followed by sickness was evident often enough, for people seldom lived perfect lives and seldom avoided all disease. When sick, they would call for a shaman, a priest-doctor who would beg the gods through prayer and incantation to restore the sick to health.

As simplistic as this approach seems to many modern peoples, the basic impetus of early peoples was epidemiologic. They had isolated a pattern of disease and sought to avoid the scourge of disease by addressing its cause, an angry god.

Gradually, exceptions to the accepted pattern of disease were noticed. Epidemics affected virtually everyone in a community, good or bad. So too, people began to notice other patterns of illness and linked aspects of their natural surroundings, such as their drinking water and certain foods, to the development of disease.

People also noticed that those in contact with a sick person often developed the same symptoms a few days or weeks later. Thus, a belief developed that disease could be transmitted somehow from person to person, perhaps by the movement of invisible particles traveling from the body of the sick person to that of the well one. The writings of Lucretius described this theory of contagious disease. With this pattern of disease noticed, the stage was set for the development of modern epidemiology, the science that looks for the pattern of diseases and the natural causes evidenced by that pattern.

Although the stage was set, many obstacles still had to be overcome. Autopsy examinations were forbidden through most of the Middle Ages, and everyday observational tools used by the modern physician, such as the clinical thermometer and the stethoscope, were not invented until the 17th and 18th centuries, respectively. Thus, it was difficult to diagnose what a person died of. Those who hazarded a guess were often wildly simplistic or incorrect.

Even in the 20th century, influenza, pneumonia, bronchitis and tuberculosis have routinely been mistaken for each other. Autopsies performed in the latter part of this century finally helped to clarify mortality from these causes.

THE DEATH CERTIFICATE

Despite today's much improved knowledge of the body and disease, the problems of relying on the information entered on a death certificate are notorious. Unfortunately, mortality data reported by countries around the world are based of necessity on death-certificate entries.

In many countries, death-certificate entries represent a physician's diagnosis. But in many other countries, the cause of death is reported by the deceased's relatives to a local clerk. Even in more sophisticated countries, listing the cause of death often obscures the real pathologic profile. For example, dying is always a dualistic event resulting from the interaction of a given host and the disease agent that afflicts the host. In one person, influenza may prove fatal because he is constitutionally weak, perhaps from age or other diseases. In another person, encounter with the influenza virus would be a minor event—in no way life threatening. But the record of influenza mortality translates simply into the ferocity or danger of influenza as a disease.

The decline in measles mortality throughout much of the 20th century is another example of the confluence of several factors. Until the recent development of the measles vaccine, nothing had changed in the incidence or severity of measles. But mortality in those stricken with pneumonia, a common fatal sequel of measles, was being reduced by sulfur drugs.

Similarly, much information and understanding are lost insofar as death certificates require a listing of only one cause of death, although secondary causes can be listed on the back. Conventions have been established that priority should be given to the cause that is most often fatal, communicable or acute. But such conventions vary from country to country.

This practice becomes increasingly problematic as populations experience greater longevity, since old people often suffer from several conditions by the time they die of any one cited cause. Someone with diabetes, poor renal function, and congestive heart failure (CHF), is taxed by a cold that develops into acute bronchitis. Medication places an added burden on their kidneys. Difficulty in breathing places an extra oxygen demand on their heart, while their blood sugar is difficult to control. After a few days, their kidneys fail as does their heart and they die. Did the cold kill them? Did the bronchitis? Or was the cause of death heart failure, kidney failure, or diabetes? The physician must make a choice. In England and Wales, the death rate from bronchitis is higher than in most other countries. But these UK countries are inclined to list cases like the one described as a bronchitis death whereas other countries tend to list it as a cardiovascular death.

When a death certificate was introduced in England that asked the physician to list death "as consequence of," the number of deaths ascribed to bronchitis doubled. Deaths from nephritis in Canada and the United States doubled as well, while one-third to one-half of the deaths typically attributed to diabetes were counted for some other cause.

DIFFICULTIES OF NOMENCLATURE AND CLASSIFICATION

Beyond these difficulties are ones of nomenclature and classification. To solve these problems, an International Classification of Diseases has been established, which has been revised from time to time. The current code represents the ninth such revision. But in its attempt to standardize diagnosis from country to country, the classification has posed other problems. As knowledge of diseases has increased, the classification has gradually changed from anatomic groupings to etiologic ones. Rheumatic fever is still listed anatomically as a heart disease because it affects the heart. But if it were true to the trend, it would be listed according to cause and would be regarded as an infectious disease because we now know that rheumatic fever is caused by a bacterium and is infectious. In the fourth revision, brain tumors were removed from the category of nervous system diseases and put with neoplasms, as we realized that these tumors are the results of cancerous growth. During the fourth revision of the code, a more mysterious change was the removal of criminal abortion from accidental death to complication of pregnancy.

Over the years, as diagnosis has become more specific, deaths due to ill-defined causes have also decreased and other heretofore ill-defined diseases, such as various neoplasms, show increased mortality. As populations have aged and physicians have become accustomed to diagnosing the cause of death in the old, several degenerative diseases, such as diabetes, nephritis, ulcer, and cirrhosis have left the ill-defined category.

CENSUS PROBLEMS

In addition to classification and nomenclature complexities, elementary census biases enter the picture when countries try to calculate their mortality and morbidity rate due to different diseases. These rates are usually expressed as the number of deaths or disease cases per 100,000 population. Sometimes the rates are calculated for men and women separately or for people in different age groups separately. But census numbers are known for their underestimates of population even in advanced countries like the United States. Young children and transient males who travel for their work are often missed in population counts. The 1960 United States census missed an estimated 3 million people, particularly blacks. Latin Americans tend to report more 5- to 9-year-old children than 0- to 4-year-olds.

Often, information on sex is missing and when asked for their age, people tend to say they are 18 or 21 when these are the ages of majority in a country and 65 when social benefits are available to 65-year-olds. Many people between age 21 and 40 years tend to lower their age when asked. On the other hand, those who do report their true age tend to round their age, especially to even numbers or to ages divisible by five. To compensate for this tendency, researchers often use age intervals when these statistics are compiled.

SURVEYS

Data on morbidity pose yet different problems in that they are usually obtained from health department reports, review of hospital records, or sample surveys of the population. In the United States, physicians are legally obligated to report a large array of diseases, particularly infectious ones, to their health departments. The latter in turn report their data to the Atlanta Centers for Disease Control. Reports come from all of the states, but data gathered independently tend to reveal an under-reporting of disease to the Centers in many instances.

Sometimes hospital records are used for gathering data but these records are often incomplete or have incorrect entries. In addition, hospitalized patients may not reflect the typical patient with a given disease because hospitalized patients are likely to be those who are more severely ill with a specific disease or those who are intractable to less extreme forms of outpatient treatments.

Sample surveys are also subject to misleading findings, depending on how the sample is chosen and how the survey questions are constructed and asked. Data from several large government surveys have been included in this volume. Elaborate statistical sampling methods have been employed to ensure that the surveys are representative. But the questions sometimes fail to elicit pertinent and interesting information. One example can be found in the discussion in *Cardiovascular Disease* that deals with cerebrovascular disease.

A sample of people were asked about their limitation of normal activity due, presumably, to illness. Some were people who had suffered a stroke; others had not. The stroke victims generally showed greater limitation of activity. But these same people were also generally older and perhaps infirm because of other health conditions. There was no indication that their limitation of activity was specifically related to their stroke event. Thus, we do not know, in light of this particular study, how much dysfunction is caused by stroke in the general population compared to other disability conditions or able-bodied people.

The operations and procedures, together with hospital utilization and physician office visits for people with various diagnoses discussed in this work, were obtained from large government studies, such as the National Ambulatory Care Survey and the National Hospital Discharge Survey, which are conducted annually or periodically. Again the focus of these surveys is not always constant from one to another. Comparison of data from an early survey, such as the NHANES I Nutrition Survey, with data on some variables measured by a later survey, such as the NHANES II Survey, is not always possible.

RANDOM VARIABILITY

The perspicacious reader must also realize that health data gathered through survey studies are always subject to a certain amount of random variability. More than a century ago, scientists found to their chagrin that whenever any entity is measured multiple times, the measurement varies. This is true even when the measurement is taken by the same person each time using the same instrument in the same way.

In astronomy, this variability came to be known as the personal equation. But this same kind of variability occurs when one obtains data from a random sample presumably representative of a population of interest. Another random sample surveyed in the same way and equally representative typically yields slightly different results. This variability is called the standard error of a particular study.

The importance of keeping in mind that every sample surveyed has a standard error comes into play when comparisons of data expressed as averages are made. Luckily, the standard error of studies is often small; hence, fairly large differences among groups can be accepted as true differences in reality and not merely the reflection of sampling variability.

When reported differences are small, however, one should not conclude that there is in fact a real difference between two groups unless one knows that the standard error of the study samples is smaller than the small reported difference. For a more detailed explanation of sampling variability, see my article, "Randomization and optimal design," *Journal of Chronic Diseases* 36:606–609, 1983.

CRUDE AND AGE-ADJUSTED DATA

Another factor that good health surveys take into account is the age of the groups compared. Clearly, if the blacks interviewed in a study sample were on average 10 years younger than white subjects, one would be mistaken to conclude that whites smoke more than blacks. Obviously, members of groups that smoke to the same degree will show one smoking longer than the other if the members of one group are older than those of the other. The way to correct for age differences when age is likely to affect whether one has an illness or has followed a particular pattern for some time is to compare age-adjusted samples. You will note throughout this volume that crude rates are given as are age-adjusted rates when they are relevant and available.

Since the rates of mortality and morbidity vary among people of different ages, sex, races, and sometimes ethnic and religious backgrounds — particularly in the United States — one has to be mindful of differences in these groups that may account for their differing disease rates. Age is clearly one of these differences that needs to be adjusted for when comparing data. The average and median ages of the black United States population is considerably lower than the white population. Thus, we would expect to see a lower rate of old-age degenerative disease among blacks than among whites when there is no age adjustment. When age is adjusted for or the rate at the same age is compared, epidemiologists have discovered that blacks actually have a higher rate of hypertension than whites.

Another factor not as easily corrected for is access to and utilization of medical resources. If a particular group, such as blacks, are economically less able or socially less inclined to seek medical care when sick, they may ultimately reflect a higher mortality rate from their diseases or a greater morbidity rate as their untreated conditions grow more severe. The higher mortality in such situations should not be regarded as an indication that the higher mortality group has the disease to a greater extent. In other words, blacks may not have more cancer than whites, but they may have a higher cancer mortality rate because they do not receive an early diagnosis or follow treatment regimens for economic or social reasons.

Some researchers speculate that males have a higher general mortality rate than females in part because they tend to seek less medical help for their ailments and fail to follow prescribed treatment regimens for psychological reasons or because it is not convenient for them to see a physician due to career demands.

Aside from the differences in the groups just discussed, differences also exist in groups that may explain why disease does indeed occur more often in some groups than in others. In fact, this is the basic logic of epidemiology and the real incentive for keeping track of vital statistics. Epidemiologists seek to isolate patterns in disease to determine possible pathologic causes.

TELLING PATTERNS

Once it is determined that members of one group are sick and those of another are not, epidemiologists study factors that may be affecting the groups differently. One of the earliest of these investigations was conducted by the physician John Snow, who investigated cholera in London between 1848 and 1854. At that time, different parts of London were supplied with water by different companies. Snow noticed that the cholera cases were confined to areas supplied by two specific water companies. In contrast to the others, these two obtained their water from a very polluted section of the Thames River.

One of the companies changed its source farther up river, and when water pipes were laid in the city, its pipes were alternated with those of the other Thames River company such that each supplied every other house in an area of London that they both served. Snow counted the number of houses in the district served by each company and the number of cholera cases that developed in houses served by each company.

The resulting rates were greatly different, with a much higher rate of cholera in the houses served by the company that was still drawing its water from the polluted source.

This classic study reflects a design referred to as the case control method. This form of research is especially important and useful when one is trying to determine the possible causes of a disease. It has been employed widely and has added to our medical knowledge in many ways from the discovery that infant deformities were in the offspring of women who had nothing in common other than ingestion of thalidomide during their pregnancy to the studies that showed a much higher incidence of lung cancer among smokers than among nonsmokers.

Much of the work that has revealed the risk factors for various cancers were obtained from case control studies that compared people with cancer to a group of people without cancer, the control group, which was matched in age, sex, and so on with the disease or case group. Middle-aged women in Aurora, Illinois were reported to have bone cancer more than women in surrounding communities. They seemed like the other women except that they had all worked at a radium dial watch factory in Aurora some years previously, whereas none of the cancer-free control group had worked with the radium. The conclusion was that exposure to radioactive material is a risk factor for developing bone cancer.

Because of modern developments in statistical analysis, researchers also determine possible risk factors when more than one is operative. Such analysis would be used with large cross-sectional community studies that record the prevalence of a disease and other characteristics of the population. The Framingham heart study was of this sort. It revealed that people with heart disease tend to have hypertension, elevated cholesterol readings, and a history of smoking more than those who do not suffer from heart disease.

A follow-up study conducted for several years is currently recording the practices of the offspring of the original study population and the development of heart disease among them. This type of study is called a cohort incidence study because it looks for the development of disease over time. Expensive and lengthy, it is also sometimes impractical.

Each of these designs is useful when one is trying to find the cause of a disease, especially a disease that develops slowly over time. Another type of design that is useful to determine the best form of treatment for a disease is the clinical trial. Some professionals erroneously regard this design as more scientific than the others because the investigator has some control over the exposure of the test sample to a given factor, a treatment of some sort, but this view is incorrect. The randomized controlled trial is subject to many of the same biases as the other designs that I discuss in my article, "The case control or retrospective study in retrospect," *Journal of Clinical Pharmacology* 21:269–274, July 1981. The debate is moot, however, because the clinical trial cannot be used to determine the cause of a disease. No one can ethically subject healthy people to a factor suspected of causing a disease.

An early example of a clinical trial that *did* test various treatments and also determined the cause of a disease was an investigation made by James Lind into the treatment of scurvy among English sailors in 1747. Sailors long away at sea were afflicted with debilitating scurvy because fresh fruits and vegetables were not storable aboard ship for long periods, and they lacked vitamin C when they went on long voyages.

Lind, on board the *Salisbury*, gathered sailors who were suffering from scurvy and divided them into several groups matched for severity and other factors. He then required that one group take 25 gutts of elixir vitriol daily, another group 2 spoonfuls of vinegar three times daily, another nutmeg, another oranges and lemons, while another group was allowed only a ration of sea water. Within days, dramatic change for the better occurred only in those eating the oranges and lemons.

Lind concluded that eating citrus fruits was essential to the diet of anyone who wished to avoid scurvy and that the disease was caused by the lack of these same fruits in the diet. The British Navy adopted the policy of serving its sailors limes and lime juice in 1795.

This experiment led Lind to the cause as well as to the treatment of scurvy, yet he did not choose to cause scurvy in the sailors by withholding citrus fruits from them. They were already sick. In this instance, he felt no compunction about giving one group only sea water, which he regarded tantamount to no treatment, a strategy employed today usually with a group of sick people that constitutes a control group.

Ethical considerations can affect such decisions, and often such experiments avoid having a no-treatment group in favor of having several groups each treated differently but all treated with some accepted treatment. The groups are called comparison groups and provide data on which treatment of several possible ones is the best.

Readers mindful of these many considerations and of the strategies used by medical researchers to determine what disease patterns exist and how they reveal possible causes of disease will better evaluate the information in this series. They will also better understand why controversy often rages within the medical community about the causes or treatment of disease. And they will better appreciate the remarkable progress achieved by epidemiologists, medical researchers, treating physicians, and policy makers in increasing average life expectancy and eliminating much pain and suffering from normal human existence.

Glossary

Age-adjusted rate: age adjustment, using the direct method, is the application of age-specific death rates in a population of interest to a standardized age distribution to eliminate the differences in observed rates resulting from differences in population composition

Adenovirus: a virus group responsible for many respiratory infections

Aerobic: applying to organisms that live only in the presence of oxygen

Agglutination: a congealing of microorganisms when a bacterial culture is mixed with an immune serum

Alveolar: pertaining to the small cavities of the lung

Anaerobic: defining microorganisms that can live in the absence of molecular oxygen

Anorexia: loss of appetite

Anuria: suppression or failure of kidney function

Bacteremia: bacteria in the bloodstream

Bronchogram: radiographic film of lungs and bronchi

Chancre: a hard primary ulcer associated with syphilis

Cohort: any group of people with a common characteristic or set of characteristics that are studied or followed over time

Conjunctivitis: inflammation of the mucous membrane which lines the eyelids

Coryza: a head cold

Death rate: a measure that divides the number of deaths in a population in a given period by the resident population at the middle of that period

Diplopia: impaired vision

Dyspnea: shortness of breath

Dysarthria: difficulty in joint articulation

Endemic: applied to a disease occurring repeatedly in a given geographical area but not in a widespread fashion; not epidemic

Eosinophilia: an above-normal level of eosinophils (typically 1% – 3% of white cell count) in the circulating bloodstream

Exotoxin: toxin produced by bacteria and discharged into surrounding medium

Hematocrit: a measure of the volume of erythrocytes in a given volume of blood

Hemoptysis: cough with blood from hemorrhage of larynx, trachea, bronchi, or lungs

Incidence: the number of cases of disease having onset during a particular time, often expressed as a rate

Infiltrate: to pass into or through a substance, as when entering a cell or lung tissue

Leukocytosis: a white cell count higher than $10{,}000/mm^3$, usually indicating an infection

Leukopenia: abnormally low white cell count below $5000/mm^3$

Lymphadenopathy: lymph gland disorder associated with many diseases

Maculopapular: Consisting of discolored spots on the skin or pimple-type lesions

Malaise: uneasiness; restlessness due often to infection

Merozite: formed by asexual reproduction via breakup of schizont, it invades cells where it transforms into a gametocyte or repeats the process of schizogony

Myalgia: pain or tenderness of muscles

Nosocomial: referring to a hospital

Oliguria: reduction in urine output from such factors as perspiration, hemorrhage, and coma

Parenteral: occurring outside the intestines

Periorbital: around the eye, i.e., the eye socket

Petechial: like a purple spot on the skin that appears during a malignant fever

Pharyngitis: inflammation of the pharynx

Polymyositis: inflammation of several muscles

Prevalence: the number of cases of a disease, infected persons, or persons with some other attribute during a particular interval, often expressed as a rate

Ptosis: a sagging of tissue, as a drooping eyelid

Purulent: filled with pus

Salpingitis: inflammation of the fallopian tube

Serotype: identification of an organism by type and configuration of its antigens

Splenomegaly: enlarged spleen

Tachycardia: rapid heart beat at abnormal rate

Bibliography

American Hospital Association: American hospital association guide to the health care field. Chicago: American Hospital Association, 1982

Anonymous. Needlestick transmission of HTLV-III from a patient infected in Africa. *Lancet* ii:1376–7, 1984

Aserkoff B, Schroeder SA, Brazhman PS: Salmonellosis in the United States—A five-year review. *Am J Epidemiol* 92:13–24, 1970

Austrian, R: Some observations on the *Pneumococcus* and on the current status of pneumococcal disease and its prevention. *Rev Infect Dis 3* (supp.): S1–S15, March–April 1981

Bell TA, Hein K. Adolescents and sexually transmitted diseases. In Holmes KK, Mardh P-A, Sparling PF, Wiesner PJ, (eds): *Sexually Transmitted Diseases.* New York: McGraw Hill (in press)

Bennett JV: Human infections: economic implications and prevention. *Ann Intern Med* 89: 761–763, Pt. 2, 1978

Black RE, Crann GE, Blake PA: Epidemiology of common-source outbreaks of shigellosis in the United States, 1961–1975. Am J *Epidemiol* 108:47–52, 1978

Broome CV: Efficacy of pneumococcal polysaccharide vaccines. *Rev Infect Dis 3* (supp.): S82–S88, March–April 1981

Brown S, Biddle J, Warnnisorn T, et al: Antimicrobial resistance of *Neisseria gonorrhoeae* in Bangkok: is single-drug treatment passe? *Lancet* 2:1366–8, 1982

Brown ST, Wiesner PJ: Problems and approaches to the control and surveillance of sexually transmitted agents associated with pelvic inflammatory disease in the United States. *Am J Obstet Gynecol* 138:1096–1100, 1980

Bryan FL: Emerging foodborne diseases. I. Their surveillance and epidemiology. II. Factors that contribute to outbreaks and their control. *J Milk Food Technol* 35: 618–625, 632–638, 1972

Bryan FL: What the sanitarian should know about salmonella and staphylococci in non-dairy foods. II. Salmonellae. *J Milk Food Technol* 31:131–140, 1968

Cares JW, Goldin WA, Lynch JJ et al: The determination of quartz in airborne respirable granite dust by infrared spectrophotometry. *Am Ind Hyg Assoc J* 34:298–305, 1973

Castro KG, Fischl MA, Landesman SH et al: Risk factors for AIDS among Haitians in the United States. Atlanta, Georgia: International Conference on AIDS, April 16, 1985

CDC. A cluster of Kaposi's sarcoma and *Pneumocystis carinii* pneumonia among homosexual male residents of Los Angeles and Orange Counties, California. *MMWR* 31:305–7, 1982

CDC. Acquired immune deficiency syndrome (AIDS): precautions for clinical and laboratory staffs. *MMWR* 31:577–80, 1982

CDC. Immunodeficiency among female sexual partners of males-with acquired immune deficiency syndrome (AIDS)—New York.MMWR 31:697–8, 1983

CDC. Acquired immunodeficiency syndrome (AIDS): precautions-for health-care workers and allied professionals *MMWR* 32:450–2, 1983

CDC. Increase in prevalence of leprosy caused by dapsone-resistant *Mycobacterium leprae. MMWR* 30: 637–638, 1982

CDC. Nosocomial Infection Surveillance, 1980–1982. In: CDC Surveillance Summaries (published four times a year). 32(No. 4SS): 1SS-16SS, 1983

CDC. Opportunistic infections and Kaposi's sarcoma among Haitians in the United States. *MMWR* 31:353–4, 360-1, 1982

CDC. Penicillinase-producing *Neisseria gonorrhoeae*—Los Angeles. *MMWR* 32:181–3, 1983

CDC. Persistent, generalized lymphadenopathy among homosexual males. *MMWR* 31:249–51, 1982

CDC. *Pneumocystis carinii* pneumonia among persons with hemophilia A. *MMWR* 31:365–7, 1982

CDC. Possible transfusion-associated acquired immune deficiency syndrome (AIDS)—California. *MMWR* 31:652–4, 1982

CDC. Prevention of secondary cases of *Haemophilus influenzae* type b disease. *MMWR* 31:672–674, 679–680, 1982

CDC. Salmonellosis traced to marijuana—Ohio, Michigan. *MMWR* 30: 77–78, 1981

CDC. STD fact sheet. Ed. 35. DHHS Publication No. (CDC) 81—8195. Atlanta Ga., 1981

CDC. Unexplained immunodeficiency and opportunistic infections in infants—New York, New Jersey, California, *MMWR* 31:665–7, 1982

CDC. Update on acquired immune deficiency syndrome (AIDS) among patients with hemophilia A. *MMWR* 31:644–6, 652, 1982

CDC. Update on Kaposi's sarcoma and opportunistic infections in previously health persons—United States. *MMWR* 31:294, 300-1, 1982

CDC. Venereal disease control laws summary (00-3553). Atlanta, Ga.: Centers for Disease Control, 1979

CDC. Venereal disease morbidity report. CDC 9.688. Statistical Services Section, Atlanta, Ga., undated

Chilman CS: Adolescent sexuality in a changing American society. DHEW Publication No. (NIH) 79–1426. U.S. Government Printing Office, Washington, D.C., 1979

Clumeck N, Van de Perre P, Carael M et al: Heterosexual promiscuity among African patients with AIDS. [Letter] *N Engl J Med* 313:182, 1985

Cohen ML, Blake PA: Trends in foodborne salmonellosis outbreaks: 1963–1975. *Food Protection* 40:798–800, 1977

Comstock GW, Palmer CE: Long-term results of BCG vaccination in the southern United States. *Am Rev Resp Dis* 93: 171–183, 1966

Comstock GW, Edwards LB, Livesay VT: Tuberculosis morbidity in the U.S., Navy: its distribution and decline. *Am Rev Resp Dis* 110: 572–580, 1974

Donadio JA, Gangarosa EJ: Foodborne shigellosis. *J Infect Dis* 119:666–668, 1969

Douglas JM, Critchlow C, Benedetti J et al: A double-blind study of oral acyclovir for suppression of recurrences of genital herpes simplex infection. *N Engl J Med* 310:1551–1556, 1984

Edwards LB et al: Height, weight, tuberculous infection, and tuberculosis disease. *Arch Environ Health* 22:106–112, 1971

Eisenberg MS, Wiesner PJ: Reporting and treating gonorrhea: results of a statewide survey in Alaska. *J Am Ven Dis Assoc:* 3:79–83, 1976

Ferebee SH: Controlled chemoprophylaxis trials in tuberculosis. A general review. *Adv Tuberc Res* 17:28–106, 1970

Haley CE, Gregory WW, Donowitz LG et al: Neonatal intensive care unit (NICU) bloodstream infections (BSI): emergence of gram positive bacteria as major pathogens. Abstract 691. Presented at the 22nd Interscience Conference on Antimicrobial Agents and Chemotherapy, Miami Beach, FL, October 4–6, 1982

Haley RW et al: Study on the efficacy of nosocomial infection control (SENIC project): summary of study design. *Am J Epidemiol* 111: 472–485, 1980.

Haley RW, Hightower AW, Khabbaz RF et al: The emergence of methicillin-resistant *Staphylococcus aureus* infections in United States hospitals. *Ann Intern Med* 97:207–308, 1982

Haley RW, Hooton TM, Culver DH et al: Nosocomial infections in U.S. hospitals, 1975–1976. Estimated frequency by selected characteristics of patients. *Am J Med* 70:947–59, 1981

Haley RW: Preliminary cost-benefit analysis of hospital infection control programs (The SENIC Project). Proceedings of an International Workshop at Baiersbronn, Germany, September 1977, pp. 93–5

Haley, RW, Schachtman RH: The emergence of infection surveillance and control programs in U.S. hospitals: an assessment, 1976. *Am J Epidemiol* 111: 574–591, 1980

Handsfield HH, Sandstrom EG, Knapp JS et al: Epidemiology of penicillinase-producing *Neisseria gonorrhoeae* infections: analysis by auxotyping and serogrouping. *N Engl J Med* 306:950–4, 1982

Harris C, Small CB, Klein RS et al: Immunodeficiency in female sexual partners of men with the acquired immunodeficiency syndrome. *N Engl J Med* 308: 1181–4, 1983

ILO U/C International Classification of Radiographs of Pneumoconioses 1971—Occupational Safety and Health Series 22 (rev). Geneva, International Labour Office, 1972, 37 pp

Ingerham NR: The value of penicillin alone in the prevention and treatment of congenital syphilis. *Acta Derm Venereol* (suppl.) (Stockh) 24: 60–88, 1951

Jaffe HW, Biddle JW, Thornsberry C et al: National gonorrhea therapy monitoring study. In vitro antibiotic susceptibility and its correlation with treatment results. *N Engl J Med* 294:5–9, 1976

Jaffe HW: Infections due to penicillinase-producing *Neisseria gonorrhoeae* in the United States: 1976–1980. *J Infect Dis* 141:191–197, 1981

Kaplan GJ, Fraser RI, Comstock GW: Tuberculosis in Alaska, 1970. The continued decline of the tuberculosis epidemic. *Am Rev Resp Dis* 105: 920–926, 1972

Kreiss JK, Kitchen LW, Prince HE et al: Antibody to human T-lymphotropic virus type III in wives of hemophiliacs. Evidence for heterosexual transmission. *Ann Inter Med* 102:623–6, 1985

Kornfeld H, Vande Stouwe RA, Lange M et al: T-lymphocyte subpopulations in homosexual men. *N Engl J Med* 307:729–31, 1982

Lederman MM, Ratnoff OD, Scillian JJ et al. Impaired cell-mediated immunity in patients with classic hemophilia. *N Engl J Med* 308: 79–83, 1983

Medical and Scientific Advisory Council Recommendations to prevent AIDS in patients with hemophilia. New York National Hemophilia Foundation, January 14, 1983

Menitove JE, Aster RH, Casper JT et al: T-lymphocyte subpopulations in patients with classic hemophilia treated with cryoprecipitate and lyophilized concentrates. *N Engl J Med* 308:83–6, 1983

Mindel A, Faherty A, Hindley D et al: Prophylactic oral acyclovir in recurrent genital herpes. *Lancet* 2:57–59, 1984

Naeye RL, Dellinger WS: Lung disease in Appalachian soft-coal miners. *Am J Pathol* 58:557–64, 1970

National Center for Health Statistics: Mortality trends for leading causes of death, United States, 1950–69, by A. Joan Klebba, Jeffrey D. Maurer, and Evelyn J. Glass. *Vital and Health Statistics.* Series 20-No. 16. DHEW Pub. No. (HRA) 74–1853. Health Resources Administration. Washington. U.S. Government Printing Office, March 1974

National Center for Health Statistics: Mortality from diseases associated with smoking: United States, 1950–64, by A. Joan Klebba, M.A. *Vital and Health Statistics*. PHS Pub. No. 1000–Series 20-No. 4. Public Health Service. Washington. U.S. Government Printing Office, Oct. 1966

Nilsen AE, Aasen T, Halsos AM et al: Efficacy of oral acyclovir in the treatment of initial and recurrent genital herpes. *Lancet* 2:571–573, 1982

Nottay BK et al: Molecular variation of Type 1 vaccine-related and wild polioviruses during replication in humans. *Virology* 108: 405–423, 1981

Palmer CE, Shaw DW, Comstock GW: Community trials of BCG vaccination. *Am Rev Tuberc* 77: 877–907, 1958

Piot P, Quinn TC, Taelman H et al: Acquired immunodeficiency syndrome in a heterosexual population in Zaire. *Lancet* ii: 65–9, 1984

Pitchenik AE, Cole C, Russell BW et al: Tuberculosis, atypical mycobacteriosis, and the acquired immunodeficiency syndrome among Haitian and non-Haitian patients in South Florida. *Ann Intern Med* 101:641–5, 1984

Pitchenik AE, Shafron RD, Glasser RM et al: The acquired immunodeficiency syndrome in the wife of a hemophiliac. *Ann Intern Med* 100:62–5, 1984

Pneumococcal polysaccharide vaccine. *MMWR* 30: 410–412, 417–419, 1981

Public Health Service: The Health Consequences of Smoking for Women. A Report of the Surgeon General. DHHS (PHS). Washington. U.S. Government Printing Office, 1980

Public Health Service: The Health Consequences of Smoking—The Changing Cigarette. A Report of the Surgeon General. DHHS (PHS) 81-50156. Washington U.S. Government Printing Office, 1981

Reichman RC, Badger GJ, Mertz GJ et al: Treatment of recurrent genital herpes simplex infections with oral acyclovir: A controlled trial. *JAMA* 251:2103–2107, 1984

Reichman LB, O'Day R: Tuberculous infection in a large urban population. *Am Rev Resp Dis* 117: 705–712, 1978

Salo OP, Lassus A, Hovi T et al: Double-blind placebo-controlled trial of oral acyclovir in recurrent genital herpes. *Eur J Sexually Trans Dis* 1:95–98, 1983

Seeff LB, Wright EC, Zimmerman HJ et al: Type B hepatitis after needle-stick exposure: prevention with hepatitis B immune globulin. *Ann Intern Med* 88:285–93, 1978

Sencer DJ, Axnick NW: Utilization of cost/benefit analysis in planning prevention programs. *Acta Medica Scandinavia* 576 (supp.): 123–128, 1975

Snider D et al: Preliminary results of 6-month regimens studied in the United States and Poland. *Chest* 80: 727–729, 1981

Stoneburner RL, Kristal A: Increasing tuberculosis incidence and its relationship to acquired immunodeficiency syndrome in New York City. Atlanta, Georgia: International conference on acquired immunodeficiency syndrome (AIDS). April 14–17, 1985

Straus SE, Takiff HE, Seidlin M et al: Suppression of frequently recurring genital herpes: A placebo-controlled double-blind trial of oral acyclovir. *N Engl J Med* 310:1545–1550, 1984

Theriault GP, Burgess WA, DiBerardinis LJ et al: Dust exposure in the Vermont granite sheds. *Arch Environ Health* 28:12–17, 1974

Theriault GP, Peters JM, Fine LJ: Pulmonary function in granite shed workers of Vermont. *Arch Env Health* 28:18–22, 1974

Theriault GP, Peters JM, Johnson WM: Pulmonary function and roentgenographic changes in granite dust exposure. *Arch Env Health* 28:23–27, 1974

Thompson S: A prospective study of chlamydia and mycoplasma infections during pregnancy: relation to pregnancy outcome and maternal morbidity. Abstract presented at the Eric K. Fernstrom Symposium III—International Symposium on Human Chlamydial Infection, Lund, Sweden, June 1982

Valenti WM, Hall CB, Douglas RG Jr et al: Nosocomial viral infections: 1. Epidemiology and significance. *Infection Control* 1:33–7, 1980

Vieira J, Frank E, Spira TJ et al: Acquired immune deficiency in Haitians: opportunistic infections in previously healthy Haitian immigrants. *N Engl J Med* 308:125–9, 1983

Weiss SH, Saxinger WC, Rechtman DJ et al: HTLV-III infection among health care workers. *JAMA*, 1985

Welliver RC, McLaughlin S: Unique epidemiology of nosocomial infection in a children's hospital. *Am J Dis Child* 138:131–5, 1984

Wiesner PJ. Magnitude of the problem of sexually transmitted disease in the United States. In: Sexually transmitted diseases, 1980 status report, NIAID Study Group. DHEW Publication No. (NIH) 81–2213. U.S. Government Printing Office, Washington, D.C., 1981, p 24.

Wiesner PJ, Thompson SE: Gonococcal diseases. *DM* 26(5):6–10, 1980

Zelnik M, Kantner JF: Sexual activity, contraceptive use, and pregnancy among metropolitan-area teenagers: 1971–1979. *Fam Plann Perspect* 12:230–7, 1980

INDEX